T0092073

DRUGS OF ABUSE, IMMUNITY, AND AIDS

ADVANCES IN EXPERIMENTAL MEDICINE AND BIOLOGY

Recent Volumes in this Series

DRUGS OF ABUSE, IMMUNITY, AND AIDS

Edited by

Herman Friedman
Thomas W. Klein
Steven Specter

University of South Florida
Tampa, Florida

SPRINGER SCIENCE+BUSINESS MEDIA, LLC

Library of Congress Cataloging-in-Publication Data

Drugs of abuse, immunity, and AIDS / edited by Herman Friedman, Thomas W. Klein, Steven Specter.
p. cm. -- (Advances in experimental medicine and biology ; v. 335)
"Proceedings of the Second International Conference on Drugs of Abuse, Immunity, and AIDS, held June 1-3, 1992, Clearwater, Florida"--T.p. verso.
Includes bibliographical references and index.
ISBN 978-0-306-44566-8 ISBN 978-1-4615-2980-4 (eBook)
DOI 10.1007/978-1-4615-2980-4
1. AIDS (Disease)--Pathophysiology--Congresses. 2. Drug abuse--Congresses. 3. Alcohol--Immunology--Congresses. 4. Cocaine--Immunology--Congresses. 5. Marihuana--Immunology--Congresses. 6. Cannabinoids--pharmacology--congresses. I. Friedman, Herman, 1931- . II. Klein, Thomas W. III. Specter, Steven. IV. International Conference on Drugs of Abuse, Immunity, and AIDS (2nd : 1992 : Clearwater, Fla.) V. Series.
[DNLM: 1. Immune System--drug effects--congresses. 2. Immunity--drug effects--congresses. 3. Acquired Immunodeficiency Syndrome--immunology--congresses. 4. Stress, Psychological--congresses. 5. Immunosuppression--congresses. 6. Cocaine--pharmacology--congresses. W1 AD559 v.335 1993 / QW 504 D7943 1992]
RC607.A26D78 1993
616.07'9--dc20
DNLM/DLC
for Library of Congress 93-5821
CIP

Proceedings of the Second International Conference on Drugs of Abuse, Immunity, and AIDS, held June 1–3, 1992, in Clearwater, Florida

ISBN 978-0-306-44566-8

PREFACE

This volume is based on the program of the Second International Conference on Drugs of Abuse, Immunity and AIDS, held in Clearwater Beach, FL in June 1992. The Conference was supported in part by the University of South Florida College of Medicine with financial assistance from the National Institute on Drug Abuse. The focus of this conference was the effects of drugs of abuse on immunity. It is now widely recognized that psychoactive drugs of abuse, including marijuana, cocaine, and opiates, as well as alcohol, have marked effects in an individual, including effects on their nervous system and behavior. In the past two decades, the scope of studies concerning the effects of some drugs of abuse have also involved investigations of alterations of various physiologic parameters including effects on the immune system, and the influence of such immune alterations on normal physiological responses. In this regard, participants in this Second International Conference provided newer information concerning both basic and clinical aspects of drugs of abuse and immunity, especially immunodeficiencies. In this regard, advances have been made in recent years concerning the nature and mechanisms whereby the immune system is regulated and the possible mechanisms by which drugs of abuse influence such immune systems. In particular, the emergence of psychoneuroimmunology as a new discipline the last decade has heightened interest in the immune responses influenced by psychoactive drugs. This has resulted in interdisciplinary investigations involving both clinical and basic scientists, including microbiologists, immunologists, physiologists, psychiatrists, oncologists, psychologists, etc.

The recreational use of drugs of abuse such as marijuana, cocaine and opiates, as well as alcohol, by large numbers of individuals has aroused serious concern about the consequences of this activity. As an example, it is well known that marijuana is widely used as a recreational drug in this as well as in other countries. In addition, cocaine use, especially crack cocaine, is considered epidemic in this country, as well as elsewhere. The "war on drugs" by the U.S. government is directly aimed at the use of marijuana and cocaine, as well as opiates and other illicit drugs. Alcohol is also known to be a major problem in this country, as it is in many other countries. It is estimated there are at least 10,000,000 alcoholics in the U.S. alone. A significant portion of those who are hospitalized for infectious diseases, as well as many chronic diseases, are alcoholics. Recently there have been reports of an association between the use of marijuana and development of certain types of cancer. Clinical observations and various clinical studies have spurred laboratory studies aimed at determining the nature and mechanism whereby such drugs affect immune function. There are strong concerns by a number of investigators that recreational drugs depress immunity and that individuals who use such drugs may be prone to infectious diseases, showing both increased morbidity and mortality due to infections. However, increased incidence of active infections has not been reported clinicially or even experimentally in terms of acute infections. Nevertheless, there have been several observations in laboratory as well as in clinical studies suggesting that chronic diseases, including infections by opportunistic pathogens, are often more frequent in drug abusers.

In the beginning of the 1970s, systematic studies were begun to determine whether recreational drugs such as marijuana and its components or opiates, like morphine, can influence immune responses in a negative manner. Similar studies were also performed with alcohol. Since then the number of these types of studies has increased, along with increased federal funding for the study of effects of drugs or alcohol on immunity. With the onset of the acquired immunodeficiency syndrome (AIDS) in the early 1980s in the United States and throughout the world, attempts were made to search for possible "co-factors" which interact with either the immunodeficiency virus or make an individual more susceptible to this virus. Approximately one fifth of all AIDS patients in this country are intravenous drug abusers and it has been shown that the AIDS virus can be spread by contaminated needles or equipment used by drug users. In addition, it is now widely recognized that such drugs may be immunosuppressive. Many AIDS patients, however, are not intravenous drug abusers but often abuse other drugs like marijuana, cocaine, or alcohol. Thus, many biomedical scientists believe it is possible that use of such drugs may serve as a co-factor in AIDS progression. Therefore, there has been a concerted effort by a number of investigators to examine in detail the mechanisms whereby these drugs compromise the immune system in general and, in particular, in concert with immunosuppressive viruses including retroviruses.

The first chapter of this volume deals with an overview of the relationship of the brain, stress, and immune function. The second chapter deals with an overview of psychological stress, immunity and immune depression. These chapters provide background information concerning the relationship between stress, immunity and the nervous system. The volume is then divided into groups of chapters dealing with individual categories of psychoactive drugs, such as studies dealing with marijuana and its components, cocaine and alcohol, as well as chapters dealing with miscellaneous drugs and human immunodeficiency virus (HIV) infection. The group of papers concerning marijuana and immunomodulation also includes a description of binding sites for marijuana on human lymphocytes. In this group of papers there is also a report dealing with marijuana and microbial infection including the effects of marijuana on *Legionella pneumophila* infection, syphilis infections, etc. The effects of marijuana on lymphocytes from individuals of different ages are also discussed and age is shown to be an important factor in immunomodulation.

The next group of papers describes results of studies concerning the emerging area of immunomodulation induced by cocaine. One paper presents a discussion of cocaine and immunocompetence as related to reactive metabolites of this drug. Cocaine-induced immunomodulation of human T lymphocyte proliferation is then presented, as well as the effects of cocaine on specific pathways of immune function, including the respiratory burst of murine macrophages. The effects of cocaine on parasitic infections and murine AIDS is then described.

The effects of alcohol on the immune response is discussed in the next group of papers. For example, the effects of ethyl alcohol on cytokine formation and infection by an opportunistic pathogen are described in one contribution. Another discusses the effects of alcohol on tumor necrosis factor and shows that alcohol has a major depressive effect. The depressive effect of alcohol on resistance to a parasitic infection during murine AIDS is then described. The marked depressive effect of ethanol on host defense mechanisms *in vivo* against bacterial infections is also described. The effects of other drugs of abuse, including inhalants, on antibody formation is presented as well as the effects of stress on natural killer cells in humans. There are then papers dealing with the AIDS epidemic and HIV infection, including the effects of stress and neurohormonal responses, as well as various factors related to malignancy associated with AIDS. The infectious complications in AIDS patients and HIV-positive individuals are also presented.

It is apparent that although many of the immune alterations induced by drugs of abuse have been defined, little is known concerning the molecular and cellular basis for these effects. Furthermore, acute and chronic public health implications are not fully appreciated or understood at the present time. Thus, the presentations of these papers by participants of this conference on drugs of abuse and immunity should be of interest to immunologists, pharmacologists, toxicologists and public health workers as well as others who care for and rehabilitate drug abusers. It is the hope of the editors that publication of this volume will inspire continued interest in the field of drugs of abuse and immunomodulation and will also result in a better definition of the true public health impact of drugs of abuse and immunity.

The editors take this opportunity to express gratitude to Ms. Ilona Friedman for outstanding assistance as the Conference Coordinator and excellent secretarial assistance in preparation of this volume. The editors also express gratitude to Ms. Sally Baker and Ms. Judy Flynn for secretarial assistance in the preparation of the conference and this volume. The editors thank NIDA staff members, Dr. Charles Sharp and Ms. Iris O'Brien, for helpful advice and suggestions in construction of the meeting program and their assistance in obtaining partial financial support. The editors thank the financial supporters of this Conference on which this book is based, including the Departments of Neurology and Anesthesiology at the University of South Florida, the University of South Florida Office of Sponsored Research, the H. Lee Moffitt Cancer Center and Research Institute and the several pharmaceutical companies which generously provided funds for travel expenses of many of the invited speakers.

H. Friedman
T. W. Klein
S. C. Specter

Tampa, FL

DRUGS OF ABUSE, IMMUNITY AND AIDS

Conference Organizers
(Department of Medical Microbiology and Immunology)

Herman Friedman, Ph.D., Professor and Chairman
Thomas W. Klein, Ph.D., Professor and Vice Chairman
Steven Specter, Ph.D., Professor
Gerald Lancz, Ph.D., Professor
Peter Medveczky, M.D., Associate Professor
Lois J. Paradise, Ph.D., Associate Professor
Susan Pross, Ph.D., Assistant Professor

Conference Coordinator

Ilona Friedman

Conference Co-Sponsors

Division of Sponsored Research - University of South Florida
Department of Medical Microbiology and Immunology - University of South Florida
Department of Anesthesiology - University of South Florida
Department of Neurology - University of South Florida
H. Lee Moffitt Cancer Center, Tampa, FL
Genetic Systems Corp., Redmond, WA
Sandoz Pharmaceutical, East Hanover, NJ
The Upjohn Company, Marietta, GA
National Institute on Drug Abuse, Rockville, MD

CONTENTS

Stress, the Hypothalamic-Pituitary-Adrenal Axis, and Immune Function 1
Marvin Stein and Andrew H. Miller

Psychological Stress, Immunity, and Immune Depression 7
Arthur Falek

Opioids, Receptors, and Immunity 13
Martin W. Adler, Ellen B. Geller, Thomas J. Rogers, Earl E. Henderson and Toby K. Eisenstein

Consequences of Opiate-Dependency in a Monkey Model of AIDS 21
Robert M. Donahoe, Larry D. Byrd, Harold M. McClure, Patricia Fultz, Mary Brantley, Frederick Marsteller, Aftab Ahmed Ansari, DeLoris Wenzel and Mario Aceto

Effects of Opioids on Proliferation of Mature and Immature Immune Cells 29
Horace H. Loh, Andrew P. Smith and Nancy M. Lee

Immune Alterations in Chronic Morphine-Treated Rhesus Monkeys 35
Daniel J.J. Carr and Charles P. France

Immunosuppressive Effects of Morphine on Immune Responses in Mice 41
Toby K. Eisenstein, Jeanine L. Bussiere, Thomas J. Rogers and Martin W. Adler

Morphine-Induced Modulation of Immune Status: Evidence for Opioid Receptor Mediation and Compartment Specificity 53
Donald T. Lysle, Mary E. Coussons, Val J. Watts, Elizabeth H. Bennett and Linda A. Dykstra

Morphine Binding Sites on Human T Lymphocytes 61
John J. Madden, David Ketelsen and William L. Whaley

Marijuana and Bacterial Infections 67
Thomas W. Klein, Catherine Newton, Raymond Widen and Herman Friedman

Effects of Marijuana on Spleen Lymphocytes from Mice of Different Age Groups 73
Susan Pross, Yasunobu Nakano, Sharon Bowen, Ray Widen and Herman Friedman

Syphilis and Drugs of Abuse 81
Lois J. Paradise and Herman Friedman

Serum Proteins Affect the Inhibition by Delta-Tetrahydrocannabinol of Tumor Necrosis Factor Alpha Production by Mouse Macrophages 89
Zhi-Ming Zheng, Steven Specter and Herman Friedman

Marijuana and Host Resistance to Herpesvirus Infection 95
G.A. Cabral, D.A. Dove Pettit and K. Fischer-Stenger

Marijuana and Head and Neck Cancer 107
James N. Endicott, Paulette Skipper and Lizette Hernandez

Evidence for a Cannabinoid Receptor in Immunomodulation by Cannabinoid Compounds 115
Norbert E. Kaminski

Cocaine and Immunocompetence: Possible Role of Reactive Metabolites 121
Michael P. Holsapple, Ray A. Matulka, Eric D. Stanulis and Stephen D. Jordan

Molecular Mechanisms Associated with Cocaine-Induced Modulation of Human T Lymphocytes Proliferation 127
Katsuhiko Matsui, Herman Friedman and Thomas W. Klein

Effects of Cocaine on the Respiratory Burst of Murine Macrophages 135
Austin Vaz, Stanley S. Lefkowitz and Doris L. Lefkowitz

Cocaine Facilitation of Cryptosporidiosis by Murine AIDS in Male and Female C57/BL/6 Mice 143
H. Darban, R.R. Watson, J. Alak and N. Thomas

Ethanol-Induced Suppression of *in Vivo* Host Defense Mechanisms to Bacterial Infection 153
Thomas R. Jerrells, A. Joe Saad and Thomas E. Kruger

Alcohol, Cytokines, and Immunodeficiency 159
John J. Spitzer and Abraham P. Baustista

Human Polymorphonuclear Leukocyte (PMN) Priming/Activation by Acute Ethanol Intoxication 165
André K. Balla, Elvira M. Doi, Paulo R. Wunder, James D. Ogle and Lawrence E. DeBault

Ethanol Affects Macrophage Production of IL-6 and Susceptibility to Infection by *Legionella pneumophila* 169
Yoshimasa Yamamoto, Thomas W. Klein and Herman Friedman

Suppression by Dietary Alcohol of Resistance to *Cryptosporidium* During Murine Acquired Immune Deficiency Syndrome 175
John I.B. Alak, Masoud Shahbazian, Dennis Huang, Yuejian Wang, Hamid Darban, Ronald R. Watson and Edward M. Jenkins

Enhancement of HIV-1 Replication by Opiates and Cocaine: The Cytokine Connection 181
Phillip K. Peterson, Genya Gekker, Ronald Schut, Shuxian Hu, Henry H. Balfour, Jr. and Chun C. Chao

Small Animal Model of AIDS and the Feline Immunodeficiency Virus 189
M. Bendinelli, M. Pistello, D. Matteucci, S. Lombardi, F. Baldinotti, P. Bandecchi, R. Ghilarducci, L. Ceccherini-Nelli, C. Garzelli, A. Poli, F. Esposito, G. Malvaldi and F. Tozzini

Current Status and Future Prospects in the Immunotherapy of Human Immunodeficiency Virus (HIV) Infection 203
John W. Hadden

Perinatal AIDS: Drugs of Abuse and Transplacental Infection 211
William D. Lyman

Solid Tumors and HIV-Infected Patients Other Than AIDS-Defining Neoplasms 219
Scot G. Remick, Ann Boguniewicz and Barbara Wolf

Stress, Endocrine Responses, Immunity and HIV-1 Spectrum Disease 225
Neil Schneiderman, Michael H. Antoni, Mary Ann Fletcher, Gail Ironson, Nancy Klimas, Mahendra Kumar and Arthur LaPerriere

Epidemiology and Infectious Complications of Human Immunodeficiency Virus Antibody Positive Patients 235
Bienvenido G. Yangco and Vicki S. Kenyon

Immune Function and Drug Treatment in Anti-Retrovirus Negative Intravenous Drug Users 241
Mary Ann Fletcher, Nancy G. Klimas and Robert O. Morgan

Psychosocial Stress and NK Cells among Members of a Communal Settlement 247
M. Schlesinger, Y. Yodfat, R. Rabinowitz, S. Bronner and J.D. Kark

Multiple Pathogens May Induce Growth Factor Cascade Resulting in KS 255
J.G. Sinkovics, J.E. Szakacs and F. Gyorkey

Exposure to the Abused Inhalant, Isobutyl Nitrite, Compromises both Antibody and Cell-Mediated Immunity 265
Lee S.F. Soderberg and John B. Barnett

Natural Killer Cells and *Cryptococcus neoformans* 269
Juneann W. Murphy

Index 277

STRESS, THE HYPOTHALAMIC-PITUITARY-ADRENAL AXIS, AND IMMUNE FUNCTION

Marvin Stein and Andrew H. Miller

Department of Psychiatry, Mount Sinai School of Medicine
Box 1229, One Gustave L. Levy Place, New York, NY 10029

A variety of stressors have been shown to alter both humoral and cell-mediated immune responses. Over the past decade the pathways by which stress may influence the immune system has been the focus of intense study. One of the most important pathways is the hypothalamic-pituitary-adrenal (HPA) axis (1, 2). It has been known for some time that glucocorticoids, the final product of HPA axis activation, have a wide range of effects on immune and inflammatory responses in humans and animals. In addition, other HPA hormones such as corticotropin releasing hormone (CRH) and corticotropin (ACTH) can directly and indirectly influence immune function.

Only recently have investigators come to appreciate the complex nature of the relationship between glucocorticoids and the immune system under physiologic conditions. In contrast to the widespread, almost invariably inhibitory immunologic effects of synthetic glucocorticoids, mounting evidence indicates that endogenous adrenal steroids have much more selective and specific effects on the immune system, allowing for not only suppression of immune responses but also enhancement of certain aspects of immune function. Therefore, endogenous glucocorticoids may not be limited solely to providing negative feedback on an evolving immune response as has been suggested, but may play a more comprehensive role in modulating the immune response. This reconceptualization of the role of adrenal steroids in immune regulation has developed from research in at least three major areas including studies from our laboratories and others on animal stress, adrenal steroid receptor expression in immune cells and tissues, and cytokine production by T helper cell subsets. Each of these areas of research will be discussed.

In our laboratory unpredictable and unavoidable electric tail shock in rats was found to suppress measures of the immune system, as determined by the number of circulating lymphocytes and phytohemagglutinin (PHA) induced lymphocyte proliferation in the peripheral blood (3). In an effort to determine adrenal involvement in these stress-induced alterations of immune parameters in the rat, we studied the effect of tail shock in adrenalectomized animals (4). The previously noted stress-induced lymphopenia was no longer apparent in adrenalectomized animals. Furthermore, despite the absence of adrenal hormones, isolated lymphocytes from the peripheral blood of stressed, adrenalectomized rats, like non-operated controls, continued to exhibit a

Drugs of Abuse, Immunity, and AIDS, Edited by
H. Friedman *et al.*, Plenum Press, New York, 1993

significant decrease in PHA-induced lymphocyte proliferation. These findings demonstrated that stress-induced lymphopenia in the rat occurs in association with the secretion of corticosteroids and can be prevented by adrenalectomy. Stress-induced adrenal secretion of corticosteroids was not required for stress-related suppression of peripheral lymphocyte stimulation by the T cell mitogen, PHA, in the rat. The suppression of T cell proliferation may be due to an adrenal-independent stress-induced depletion of functional subpopulations of T cells or a selective redistribution of T cells in lymphoid tissues. In addition, a variety of other hormonal, neurosecretory, and immunologic mechanisms may be involved in the adrenal-independent stress-induced modulation of T cell function. Nevertheless, the findings of adrenal-dependent stress-induced lymphopenia and of adrenal-independent effects on lymphocyte stimulation indicated that stress-induced modulation of the immune system is a complex phenomenon involving several, if not multiple, mechanisms. Changes in thyroid hormones, growth hormones, and sex steroids have been associated with exposure to stressors, and all have been reported to modulate immune function (5). Further, it has been shown that the hypothalamus, which plays a central role in neuroendocrine function, modulates both humoral and cell-mediated immunity (6, 7) These findings suggested that a range of neuroendocrine processes may be involved in stress-induced alterations of the immune system.

Since a variety of hormones under pituitary control have been associated with immunoregulatory processes, our laboratory (8) investigated the role of the pituitary in mediating stress-induced alterations of immunity. We studied the effects of tail shock on immune function in hypophysectomized rats. Plasma ACTH and corticosterone were increased in the stressed groups with pituitaries but were below detectable levels in the stressed hypophysectomized animals. In both the non-operated and sham-hypophysectomized animals there was a stress-induced decrease in the number of lymphocytes in the peripheral blood as well as a stress-related decrease in the number of T lymphocytes and T helper cells. Because the number of T suppressor cells and B lymphocytes was not altered by the stressful conditions, stress-induced lymphopenia in the rat is selective for T cells and specifically for T helper cells. In the hypophysectomized animals, however, no stress-related changes were found in the absolute number of lymphocytes or lymphocyte subsets. These results demonstrate that the stress-induced lymphopenia is pituitary-dependent, consistent with the observation that the number of circulating immunocompetent cells in response to a stressor is regulated by the HPA axis. The mechanism of this stress-related decrease in peripheral blood lymphocytes is unknown but may be related to vascular margination or migration of cells into the interstitial compartment, the lymphatics, or lymph nodes.

In contrast to the effects of hypophysectomy on lymphocytopenia, hypophysectomy did not reverse the effects of stress on PHA-induced lymphocyte proliferation in the peripheral blood. These findings demonstrated that factors not of pituitary origin mediate the stress-induced suppression of peripheral blood lymphocyte proliferative responses.

Another interesting finding in these studies was that the magnitude of the stress-induced suppression of lymphocyte function in the hypophysectomized animals was significantly greater than in control animals with intact pituitaries. These findings demonstrate that pituitary processes may be involved in countering stress-induced immunosuppressive mechanisms. The specific pituitary-dependent mitigating or compensating processes are not known, but probably involve multiple hormones including those with immunoenhancing properties, including growth hormone and prolactin (9,10). The findings suggest that a regulatory network of hormonal and non-hormonal systems is involved in the maintenance of immunologic capacity following exposure to stressors. The restraining influence of the pituitary on stress responses may be of relevance to the understanding of homeostatic maintenance of critical body functions.

It is of note that in all of the stress research with rats conducted in our laboratory (3, 4, 8), including the hypophysectomy study, in contrast to the findings with peripheral blood lymphocytes, there were no stress effects on splenic lymphocyte stimulation by PHA. The lack of a stress effect on the stimulation of splenic lymphocytes in contrast to peripheral blood lymphocytes may reflect differences in the various compartments of the immune system, each with its own microenvironment and subject to specific modulators and regulators.

Cunnick and co-workers (11) have also found that there are stress-induced (mild foot shock) differences in the endocrine mechanisms which mediate suppression of T lymphocyte responses in the spleen versus the peripheral blood. While adrenalectomy prevented the shock-induced suppression of the mitogenic response of the peripheral blood lymphocytes, adrenalectomy did not modify the suppression of splenic lymphocytes. In addition, while beta-adrenergic receptor antagonists attenuated the stress-induced suppression of splenic lymphocytes, these agents did not alter the suppression of peripheral blood lymphocyte mitogen responses. These findings suggest that specific and distinct mechanisms are involved in the stress-induced suppression of lymphocyte responses to mitogens in the peripheral blood and spleen. Catecholamines and the autonomic nervous system (ANS) appear to play a large role in the splenic mitogen response, and adrenal steroids appear to be responsible for the suppression of peripheral blood lymphocyte responses to mitogens.

As a means of further understanding the relationship between adrenal steroid hormones and lymphocyte function, our recent studies have focused on receptors for adrenal steroids in immune cells and tissues. Two separate high-affinity receptors for glucocorticoids have been characterized (12, 13,14): type I receptors, which are commonly referred to as mineralocorticoid receptors and type II receptors, which are also known as glucocorticoid receptors. There is heterogeneity in the expression of type I and II receptors in the brain and a unique distribution of these receptor subtypes within various brain regions (12). For example, the highest concentration of type I receptors is found in the granule and pyramidal cells of the hippocampus (12, 15). Moreover, within the hippocampus, type II receptors have the highest level of expression in the CA1 and CA2 regions (12,15). In terms of HPA axis regulation, type I receptors, which have a high affinity for endogenous adrenal steroid hormones, are believed to play a role in the regulation of circadian fluctuations in corticosteroids (13, 14). On the other hand, type II receptors have a lower affinity for endogenous adrenal steroids than type I receptors and therefore are believed to be more important in termination of the corticosteroid response to stress when endogenous levels of glucocorticoids are high (13, 14). It is important to note that unlike neurotransmitter receptors, for example, which primarily act through second messenger pathways, steroid hormone receptors when bound to their ligand serve as transcription factors and directly regulate the expression of multiple genes (16).

Several important findings have emerged from our studies on adrenal steroid receptors in the immune system. First, like in the brain, there is heterogeneity of receptor expression in immune tissues (17). For example, the thymus exhibits the highest amount of type II receptors followed by the spleen and peripheral blood. In addition, while both type I and type II receptor binding was present in the spleen, only type II binding was detected in the thymus (17). This differential expression of receptors may confer on these tissues different sensitivity or responsivity to glucocorticoids and, thereby, explain why one immune compartment or cell type may respond differently following stress compared to another.

Of great interest is our observation that while synthetic hormones like dexamethasone almost exclusively activate type II adrenal steroid receptors, naturally occurring hormones activate both type I and type II receptors depending on the concentration (17). Furthermore, pharmacological doses of synthetic glucocorticoids access and activate adrenal steroid receptors equally in all immune compartments, while endogenous glucocorticoids have a more selective and specific access to adrenal steroid receptor subtypes in the various immune tissues (17, 18). Consistent with the adrenal-dependent effects of stress on peripheral blood immune responses, endogenous glucocorticoids access and activate type II adrenal steroid receptors in the peripheral blood and thymus more readily than receptors in the spleen (18). We have recently shown that receptor activation is highly correlated with decreases in immune function, and therefore evidence of receptor activation appears to be critical for determining when and in which tissues adrenal steroid stress effects modulate the immune response (19).

One of the most intriguing findings which supports the notion of a comprehensive role of glucocorticoids in the modulation of the immune response is the existence of subsets of T helper cells which secrete specific profiles of cytokines and are differentially affected by glucocorticoids (20). These T helper (or Th) subsets have been best characterized in the mouse and have been shown to play an important role in immune regulation. Thl cells synthesize IL-2 and IFN-gamma, resulting in enhancement of cell-mediated immune responses such as delayed type hypersensitivity, and Th2 cells secrete IL-4, IL-5, and IL-6 which primarily enhance B cells and humoral immune responses. There is evidence that Th1 and Th2 clones are mutually antagonistic and hinder the development of the other (21, 22).

Interestingly, glucocorticoids enhance the production of IL-4 and suppress the synthesis of IL-2 (23) and thereby promote antibody synthesis and suppress cell-mediated responses. A glucocorticoid influence can thus be beneficial in some autoimmune states while at the same time be a risk factor when a cell-mediated immune response is needed to eliminate a pathogen. Th1 and Th2 subsets have not been demonstrated in humans. However, stages of resistance and susceptibility to lesions in leprosy has been shown to be associated with specific patterns of cytokine production and T cell subsets (24, 25).

In summary, the relationship between glucocorticoids and the immune system is complex and involves many factors. From the findings presented in this review, it is evident that endogenous glucocorticoids have selective and specific effects on the regulation of the immune system including enhancement as well as suppression of immune responses. These modulatory influences of glucocorticoids have important implications for health and illness.

Acknowledgements

This research was supported in part by Research Scientist Development Award (MH00680) to AHM and research grant (MH47674) to AHM. We wish to thank Richard Rhee for his assistance in preparation of the manuscript.

REFERENCES

1. V. Riley, Psychoneuroendocrine influences on immunocompetence and neoplasia, *Science* 212:1100 (1981).
2. H. Selye, "Stress in Health and Disease", Butterworth's, Boston (1976).
3. S. E. Keller, J.M. Weiss, S.J. Schleifer, N.E. Miller, M. Stein, Suppression of immunity by stress: effect of a graded series of stressors on lymphocyte stimulation in the rat, *Science* 213: 1397 (1981).
4. S. E. Keller, J.M. Weiss, S.J. Schleifer, N.E. Miller, and M. Stein: Stress-induced suppression of immunity in adrenalectomized rats, *Science* 221:1301 (1983).

5. R. Ader, D.L. Felten, and N. Cohen, "Psychoneuroimmunology", Second Ed., Academic Press, San Diego (1991).
6. M. Stein, S.E. Keller, and S.J. Schleifer, The hypothalamus and the immune response, *in*: "Brain, Behavior, and Bodily Disease", H. Weiner, M.A. Hofer and A. J. Stunkard, eds., Raven Press, New York (1981).
7. R. J. Cross, W.H. Brooks, H.L. Roszman, and R. Markesbery, Hypothalamic-immune interactions, *J. Neurol. Sci.* 53:557 (1982).
8. S. E. Keller, S.J. Schleifer, A S. Liotta, R.N. Bond, N. Farhoody, and M. Stein, Stress induced alterations of immunity in hypophysectomized rats, *Proc. Nat. Acad. Sci* 85:557 (1988).
9. E. W. Bernton, H.V. Bryant, and J.W. Holaday, Prolactin and immune function, *in*: "Psychoneuroimmunology", Second Ed., R. Ader, D.L. Felten, and N. Cohen, eds., Academic Press, San Diego (1991).
10. K. W. Kelley, Growth hormone in immunobiology, *in*: "Psychoneuroimmunology", Second ed., R. Ader, D.L. Felten, and N. Cohen, eds., Academic Press, San Diego (1991).
11. J. E. Cunnick, D.T. Lysle, B.J. Kucinski, and B.S. Rabin, Evidence that shock-induced immune suppression is mediated by adrenal hormones and peripheral beta adrenergic receptors, Pharmacol. *Biochem. and Behavior* 36:645 (1990).
12. J. M. Reul, E.R. deKloet, Two receptor systems for corticosterone in rat brain: Microdistribution and differential occupation, *Endocrinol.* 117:2505 (1985).
13. J. M. Reul, F.R. van den Bosch, E.R. deKloet, Relative occupation of type I and type II corticosteroid receptors in rat brain following stress and dexamethasone treatment: Functional implications, *J. Endocrinol.* 115:459 (1987).
14. A. Ratka, W. Sutanto, M. Bloemers, E.R. deKloet, On the role of brain mineralocorticoid (type I) and glucocorticoid (type II) receptors in neuroendocrine regulation, *Neuroendocrinol.* 50:117 (1989).
15. B. S. McEwen, J. Angulo, H. Cameron et al., Paradoxical effects of adrenal steroids on the brain: Protection versus degeneration, *Biological Psychiatry* 31:177 (1992).
16. R. L. Miesfield, Molecular genetics of corticosteroid action, *Amer. Review of Resp. Dis.* 141:11 (1990).
17. A. H. Miller, R.L. Spencer, M. Stein, B.S. McEwen, Adrenal steroid receptor binding in spleen and thymus after stress or dexamethasone, *Amer. J. Physiol.* 259:405 (1990).
18. R. L. Spencer, A.H. Miller, S.S. Kang, M. Stein, B.S. McEwen, Diurnal comparison of adrenal steroid receptor activation in brain, pituitary and immune tissue, Presented at the annual meeting of the Soc. Neuroscience, New Orleans, LA (1991).
19. A H. Miller, R.L. Spencer, R.L. Trestman, C. Kim, B.S. McEwen, M.S. Stein, Adrenal steroid receptor activation *in vivo* and immune function, *American J. Physiol.* 261:126 (1991).
20. T. R. Mosmann and R.L. Coffman, Two types of mouse helper T-cell clones: implications for immune regulation, *Immunol. Today* 8:223 (1987).
21. T. R. Mosmann and R.L. Coffman, Th1 and Th2 cells: Different patterns of Iymphokine secretion lead to different functional properties, *Ann. Rev. Immunol.* 7:145 (1989).
22. T. F. Gajewski, S.R. Schell, G; Nau, and F.W. Fitch, Regulation of T-cell activation: differences among T cell subsets, *Immunol. Rev.* 111:79 (1989).
23. R. A. Daynes, B.A. Araneo, Contrasting effects of glucocorticoids on the capacity of T cells to produce the growth factors interleukin 2 and interleukin 4, *Eur. J. Immunol.* 19:2319 (1989).
24. M. Yamamura, K Ugemura, R.J. Deans, K Weinberg, T.H. Rea, B.R. Bloom, and R.L. Modlin, Defining protective responses to pathogens: cytokine profiles in leprosy lesions, *Science* 254:277 (1991).
25. P. Salgame, J.S. Abrams, C. Clayberger, H. Goldstein, J. Convit, R.L Modlin, and B.R. Bloom, Differing Iymphokine profiles of functional subsets of human CD4 and CD8 T cell clones. *Science* 254:279 (1991).

PSYCHOLOGICAL STRESS, IMMUNITY AND IMMUNE DEPRESSION

Arthur Falek

Human and Behavioral Genetics Research Laboratory
Department of Psychiatry and Behavioral Sciences
Emory University, Georgia Mental Health Institute
Atlanta, Georgia 30306

The opportunity to present a Special Lecture at this International Conference on Drugs of Abuse, Immunity and AIDS is a privilege, and I am most grateful to Drs. Friedman, Klein and Specter for the honor they have accorded me. However, to ferret out an area for presentation that does not contain information presented by other speakers in this session, or to just review their published findings, would be a waste of time for this presentation. Certainly, I do not want to use my time to discuss in any part, the information provided by my colleagues - Drs. Robert Donahoe and John Madden - in their presentations. I have decided, therefore, to focus on an issue of long-standing interest to me which also may have relevance to upcoming discussions of other presentations in this section of the publication.

The new textbook on **Stress and Immunity** by Plotnikoff, Murgo, Faith and Wybran, (1) published by CRC Press last year, provides a detailed and thoughtful review by Hillhouse, Kiecolt-Glaser and Glaser (2) on Stress-Associated Modulation of the Immune Response in Humans. These scientists and others who authored chapters in **Stress and Immunity**, authored chapters in the 2nd edition of **Psychoneuroimmunology** by Ader, Felten and Cohen, (3) published by Academic Press also in 1991, and authors of papers published elsewhere, have reported mostly the down-regulation of immune cell responses measured in a variety of ways with a variety of psychological stressors. Almost all have noted the complex nature of these responses. For more than a decade there has been identification of the role played by the endocrine system and how high or low levels of endocrine hormones enhance or suppress immune functions. In a series of carefully designed experiments in rats, Weiss (4) and associates at Duke University, elucidated physiological mechanisms underlying a number of cellular immune responses. They demonstrated that stressful conditions significantly suppressed blood and spleen lymphocyte immune responses and reported on multiple physiologic pathways that mediated these responses. These pathways include adrenal hormones, small molecules in the blood (e.g., steroids and catecholamines) and, in addition, a large peptide (> 10 kilodalton) produced by the animal. These investigators also showed that stressful conditions of moderate intensity enhanced rather than suppressed cellular immune responses providing initial evidence that very small quantities of interlukin 1, acting in the animal brain, suppressed cellular immune responses rapidly and without rebound for up to 24 hours. Furthermore, there are the findings by Irwin and his group

Drugs of Abuse, Immunity, and AIDS, Edited by
H. Friedman *et al.*, Plenum Press, New York, 1993

(5) at the San Diego Veterans Administration Medical Center as well as Jain and colleagues (6) at New York University Medical Center, affirming, at least in rodents, an initiating role of the corticotropin releasing factor (CRF) of the hypothalamus in modulating the immune system response to stress largely by adrenal independent mechanisms through pathways that regulate the autonomic nervous system.

However, while the physiological mechanisms underlying stress responses in animals are being described in ever increasing detail, there is only limited discussion among psychoneuroimmunologists of the apparently more complex way humans, in particular, cope with a stressful/threatening event psychologically. What is at issue is whether the more complex processing of the psychological response to a stressor observed in humans introduces an increased variability that is currently being overlooked at the physiological and, particularly for this conference, at the immunological level. This is the issue I wish to address in this presentation.

It is most appropriate at the outset to acknowledge the importance that Hillhouse, Kiecolt-Glaser and Glaser (2) gave to this topic in their chapter in **Stress and Immunity** and to commend them as well for their ever-increasing compendium of findings in humans of the effects of stressful life events on immunological modulation and disease. In the context of a scientific discussion about this area of investigation, it is also appropriate to focus on apparent limitations of those findings. Let me also put aside for the moment the evidence that there are strain differences in research animals, as well as personality differences in humans, implicating genetic factors that result in variations of response in subtypes of a species to a specific stressor.

In addition to studies indicating subtypes of individuals with identified immunologic differences in response to psychological stress, Hillhouse, Kiecolt-Glaser and Glaser (2) also provide a conceptual foundation for the cross-sectional model they employ to measure the immunological modulation that occurs when an individual responds to a psychologically stressful event. This issue has been of interest to psychologists and psychiatrists for many years who have reported on the complexity of the stress response process, e.g., Janis, (7) Coelho, (8) Lazarus and Folkman, (10). In fact, Hillhouse, Kiecolt-Glaser and Glaser (2) point out that Lazarus and Folkman (10) in their well-known text on **Stress, Appraisal and Coping**, conceptualized that the interactions of a psychological stressor are components of its introduction as an external threat, its internal evaluations by the individual, the individual's marshalling of personal resources to deal with the threat, and the individual's assessment of the stressor's potential to significantly modulate physical and psychological outcomes. It is there opinion that these factors result in the cognitive, emotional, physiological and behavioral manifestations of stress. To this point I am in agreement with the comment.

However, in the section of their chapter, entitled **"Overview of the Stress-Immuno Relationship"** in **Stress and Immunity** Hillhouse and colleagues (2) describe the physiological effects of stress as categorized under the "rubric of arousal" while the interrelated emotional presentations are under the heading of anxiety. What is meant by anxiety? Hillhouse and colleagues (2) ascribe to the definition of anxiety presented by Paterson and Neufeld (11) who describe anxiety as a state of general arousal related to the emotions of anger, fear, excitement or depression. What is not included is Paterson and Neufeld's further statement in their chapter that anxiety is a "generic emotional concomitant of arousal" that may be expressed as <u>any</u> of the above-stated emotions. Although several of these emotions are thought to differ psychologically, what this definition does, unfortunately, is smooth out the variability encompassed in the above-mentioned cognitive and emotional components that comprise different aspects of the coping response. Furthermore, as Paterson and Neufeld (11) regard anxiety as a generic expression of anger, fear, excitement and depression, this would seem to imply that one set of physiological outcomes expressed in response to a stressful event is equivalent to that obtained by measuring the physiological effects at any other time in the pattern of responses. The implication is that what is being identified is a global effect rather than a state effect. There are many publications including that of Folkman and Lazarus (12) that would contest this point of view with evidence that in humans, and in at least some lower primates, there is a more complex response as the individual processes through a psychologically stressful event. The authors of these publications would point out that it is not only important to keep in mind the fluctuations and changes that are exhibited when processing through a stress response, but that the design of experiments to assess the neuroendocrine and immune consequences of stress need to incorporate such measurements into each of the identified phases in the process.

This, in fact, is also stated by Hillhouse and colleagues (2) towards the end of their chapter when they point out that "no single point measure provides the 'true' picture of this complex relationship", "that longitudinal studies with many data points across the different systems are needed to understand these processes" and that "it will not be possible to understand these systems until the time and effort is extended to map out these interactions." I commend them for these statements as this is an appropriate approach to this issue. What is unsatisfactory, is that while these responses are expressed, there is no evidence of current programs to develop new approaches to overcome the previously identified limitations. As indicated by Martin (13) in his chapter in **Advances in the Investigation of Psychological Stress** what is consistently presented in the literature are cross-sectional findings.

My knowledge about the various aspects of coping in response to a stressful event and a conceptualization of the content in each of the stages was based initially on experiences in providing help to family members of patients newly diagnosed with Huntington's disease. In genetic counseling sessions with these family members, I became aware of an identifiable pattern of responses in these individuals as they coped with this obviously stressful situation. As many of you may know, Huntington's disease is a inherited neuropsychiatric disorder with onset usually in the late 30's or early 40's resulting in chronic mental and physical deterioration with ever increasing choreiform movements as well as dementia and an early death 15 to 20 years after onset. As it is an autosomal dominantly inherited disorder, each child of an affected parent has a 50% chance of also developing the disorder sometime in his/her lifetime. A review of the literature about coping responses to a variety of stress-producing situations including bereavement, self-dying, physical trauma as well as environmental trauma provided evidence of similar patterns of response to these different stress-producing situations [Falek and Britton] (14).

After interviewing many parents of young people who had died in a fire while attending a dance in Boston, this pattern of responses to a stressful event was first described by Lindeman (15) in 1944. This pattern of responses was described as the dynamics of grief as applied to the dying by Schilder (16) in 1951, and was later described as the coping responses of terminal cancer patients by Kubler-Ross (17) in 1969. Since then this pattern of responses has been associated with many other stressful situations. Most commonly, investigators report a pattern of four general responses to individuals under stress: 1) shock and denial, 2) anxiety, 3) anger and/or guilt and 4) depression. These basic responses to a stressor are not particular to the trauma, but appear to be a general adaptation reaction to any situation of severe stress and is considered the phenotypic expression of psychological mechanisms attempting to reestablish the steady state. The importance of these observations to this Conference is that this four-part coping sequence to regain homeostasis is the behavioral expression in the ongoing process of cognitive and emotional incorporation of any traumatic event leading to psychological readjustment. If the behavioral responses reflect to any degree what is occurring at the physiological level, it is most unlikely that the neuroendocrine and immunological findings detected at an early stage of the coping process, as for example the stage of shock/denial, will be similar to what is observed during the periods of anxiety or depression.

A psychological interpretation of the stage of shock/denial is that the individual does not acknowledge the stressful situation at either the cognitive or emotional level and is not motivated at this point to initiate the behavioral changes necessary to adjust to the new reality. The second stage in the coping sequence is that of anxiety as the individual perceives the change produced by the stress and experiences realistic fear manifested as anxiety in attempts to deal with the new situation on an intellectual level. As attempts to resolve the problem at the cognitive level repeatedly fail, the individual becomes frustrated and angry, and as habituation occurs the symptoms of depression appear. As a normal person cannot function in a continued state of depression, he will begin trying new behaviors in an attempt to adjust to the current situation. This is an approach to a realistic adjustment, since the behavioral changes emanate from both the emotional and cognitive realization of the stressful event.

I have taken the time to outline some of the components of the coping response to a stressful situation to point out that the psychodynamic changes observed at different stages in the coping response may be indicative of variability in response at the immune and other physiological levels as individuals progress through the process of coping. While some of the terms used to describe different aspects in the process of coping with a stressful event may have changed over time, it is evident that the conceptual model continues to focus on the coping response as a process (Lazarus and Folkman, (10); Folkman and Lazarus, (12); Martin) (13). What is required for the development of this model are: 1) tools for data acquisition that most clearly identify components of specific stages in the pattern of processing in response to a stressor and 2) method(s) of assessment that confirm the generation of an accurate, predictive model of change from one stage to another as the individual processes through the phases of this psychoneurobiological system.

These objectives need to be incorporated into the rapidly growing program of research in psychoneuroimmunology as well as studies of psychological stress. A recent review of scales to assess coping strategies by Martin (13) indicates less than a handful of measures have been proposed with little evidence of their validity or usefulness in specifying stages in the process. Until appropriate psychological scales are devised, neuroendocrine and immunological assessments will only be based on subjective determinants of an individual's stage in the coping process for comparison with physiological findings. On the one hand, what is so remarkable is that in spite of this limitation most, if not all, of us with clinical skills believe we are able to recognize the behavioral presentation when individuals are in one or another stage in the process. On the other hand, there is no indication when an individual is in the process of moving from one stage to another, and we do not know whether there is a behavioral or a physiological indicator that signals the occurrence of a behavioral change, or if both the behavioral and physiological signals of change occur simultaneously.

Furthermore, as mentioned in the early part of this presentation, it may be that subtypes identified as depressed or anxious with evidence of neuroendocrine alterations and immunologic depression are more consistent both psychologically and immunologically because the test subjects are at one or another intermediate stage of the coping sequence and unable to achieve homeostasis. This would also fit with the implication that these subtypes are the consequence of some genetic factor(s) that inhibit completion in the processing of the coping response.

As progression through the stages of coping appears to be complex and nonlinear, a model of evaluation based on simple regression analyses would be inappropriate. An accurate and predictive model to explore this psychoneurobiological system may be through the stochastic Markov process, e.g., Feller, (18) in which future values of a random variable are statistically determined by present events and dependent only on the immediately preceding one. At a more complex level are the chaos type models that provide a new way of seeing order and pattern in a system that formerly seemed only random, erratic and unpredictable, e.g. Gleick, (19).

What is evident at present is that to investigate the dynamic interrelations of the immunological, neuroendocrine and psychological components of psychological stress in humans so as to account for the apparent ordered complexity of these associations over time will require the development of procedures for evaluation and the structuring of research designs that are not currently available.

REFERENCES

1. N. Plotnikoff, A. Murgo, R. Faith, and J. Wybran, *Stress and Immunity*, CRC Press, Boca Raton (1991).
2. J. E. Hillhouse, J. K. Kiecolt-Glaser, and R. Glaser, Stress associated modulation of the immune response in humans, Chap.1 *in*: "Stress and Immunity", N. Plotnikoff, A. Murgo, R. Faith, and J. Wybran, eds., CRC Press, Boca Raton (1991).
3. R. Ader, D. L. Felten, and N. Cohen, *Psychoneuroimmunol.* (2nd Ed), Academic Press, New York (1991).
4. J. M. Weiss, S. K. Sundar, K. J. Becker, and M. A.Cierpial, Behavioral and neural influences one cellular immune responses: Effects of stress and interlukin-1, *J. Clin. Psychiatry* 50:5, Suppl.) 43 (1989).
5. M. Irwin, R. L Hauger, L. Jones, M. Provencio, and K. Britton, Sympathetic nervous system mediates central corticotropin-releasing factor induced suppression of natural killer cell cytotoxicity, *J. Pharm. Exper. Therapeut.* 255:101 (1990).
6. R. Jain, D. Zwickler, C. S. Hollander, H. Brand, A. Saperstein, B. Hutchinson, C. Brown, and T. Audhya, Corticotropin-releasing factor modulates the immune response to stress in the rat, *Endocrinol.* 128:1329 (1991).
7. I. Janis, *Psychological Stress*, John Wiley, New York (1958).
8. G. V. Coelho, D. A. Hamburg, and J. E. Adams, "Coping and Adaptation", Basic Books, New York (1974).
9. J. K. Kiecolt-Glaser, and R. Glaser, Stress and immune functions in humans, *in*: "Psychoimmunology", (2nd Edition), Academic Press, New York pp. 849 (1989).
10. R. S.Lazarus, and S. Folkman, "Stress, Appraisal and Coping", Springer, New York (1984).
11. R. J. Paterson, and R. W. J. Neufeld, The stress response and parameters of stressful situations, Chap. 1. *in*: "Advances in Investigations of Psychological Stress, R. W. J. Neufeld, ed., John Wiley, New York, pp. 7 (1989).
12. S. Folkman, and R. S. Lazarus, If it changes it must be a process: Study of emotion and coping during three sages of a college examination, *J. Personality and Social Psychol.* 48:150 (1985).
13. R. A. Martin, Techniques for data acquisition and analysis in field investigations of stress, Chap. 6 *in*: "Advances in Investigations of Psychological Stress," R. W. J. Neufeld, ed., John Wiley, New York pp. 195 (1989).
14. A. Falek, and S. Britton, Phases in coping: The hypothesis and its implications, Social Biology 21:1 (1974).
15. E. Lindemann, "Symptomatology and management of acute grief", *Amer. J. Psychiat.* 101:141 (1944).
16. P. Schilder, *Psychotherapy,* W.W. Norton, New York (1951).
17. E. Kubler-Ross, "On death and dying", Macmillan, New York (1969).
18. W. Feller, *in*: "An Introduction to Probability Theory and its Applications", Vol 1, 3rd Edition. John Wiley, New York, "Markov Chains", Chapter XV pp. 372 (1968).
19. J. Gleick, "Chaos". Viking, New York (1987).

OPIOIDS, RECEPTORS, AND IMMUNITY

Martin W. Adler[1], Ellen B. Geller[1], Thomas J. Rogers[2], Earl E. Henderson[2], and Toby K. Eisenstein[2]

[1]Department of Pharmacology
[2]Department of Microbiology and Immunology
Temple University School of Medicine
Philadelphia, PA 19140

INTRODUCTION

One property common to all drugs that are abused is that they act on the central nervous system to produce feelings that are deemed desirable. Along with producing these so-called desirable effects, however, the drugs produce many other effects. These may be due to indirect actions resulting from the fact that all systems interact, or they may be due to the presence of specific receptors for a particular drug in many parts of the body. Receptors may be defined as chemical structures that first bind the drug and then produce an effect when they are activated. This definition is in contradistinction to a binding site or acceptor site, which binds the drug but does not produce a biological effect.

It was not until 1973 that specific receptors for an abused class of drugs were identified. At that time, the opiate receptor was discovered (1-3). We now know that there are several types of opioid receptors and the ones generally accepted are mu, kappa, and delta. Furthermore, each of these types is believed to have subtypes, similar to the picture seen with other endogenous systems. The endogenous opioid system consists not only of the receptors, but of several endogenous opioid peptides. These compounds arise from 3 precursor molecules: proopiomelanocortin gives rise primarily to ß-endorphin; proenkephalin, to the 5-amino-acid peptides, met- and leu-enkephalin; and prodynorphin, to dynorphin.

This paper is concerned with the effects of opioids on the immune system. In order to properly evaluate the effects of drugs on any system and to determine if the actions are receptor-mediated, certain basic pharmacological principles should be followed (Table 1).

STUDYING RECEPTOR-MEDIATED INTERACTIONS

Although all of the principles listed in Table 1 are important, time of testing and pharmacokinetics are particularly critical when determining if an antagonist is effective

Drugs of Abuse, Immunity, and AIDS, Edited by
H. Friedman *et al.*, Plenum Press, New York, 1993

Table 1. Pharmacological principles applied in determining responses to opioids

Use both *in vivo* and *in vitro* administration
Use different routes of drug administration
Do full dose-response curves
Choose time of testing based on latency and duration of drug action
Consider pharmacokinetics, especially if more than one drug is used
Consider species and strain differences of test animals
Use selective agonists and antagonists
Use acute and chronic drug administration

in vivo. The antagonist has to be administered at a time when its action coincides with the action of the agonist. For example, if naloxone is given 20 or 30 or more minutes prior to morphine, the effect of the naloxone has diminished markedly and is almost over before the peak effect of morphine is reached, and the conclusion that naloxone does not block the effect may not be warranted. In other words, the half-life of the drugs has to be considered. In the case of naloxone, the half-life is in the range of 16-20 minutes (4-6), meaning that only one-half of the amount of naloxone is still present at that time and the remainder disappears according to first-order kinetics in a logarithmic fashion. Basic pharmacological principles such as these become even more important when dealing with interactions among different chemicals and different systems.

INTERACTIONS BETWEEN OPIOIDS AND IMMUNE SYSTEM

In recent years, we have begun to appreciate that there is a close interaction between the brain and the immune system. It has been known for many years that there is an interrelationship between the pituitary, the hypothalamus, and the adrenal gland. In situations producing marked stress, there is analgesia and the brain can cause the release of hormones in the body, such as the glucocorticoids, that can produce suppression of the immune system. In addition, the chemical products (i.e., cytokines) released by immune cells can have a marked effect on the nervous system. For example, interferon-α, tumor necrosis factor, and interleukin-6 can induce a fever that is partly blockable by the opiate antagonist naloxone (7), and interferon-α can affect the firing rate in various brain loci (8). Other cytokines have been reported to have a variety of actions on neuronal systems [for review, see (9).] Because of the relationship between the two systems, it is logical to assume that a drug acting on the central nervous system might well have effects on the immune system.

What provided the impetus for the studies of the effects of centrally acting abused drugs on the immune system was the close relationship between intravenous drug use and HIV infection. Although it certainly appeared (and has since been proven) that the infection could be spread by needle-sharing, a number of investigators believed that it was possible that there might be a more direct link between the drugs and the immune system. For example, it was well known that heroin addicts were subject to many more cases of serious infection than others in the population. This had generally been attributed to malnutrition and/or lack of sanitation (10), but could it have been something else as well? Our laboratory was one of several that began to investigate whether there could be a direct effect of abused drugs on the immune system. Based on reports from a number of groups, including some that are represented in this symposium, it is now known that morphine suppresses a number of components of the immune system, including T-cell rosetting (11,12), macrophage function (13), responses to PHA and Con A (14,15), delayed-type hypersensitivity (16), and NK activity (17,18). In those experiments where naloxone was used, it blocked the actions of morphine. Morphine can decrease antibody formation and increase susceptibility to certain infections (19-21). When given in an adequate regimen and at an appropriate time with regard to pharmacokinetics, naloxone can block these effects. Of great interest is the finding that morphine and heroin appear to enhance proliferation of the HIV virus and that this effect is blockable by naloxone (22,23). Somewhat paradoxically, studies with the endogenous opioid ß-endorphin have generally reported naloxone-antagonizable enhancement of the activity of NK cells (24,25). The C-terminal fragments of the peptide decrease activity of NK cells, however, and this action is not blocked by naloxone (26). Despite the fact that binding studies have been relatively unsuccessful (27), the pharmacological evidence is quite conclusive that most of the receptors involved in the immune system responses to opioids are similar to those in the nervous system. Mu and kappa opioid receptors appear to be present on immune cells and are involved in the regulation of lymphoid cell production of antibodies (28).

In order to determine the effects of opioids on the immune system, we have utilized 3 paradigms and these are shown in Table 2. Such paradigms yield data that allow determination of whether the effects are direct, indirect, or, possibly, both.

One of the standard approaches to determining if morphine produces a demonstrable effect on the immune system of a mouse is to administer the drug at a high dose for several days. This can be accomplished by the subcutaneous implantation of a pellet containing 75 mg of morphine base. With respect to the formation of antibody to tetanus toxin, our studies found that there was no significant difference between mice that received the primary dose of tetanus toxoid 24 hrs after pellet implantation and

Table 2. Paradigms for determining effects of opioids on immune system

PARADIGM	TREATMENT	ASSAY
In vivo, in vivo	Morphine, naltrexone, or placebo pellets implanted *in vivo*	Serum response to tetanus toxoid
In vivo, in vitro	Morphine, naltrexone, or placebo pellets implanted *in vivo*	*In vitro* primary splenic PFC responses
In vitro, in vitro	Opioids administered *in vitro*	Normal spleen cells cultured with or without opioids

those in the placebo group. If, however, an interval of 72 hrs elapsed between the time of pellet implantation and the time at which a primary dose of tetanus toxoid was injected, there was a 10-fold reduction in the titer of antibody to tetanus toxoid (20) in the secondary response.

We have also found that when morphine is administered to a mouse by pellet implantation, there is a suppression of the *in vitro* primary antibody response to sheep red blood cells which is reversed by naltrexone. The results are shown in Figure l, taken from the data of Bussiere et al., (29). It is readily apparent that the marked suppression produced by morphine is completely antagonized by naltrexone, indicating a classical opioid-receptor-mediated effect.

The effects just discussed could be explained either by a direct action on cells of the immune system or an indirect effect due to the release of corticosteroids by morphine. To eliminate the possibility of indirect effects on immune cells, studies involving *in vitro* drug exposure are particularly useful. Another of the pharmacological principles shown in Table 1 is that selective agonists should be used, a relatively simple principle when studying drug effects *in vitro*. In addition to using morphine, therefore, the effects of selective agonists for the mu, kappa, and delta opioid receptors can be evaluated since morphine can affect all three types of receptors. As reported by Taub et al., (28), it was found that the mu-selective agonist, Tyr-D-Ala-Gly-N-Me-Phe-Gly-ol (DAMGO), and the kappa-selective opioid agonists, U50,488H and U69,593, in concentrations as low as 10^{-10} M, inhibited the capacity of murine lymphoid cells to generate antibody. The delta-selective agonist D-Pen^{2,5}-enkephalin (DPDPE), at concentrations ranging from 10^{-12} to 10^{-5} M, had no detectable effect on antibody response. In order to confirm the specificity of the agonist effect on the particular type of opioid receptor, selective antagonists were used. Nor-binaltorphimine (Nor-BNI), the highly selective antagonist for the kappa opioid receptor, blocked the suppression produced by U50,488H. Morphine, which acts primarily at the mu receptor, was not blocked.

STRAIN DIFFERENCES

The CxBk/By mouse is a strain of mouse that is deficient in the mu receptor. If morphine and DAMGO, both of which are selective for the mu opioid receptor, exerted their immunosuppressive effects by way of the mu receptor, neither should suppress

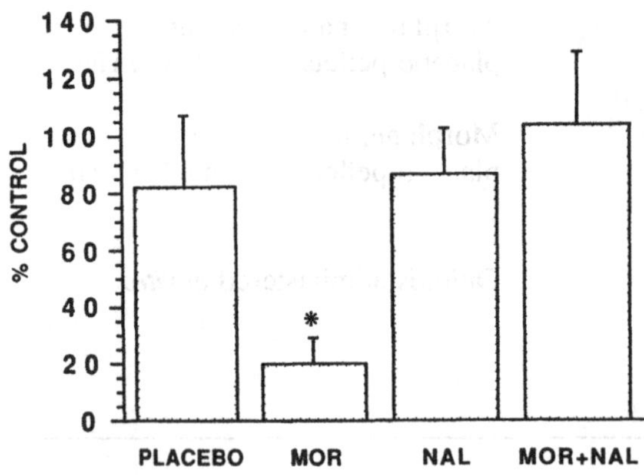

Fig. 1. Morphine-induced suppression of antibody response and antagonism by naltrexone in C3HeB/FeJ mice.

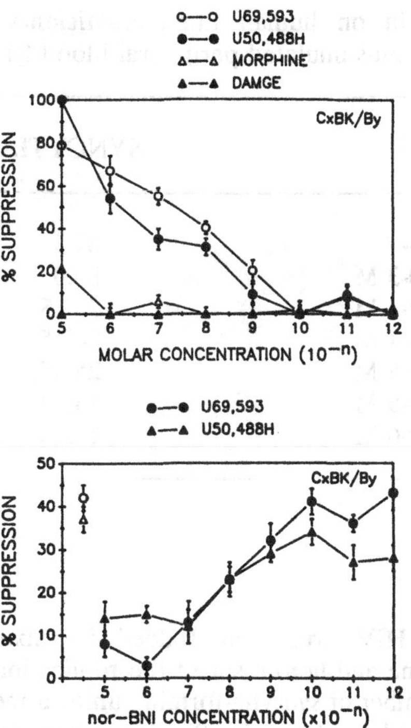

Fig. 2. **Lack of antibody suppression by mu agonists in mu-deficient mouse strain (upper). Suppression by kappa agonists and blockade of effect by kappa-selective antagonist (lower). (From Taub et al., 1991.)**

antibody formation in that strain. This prediction was confirmed *in vitro* (28) and *in vivo*. The *in vitro* studies demonstrated that the kappa-selective agonists still produced a suppression and the kappa-selective antagonist, nor-BNI, blocked the effect. The results are shown in Fig. 2.

In pharmacologically defined systems, morphine's effects often vary with the species and the strain tested. For example, although analgesia appears to be produced in all species and all strains within a species, there may be both quantitative and qualitative differences in the effects of morphine on body temperature and pupillary size (30,31). Although we have found that morphine produces immune suppression in all mouse strains tested except the μ-deficient CxBK mice, the effect of the opioid antagonist naltrexone varies with the strain. In some strains, naltrexone not only fails to antagonize the immunosuppressive effects of morphine, but it produces agonist-like effects of its own (29). Eisenstein discusses strain differences in some detail in her paper in this volume.

OPIOIDS AND HIV

It is quite clear from the work reported from our laboratory and others that morphine and related alkaloids and endogenous and exogenous peptides have marked effects on a variety of parameters of immune function. Although such results are consistent with the notion that the drugs act as cofactors in the progression of the HIV symptom complex, they do not preclude the possibility that morphine and heroin might

Table 3. Effects of heroin on human immunodeficiency virus-1 replication in phytohemagglutinin-stimulated peripheral blood lymphocytes

DRUG	DOSE	SYNCYTIA/10^5 CELLS
None	-------	87.5
Heroin	1x10-3 M	86.0
	5x10-4 M	219.5
	1x10-4 M	307.5
	5x10-5 M	257.5
	1x10-5 M	138.0
	5x10-6 M	153.0

have some effect on the HIV virus itself. Indeed, in subsequent studies we have demonstrated that morphine and heroin speed the replication of the HIV virus (32). Table 3 shows that the number of syncytia-forming units, a measure of the number of HIV viruses, increase markedly with heroin. Similar results in terms of HIV replication were reported by Peterson and Sharp and their group at the University of Minnesota (22).

We are now trying to learn something about the mechanisms involved. There are several reasons to believe the opioids may be involved in the onset of symptoms and the severity of AIDS: 1) incubation period shorter for HIV-induced disease in intravenous drug abusers; 2) *in vitro* assays of HIV replication are affected by opioids; 3) opioid effects on HIV replication are blocked by opioid antagonists.

SUMMARY

The results achieved by those seeking to determine whether opioids and other drugs of abuse can affect immunity are quite astonishing given the short period of time that research has focused on this area. Despite the fact that there is no longer any question that opioids produce a variety of effects on the immune system, the extent and significance of these changes in the drug-abusing population remains to be determined. Whether or not the findings in mice and in *in vitro* preparations can be extrapolated to man is not yet known. Of major significance is the question of whether the endogenous opioid system is involved in immunoregulation. Given the multitude of drugs taken by drug abusers and the varying patterns of drug administration, the significance of the findings in the literature is still an open question. However, it is only by continuing studies such as those discussed at this meeting that we will find the answers.

Acknowledgements

The work was supported by grants DA00376, DA06650 and T32 DA07237 from the National Institute on Drug Abuse.

REFERENCES

1. E. J. Simon, J.M. Hiller, and I. Edelman, Stereospecific binding of the potent narcotic analgesic [^{3}H]-etorphine to rat-brain homogenate, *Proc. Natl. Acad. Sci.* USA 70:1947 (1973).
2. C. B. Pert and S.H. Snyder, Opiate receptor: Demonstration in nervous tissue, *Science* 179:1011 (1973).
3. L. Terenius, Stereospecific interaction between narcotic analgesics and a synaptic plasma membrane fraction of the rat cerebral cortex, *Acta Pharmacol. Toxicol.* 32:317 (1973).
4. H. W. Kosterlitz and A.J. Watt, Kinetic parameters of narcotic agonists and antagonists, with particular reference to naloxone, *Brit. J. Pharmacol. Chemother.* 33:266 (1968).
5. R. J. Tallarida, C. Harakal, J. Maslow, E.B. Geller, and M.W. Adler, The relationship between pharmacokinetics and pharmacodynamic action as applied to *in vivo* pA2: Application to the analgesic effect of morphine, *J. Pharmacol. Exp. Ther.* 206:38 (1978).
6. S. H. Weinstein, M. Pfeffer, and J.M. Schor, Metabolism and pharmacokinetics of naloxone, *in*: "Narcotic Antagonists", M.C. Braude et al., eds., Raven Press, New York (1974).
7. C. M. Blatteis, L. Xin, and N. Quan, Neuromodulation of fever: apparent involvement of opioids, *Brain Res. Bull.* 26:219 (1991).
8. N. Dafny, B. Prieto-Gomez, and C. Reyes-Vazquez, Does the immune system communicate with the central nervous system? Interferon modifies central nervous activity, *J. Neuroimmunol.* 9:1(1985).
9. D. L. Felten, N. Cohen, R. Ader, S.Y. Felten, S.L. Carlson, and T.L. Roszman, Central neural circuits involved in neural-immune interactions, *in*: "Psychoneuroimmunology," R. Ader, D.L. Felten, and N. Cohen, eds., Academic Press, San Diego (1991).
10. J. H. Jaffe, Drug addiction and drug abuse, *in*: "Goodman & Gilman's The Pharmacological Basis of Therapeutics", A.G. Gilman et al., eds., Macmillan, New York (1985).
11. J. Wybran, T. Appelboom, J.-P. Famaey, and A. Govaerts, Suggestive evidence for receptors for morphine and methionine-enkephalin on normal human blood T lymphocytes, *J. Immunol.* 123:1068 (1979).
12. R. M. Donahoe, C. Bueso-Ramos, F. Donahoe, J.J. Madden, A. Falek, J.K.A. Nicholson, and P. Bokos, Mechanistic implications of the findings that opiates and other drugs of abuse moderate T-cell surface receptors and antigenic markers, *Ann. N. Y. Acad. Sci.* 496:711 (1987).
13. S. Roy, S. Ramakrishnan, H.H. Loh, and N.M. Lee, Chronic morphine treatment selectively suppresses macrophage colony formation in bone marrow, *Eur. J. Pharmacol.* 195:359 (1991).
14. H. U. Bryant, E.W. Bernton, and J.W. Holaday, Morphine pellet-induced immunomodulation in mice: Temporal relationships, *J. Pharmacol. Exp. Ther.* 245:913 (1988).
15. T. K. Eisenstein, D.D. Taub, M.W. Adler, and T.J. Rogers, The effect of morphine and DAGO on the proliferative response of murine splenocytes, *in*: "Drugs of Abuse, Immunity, and Immunodeficiency", H. Friedman., ed., Plenum, New York (1991).
16. N. R. Pellis, C. Harper, and N. Dafny, Suppression of the induction of delayed hypersensitivity in rats by repetitive morphine treatments, *Exp. Neurol.* 93:92 (1986).
17. Y. Shavit, A. Depaulis, F.C. Martin, G.W. Terman, R.N. Pechnick, C.J. Zane, R.P. Gale, and J.C. Liebeskind, Involvement of brain opiate receptors in the immune-suppressive effect of morphine, *Proc. Natl. Acad. Sci.* USA 83:7114 (1986).
18. R. J. Weber and A. Pert, The periaqueductal gray matter mediates opiate-induced immunosuppression, *Science* 245:188 (1989).
19. E. Tubaro, G. Borelli, C. Croce, G. Cavallo, and C. Santiangeli, Effect of morphine on resistance to infection, *J. Infec. Dis.* 148:656 (1983).
20. T. K. Eisenstein, J.J. Meissler,Jr., E.B. Geller, and M.W. Adler, Immunosuppression to tetanus toxoid induced by implanted morphine pellets, *Ann. N. Y. Acad. Sci.* 594:377 (1990).
21. C. C. Chao, B.M. Sharp, C. Pomeroy, G.A. Filice, and P.K. Peterson, Lethality of morphine in mice infected with Toxoplasma gondii, *J. Pharmacol. Exp. Ther.* 252:605 (1990).
22. P. K. Peterson, B.M. Sharp, G. Gekker, P.S. Portoghese, K. Sannerud, and H.H. Balfour,Jr., Morphine promotes the growth of HIV-1 in human peripheral blood mononuclear cell cocultures, *AIDS* 4:869 (1990).
23. E. E. Henderson, T.K. Eisenstein, J.J. Meissler,Jr., J.-Y. Yang, T.J. Rogers, E.B. Geller, and M.W. Adler, Increased proliferation of HIV by heroin *in vitro,* reported at the annual meeting of the College on Problems of Drug Dependence, Palm Beach, FL (1991).
24. R. N. Mandler, W.E. Biddison, R. Mandler, and S.A. Serrate, β-Endorphin augments the cytolytic activity and interferon production of natural killer cells, *J. Immunol.* 136:934 (1986).
25. P. M. Mathews, C.J. Froelich, W.L. Sibbitt,Jr., and A.D. Bankhurst, Enhancement of natural cytotoxicity by ß-endorphin, *J. Immunol.* 130:1658 (1983).
26. S. A. Williamson, R.A. Knight, S.L. Lightman, and J.R. Hobbs, Differential effects of ß-endorphin fragments on human natural killing, *Brain Behav. Immun.* 1:329 (1987).

27. N. E. S. Sibinga and A. Goldstein, Opioid peptides and opioid receptors in cells of the immune system, *Ann. Rev. Immunol.* 6:219 (1988).
28. D. D. Taub, T.K. Eisenstein, E.B. Geller, M.W. Adler, and T.J. Rogers, Immunomodulatory activity of μ- and K-selective opioid agonists, *Proc. Natl. Acad. Sci.* USA 88:360 (1991).
29. J. L. Bussiere, M.W. Adler, T.J. Rogers, and T.K. Eisenstein, Differential effects of morphine and naltrexone on the antibody response in various mouse strains, *Immunopharmacol. Immunotoxicol.* 14:657 (1992).
30. M. W. Adler and E.B. Geller, Physiological functions of opioids: Temperature regulation, *in*: "Handbook of Experimental Pharmacology, Vol. 104/II, Opioids II", A. Herz, et al., eds., Springer-Verlag, Berlin (1992).
31. R. B. Murray, M.W. Adler, and A.D. Korczyn, The pupillary effects of opioids, *Life Sci.* 33:495 (1983).
32. E. E. Henderson, T.K. Eisenstein, M.W. Adler, E. B. Geller, and J.-Y. Yang, Effects of opioids on human immunodeficiency virus (HIV-1) replication *in vitro*, *in*: "The Second International Conference on Alcohol, Drugs of Abuse and Immunomodulation (AIDS)", Advances in Biosciences, R. Watson, ed., Pergamon, Oxford, in press.

CONSEQUENCES OF OPIATE-DEPENDENCY IN A MONKEY MODEL OF AIDS

Robert M. Donahoe[1,2], Larry D. Byrd[2], Harold M. McClure[2], Patricia Fultz[2], Mary Brantley[1], Frederick Marsteller[1], Aftab Ahmed Ansari[2], DeLoris Wenzel[2], and Mario Aceto[3]

[1]Dept. of Psychiatry,[2]Yerkes Regional Primate Res. Ctr., Emory Univ., G.M.H.I., Atlanta, GA 30306, [3]Dept. of Pharmacol. and Toxicol., Med. College of VA, VA Commonwealth Univ., Richmond, VA 23298

INTRODUCTION

In 1898, Cantacuzene (1) reported that rodent phagocytes exposed to morphine had reduced phagocytic and chemotactic activity in both *in vitro* and *in vivo* experimental systems. This work was carried out in the laboratory of the father of cell-mediated immunology, Elie Metchnikoff, and represents the first rigorous scientific study aimed at characterizing the immunological effects of opiates. About 10 years later, Archard et al., (2) corroborated the findings of Cantacuzene (1). By 1928, evidence indicating the immunomodulatory potential of opiates was reviewed by Terry and Pellens (3).

After this early interest in the immunological properties of opiates, a variety of clinical observations appeared in the literature which documented that heroin addicts suffer from inordinate levels of opportunistic disease indicative of immune deficits (4-6). By the late 1960s', the association of opportunistic disease with opiate abuse assumed considerable public-health importance when it became evident that heroin addicts were at high risk for infectious hepatitis and served as a reservoir for this disease (7). Today the same set of circumstances as applied to the association between i.v. drug abuse and hepatitis are seen in the association of i.v. drug abuse with AIDS. As a consequence of such associations, there has been an intense interest over the past two decades in characterizing the immunological properties of opiates.

Contemporary Experimental Evidence that Opiates Affect Immune Function

In 1974, Brown et al., (8) examined the status of the cell-mediated and humoral branches of immunity in heroin addicts and found that polyclonal activation of T-cells through stimulation by plant lectins was depressed in cells from heroin addicts relative to controls. They also showed that levels of circulating immunoglobulins in addicts were higher than normal. Around this same time, Falek et al., (9) showed that heroin addicts experienced increased susceptibility to chromosomal damage as assessed cytogenetically.

Since cytogenetic analyses are done with leukocyte preparations stimulated *in vitro* by T-cell mitogens, the studies of Falek et al., (9) provided another indication of disturbance of T-cell function in heroin addicts. A later study by McDonough et al., (10) from the Falek laboratory showed that heroin addicts had depressed levels of T-cells as measured by the formation of T-cell E-rosettes. Importantly, this study also revealed that the immunomodulating effects of opiates appeared to be directed specifically at the T-cell since the depressed E-rosette formation that was seen was reversible by the opiate receptor antagonist, naloxone (10). Moreover, this finding came nearly simultaneously with the discovery by Wybran et al., (11) that T-cell E-rosette formation was depressed by opiates in a naloxone-reversible fashion after leukocytes from normal individuals were exposed to morphine *in vitro*.

The studies of McDonough et al., (10) and Wybran et al., (11) led to the conclusion that opiates could directly act upon T-Cells to influence their function. Importantly, these studies also suggested that opiates exert T-cell effects through T-cell opiate receptors. Indeed, several reports over the past decade have established that T-cells have pharmacologically relevant opiate receptors (reviewed in reference 12). In this regard, the recent report by Taub et al., (13) is most informative since it showed that generation of immune responsivity *in vitro* was directly affected by opiates through mechanisms involving specific subtypes of opiate receptors.

Since T-cell responsiveness is an essential component of host defense against opportunistic infection, observations that opiates directly affect T-cell function suggest that immune deficits of heroin addiction could be due to direct effects of opiates on T-cell functions. However, other information about the immunological effects of opiates suggest that direct effects on T-cells are unlikely to be the sole means by which opiates influence host immunocompetency. In 1986, Shavit et al., (14) reported that morphine influences NK-cell responsiveness through centrally mediated events. In 1989, Weber and Pert (15) showed that the periaqueductal gray region of the brain was responsible for opiate-induced modulation of NK-cell activity. Indeed, a number of other groups (some are presenting at the present symposium), have also found that many aspects of the immunological effects of opiates are centrally mediated-including various aspects of T-cell responsiveness.

THE POSSIBLE ROLE OF OPIATES IN AIDS: A MONKEY MODEL

Given the preceding background, it is logical to suspect that opiates might alter host susceptibility to productive infection with HIV-1, and, subsequently, development of AIDS. Epidemiologically, there is uncertainty about this issue. Des Jarlais et al., (16) and Stoneburner, et al., (17) have presented evidence that may be interpreted to indicate that heroin addicts may experience an exacerbated course of AIDS, while epidemiological assessments conducted by Kaslow et al., (18), Farizo, et al., (19), Zenilman et al., (20) and others (21) have reached an opposite conclusion. Due to such uncertainty and the fact that epidemiological assessments of heroin addiction are confounded by a great many uncontrollable variables, as well as the fact that the immunological and virological factors that affect development of AIDS remain ambiguous today, there clearly exists a need for better definition of the role of opiates in AIDS. To this end, we have conducted a study to examine effects of opiates on expression of a virus infection that causes an AIDS-like syndrome in rhesus monkeys [the opiate-AIDS-monkey (OAM) study]. The virus used in this study was the sooty managabey strain of simian immunodeficiency virus (SIVsmm) (22). SIVsmm has been shown to cause a variety of AIDS-like signs and lesions in rhesus macaques (23), including the death of approximately 40% of animals infected with virus within 2 yrs of initiation of such infections.

The design for the OAM study was relatively straightforward. Six monkeys were made opiate-dependent by injecting 3mg/kg of morphine every 6 hrs according to a protocol defined by Woods et al., (24). Two weeks after opiate-injections were begun, the monkeys were infected with SIVsmm. The monkeys were then observed for 2 yrs for the development of AIDS-like disease, including clinical observations, physical exams, and hematological, immunological and virological assessments. Opiate-dependency was maintained throughout this time also, except for brief episodes of several days when the effects of opiate withdrawal were assessed.

Four of the six monkeys used for this study were previously used in a 5-yr experiment to examine cross tolerance of opiate-dependent animals to newly synthesized drugs suspected of having opiate-like properties. These animals were a generous gift of Dr. Mario Aceto and were brought to the Yerkes Regional Primate Research Center from the Medical College of Virginia at Richmond. These monkeys had an established opiate-dependency for approximately 5 yrs with variable repeated incidences of withdrawal from opiates. Because of their history of long-term exposure to opiates, the 4 monkeys from Virginia were used in the OAM study to experimentally mimic conditions similar to chronic heroin addiction in man. Based on the hypothesis that immune deficiencies are more likely to occur in animals as their duration of opiate exposure increases [as appears to be the case with street heroin addiction (25)], the monkeys from Virginia were included in the OAM study to determine if extended prior exposure to opiates might exacerbate SIVsmm infection.

Since there was no reason to suspect that saline injections would exacerbate the course of AIDS in SIVsmm-infected monkeys, control animals receiving repeated injections of saline as a morphine-placebo were not included in the OAM study to conserve monkeys and to limit the costs of the study. The controls for this study consisted of several groups of monkeys housed in separate quarters that were infected with the same dose and lot of SIVsmm as the opiate-dependent animals but which had never been exposed to opiates.

The results of the OAM study are presently being analyzed statistically in preparation for publication. One important point that is already evident from this study is that opiates did not exacerbate the course of infection with SIVsmm and the development of AIDS-like disease in this small group of animals. In fact, the evidence tends to suggest that some AIDS symptoms that commonly develop in monkeys infected with SIVsmm were expressed to a significantly lesser extent in the opiate-dependent monkeys than expected. Consideration of death-rate in this regard is most informative. No animals died in the opiate-dependent SIVsmm-infected group during the 2-yrs following injection of SIVsmm, while the expected frequency of death from an AIDS-like syndrome during this time is approximately 40% (23). On the other hand, it was notable that 2/6 animals in the SIV-infected opiate-dependent group developed diffuse bacterial dermatitis that is not seen typically in opiate-dependent monkeys not infected with SIV. In these instances, dermatitis started at the opiate injection-site (much like what happens when heroin addicts experience dermatitis), and the SIVsmm infection appeared to promote the spread of such infection.

Despite the atypical course of AIDS-like disease that was witnessed for opiate-dependent monkeys infected with SIVsmm, the clinical signs of infection that are commonly associated with this virus were remarkably typical as long as tolerance to the opiate was well maintained by repeated injections of opiate every 6 hours. That is for opiate-dependent animals, production of anti-p24 anti-viral antibody, isolation of virus by co-culture of monkey and human lymphocytes, and expression of absolute numbers of CD4 and CD8 T-cells all occurred in expected fashion during the 2-year course of the study. Importantly, however, when opiates were briefly withdrawn from opiate-dependent SIVsmm-infected monkeys, there was an acute exacerbation of virus expression as measured by co-culture techniques. Such exacerbation was recorded at a time during the course of infection when attempts at isolating virus were repeatedly negative for 5/6 animals, i.e., at a time of persistent viral latency that is typical of immunodeficiency virus infections. In this instance, 3/5 latently-infected monkeys transiently expressed virus 2 days after initiation of opiate withdrawal.

DISCUSSION AND CONCLUSIONS

Several factors support the validity of the monkey model in the OAM study as being representative of circumstances encountered by opiate-dependent humans infected with HIV-1. One is the closeness of SIVsmm to HIV-1. Both of these viruses are lentiviruses, and they share approximately 40% genomic homology (26). Also, the course of infection and the association of development of AIDS-like disease with loss of CD4+ T-cell numbers after infection of monkeys with SIVsmm is closely akin to the pathogenesis of HIV-1 infection (23; unpublished findings). It is also important that the conditions necessary for maintaining opiate-dependency in the monkey model are much like those necessary for maintenance of opiate-dependency in humans.

In regard to immunological breakdown and influence over expression of SIVsmm infection, the effects of opiate-dependency in the OAM study may be viewed as variably detrimental, neutral or even protective. Thus, in the OAM study, it was clear that opiate-dependent monkeys infected with SIVsmm did not experience an exacerbated course of AIDS-like disease, even for the monkeys from Virginia which had a long prior history of opiate exposure. Also, the results of the major assessments of virological status of SIVsmm infection in opiate-dependent monkeys (i.e., antibody titers and viral isolation by co-culture), generally, were no different from those seen with non-opiate-dependent animals. Such observations suggest that the effects of opiates on SIVsmm infection could be regarded as essentially 'neutral'. However, in several respects, it was also apparent that the monkeys in the OAM study experienced a reduction in the rate and severity of expression of certain signs of AIDS-like disease, a phenomenon which may be viewed as a 'protective' effect. On the other hand, the effects of opiate withdrawal that were evident in the OAM study may be viewed as 'detrimental' because withdrawal caused transiently severe immune deficits (poor blastogenesis, aberrant leukocyte subtyping) in all animals involved and, for some animals (3 of 5) caused apparent induction of latent SIVsmm.

Since the OAM study did not indicate any obvious exacerbation of SIVsmm infection and AIDS-like disease as the result of opiate-dependency, it is reasonable to question whether the rather subtle indications of opiate-dependent protective effects, and the potentially detrimental effects of immunological disturbances and induction of latent SIVsmm resulting from opiate-withdrawal, that were also seen in the OAM study, are relevant to the determination of the way opiates affect the outcome of HIV-1 infections in opiate addicts. Unfortunately, the limited numbers (six) of opiate-dependent animals infected with SIVsmm in this study obviate any definitive conclusions in this regard. Still, the critical nature of this issue encourages informed speculation.

Concerning induction of virus by opiate-withdrawal, there are good reasons to suspect that such induction is genuine. Other aspects of the OAM study and other studies from our laboratory regarding the immunological effects of opiate-dependency have clearly shown that withdrawal from opiates has dramatic effects on immune status of affected hosts (manuscripts in preparation). Since activation of lymphocytes is required for integration of immunodeficiency viruses, like HIV-1, into the genome and non-integration of immunodeficiency virus is inducible in quiescent T-cells (27), it is quite possible that the immune crisis caused by opiate withdrawal is conducive to induction of such viruses. Furthermore, it is certain that the relationship of stress to opiate withdrawal is pertinent to this immune crisis and its potential to participate in viral induction since opiate-withdrawal is an extreme psycho-physiological stressor and since stress is a well known cause for induction of latent retroviruses like SIVsmm (28).

In the OAM study, induction of SIVsmm as the result of opiate-withdrawal only occurred one time, that we measured, over a 2-year course of opiate-dependency. In this instance, virus was isolated transiently and at relatively low levels. These circumstances limit the certainty with which conclusions can be made about the consequences of viral induction by opiate withdrawal. Such limitations do not, however, diminish the importance of the observation that opiate-withdrawal appeared to induce latent SIVsmm in the OAM study. Had the opportunity existed in this study to examine different sampling regimens and conditions of opiate-withdrawal, and multiple instances of opiate-withdrawal, it is possible that the phenomenon of viral induction consequent to opiate-withdrawal would have been demonstrated more robustly. Given the relationship of stress to withdrawal and viral induction as discussed previously, such a possibility is, in fact, quite probable. Because of what is known about the relationship of the expression of immunodeficiency viruses to the onset of AIDS and because opiate-withdrawal is a common and chronic occurrence for most street heroin addicts, such possibilities have very serious public-health implications.

The onset of AIDS for both humans and monkeys is associated with consistently productive expression of immunodeficiency virus (26,29,30). Expression of immunodeficiency virus in this way occurs in different temporal patterns for different individuals, but it often occurs years after initiation of infection, after extended periods of viral latency (30). AIDS onset also appears to be related to a natural viral-selection process that, over time, fosters the predominance of more virulent strains of immunodeficiency virus (30). Thus, it seems reasonable to conjecture that, if HIV-1 is induced as the result of opiate-withdrawal in heroin addicts, it would likely contribute to the pathogenic manifestations of AIDS.

The foregoing discussion is also relevant to consideration of reasons that opiate-dependency failed to cause any obvious exacerbation of AIDS-like disease in the OAM study. It is a classical feature of opiate-dependency that drug tolerance can be maintained and the withdrawal syndrome avoided if an appropriate drug-dosing regimen is used. The dosing-regimen for the OAM study was designed for this purpose; and, except in the few brief instances during the study when opiates were purposefully withdrawn from the study animals, this regimen was, by all measures, successful at maintaining the tolerant state. Accordingly, it is possible that the state of tolerance that was evident for the animals in the OAM study may have effectively prevented or retarded potentially deleterious stressful effects of opiate-withdrawal, such as loss of immunocompetency and viral induction. Such a possibility is supported by another study from our laboratory (manuscript in preparation) in which we showed that opiate-dependent monkeys become tolerant to a number of immunological effects of opiates over time. Indeed, earlier studies by Shavit et al., (31) have also shown that the NK-modulating effects of morphine are ameliorated in rodents at the same time that they develop pharmacological tolerance to the drug.

Reduction of stress by a well-maintained opiate-dependency may also have accounted for the fact that some of the test monkeys in the OAM study appeared to be protected against expression of certain signs of AIDS-like disease--the most prominent of which was a slowing of the death rate of SIVsmm infection. Thus, by reducing the chances for induction of latent virus by stress, a well-maintained opiate-dependency may result in retardation of virological and immunological processes that influence the onset of AIDS. Such a notion is compatible with other observations of the benefits of stress-reduction in the management of HIV-1 infected patients (32).

Recent data of Risdahl et al., (33) also support the possibility that opiate-dependency may alter expression of latent immunodeficiency viruses since they found that swine are protected from the lethal effects of swine herpesvirus by maintenance of opiate-dependency. Interestingly, Risdahl et al., (33) also showed the susceptibility of opiate-dependent swine to bacterial infection is increased relative to controls. This latter observation corresponds with the data from the OAM study as well as data from earlier studies of Tubaro et al., (34,35) who showed that an opiate-dependent host experiences reduced resistance to bacterial infection which corresponds to reductions in phagocytic activity of host macrophages/monocytes. Therefore, it seems that opiate-dependency is likely to have differing effects on infectious processes depending on the nature of the infection and the immune processes involved in fighting the infection as well as the relative effectiveness by which the state of opiate-dependency is maintained.

In conclusion, even though the limited scope of the OAM study taxes the statistical validity of some of the data from this study, the plausibility of these data is well supported by corroborating evidence. Accordingly, these data contribute to a logical and appealing conceptualization of the way opiates influence host defenses against opportunistic infections. The unique contribution of the OAM study, therefore, has been to have determined that the virological and immunological consequences of opiate-dependency are seemingly conditionally affected by the relative state of opiate-dependency in terms of maintaining tolerance and avoiding opiate-withdrawal so that a well-maintained opiate-dependency may be beneficial to the host in some aspects while a poorly-maintained dependency is likely to have detrimental consequences.

A concept that holds that the virological and immunological effects of opiates are conditionally expressed relative to the state of opiate dependency can be helpful in resolving issues that have been raised by various epidemiological studies (16-21) about the influence of opiates over expression of the pathophysiology of HIV-1-infection and development of AIDS in heroin addicts. Thus, the OAM study suggests that addicts may be variably protected from, or made more susceptible to, the consequences of HIV-1 infection depending on the relative state of maintenance of opiate-dependency among individual addicts. The conditionality of the effects of opiate-dependency may also help explain why people who use opiates therapeutically (who would be expected to have a well-maintained opiate-dependency) generally do not exhibit evidence of severe immune depression while street heroin addicts (whose maintenance of dependency is often poor) often do.

The results of the OAM study and the conclusions that it suggests indicate that stress-reduction may be a viable therapeutic goal for treatment of individuals with HIV-1 infections and other types of chronic, latent and incurable viral infections as a means of limiting or delaying the consequences of such infections. Such a consideration is compatible with the precepts of psychoneuroimmunology (36) wherein stress has long been held as a major factor in immune modulation and in dictating host response to opportunistic disease. Such considerations, however, are not made to suggest that opiates themselves should be used for this purpose -- except for treating heroin addicts, in which event methadone maintenance is often the therapy of choice. Otherwise, the addiction liabilities of opiates as well as their known immunomodulatory potential and abilities to promote bacterial infections obviate the general use of these drugs as a means of reducing stress. Presumably, various non-opiate means of reducing stress are available that would be satisfactory for addressing this therapeutic goal.

Obviously, further study is needed to validate or refute the speculation raised by the findings of the OAM study. Since there is little hope now and in the future to disconnect the harmful association between opiate abuse and AIDS, there would seem to be every reason to vigorously pursue the answers to the questions raised by this study.

Acknowledgements

This work was supported by HIH grants from the National Institutes on Drug Abuse (DA04400) and from the National Center for Research Resources to the Yerkes Regional Primate Research Center (RR-00165). The Yerkes Center is fully accredited by the American Association for Accreditation of Laboratory Animal Care. The expert secretarial assistance of Mrs. Sybil Mashburn and Mrs. Nurit Golan is gratefully acknowledged as is the technical assistance of Michael Litrel, Jennifer Patera, Protul Shrikant, Granger Sunderland, and Gabriella Thomas. The assistance of the veterinary and animal-care staff at the Yerkes Center is also gratefully acknowledged.

REFERENCES

1. J. Cantacuzene, Nouvelles recherches sur le mode de destruction des vibrions dans l'organisme. *Annals Institute de Pasteur* 12:274 (1898).
2. C. Archard, H. Bernard, and C. Gagneux, Action de la morphine sur les proprietes leucocytaires: leuka-diagnostic du morphiniseme, *Bulletin Mem. Soc. Med. Hopitauz de Paris* 28:958 (1909).
3. C. E. Terry, and M. Pellens, "The Opium Problem". New York: Bureau of Social Hygiene, (1928).
4. H. H. Hussey, and S. Katz, Infections resulting from narcotic addiction; report of 102 cases. *Am. J. Med.* 9:186 (1950).
5. J. D. Sapira, The narcotic addict as a medical patient, *Am. J. Med.* 45:555 (1968).
6. D. B. Louria, Infectious complications of nonalcoholic drug abuse, *Ann. Rev. Med.* 25:219 (1974).
7. W. E. Dismukes, A. W. Karchmer, R. F. Johnson, and W. J. Dougherty, Viral hepatitis associated with illicit parenteral use of drugs. *J.A.M.A.* 206:1048 (1968).
8. S. W. Brown, B. Stimmel, R. N. Taub, S. Kochwa, and R. E. Rosenfield, Immunological dysfunction in heroin addicts. *Arch. Intern. Med.* 134:1001 (1974).
9. A. Falek, R. B. Jordan, B. S. King, P. J. Arnold, and W. B.Skelton, Human chromosomes and opiates. *Arch. Gen. Psychiat.* 27:511 (1972).
10. R. J. McDonough, J. J. Madden, A. Falek, D. A. Shafer, M. Pline, D. Gordon, P. Bokos, J. C. Kuehnle, and J. Mendelson, Alteration of T and null lmphocyte frequencies in the peripheral blood of human opiate addicts: *in vivo* evidence of opiate receptor sites on T-lymphocytes, *J. Immunol.* 124: 2539 (1980).
11. J. Wybran, T. Appelboom, J. P. Famaey, and A. Goverts, Suggestive evidence for receptors for morphine and methionine-enkephalin on normal human blood T-lymphocytes. *J. Immunol.* 123:1068 (1979).
12. J. J. Madden and R. M. Donahoe, Opiate binding to cells of the immune system, *in*: "Drugs of abuse and immune function," Watson, R.R. (ed), CRC Press, Inc., Boca Raton, FL, pp. 213-228, (1980).
13. D. D. Taub, T. K. Eisenstein, E. G. Geller, M. W. Adler, and T. J.Rogers, Immunomodulatory activity of mu- and kappa-selective opioid agonist, *Proc. Natl. Acad. Sci.*, U.S.A. 88:360 (1991).
14. Y. Shavit, A. Depaulis, R. D. Martin, G. W. Terman, R. N. Pechnick, C. J. Zane, R. P. Gale, and J. C. Liebeskind, Involvement of brain opiate receptors in the immune-suppressive effects of morphine, *Proc. Natl. Acad. Sci.*, U.S.A. 83: 7114 (1986).
15. R. J. Weber, and A. Pert, The periaqueductal gray matter mediates opiate-induced immunosuppression. *Science* 245:188 (1989).
16. D. C. Des Jarlais, S. R. Friedman, M. Marmor, H. Cohen, D. Mildran, S. Vancovitz, U. Mathur, W. El-Sadr, T. J. Spira, J. Garber, S. T. Beatrice, A. S. Abdul-Quader, and J. L. Sotheran, Development of AIDS, HIV seroconversion, and potential cofactors for T4 cell loss in a cohort of intravenous drug users, *AIDS* 1:105 (1987).
17. R. L. Stoneburner, D. Des Jarlais, D. Benezra, L. Gorelkin, J. L. Sotheran, S. R. Friedman, S. Schultz, M. Marmor, D. Mildvan, and R. Maslansky, A larger spectrum of severe HIV-1-related disease in intravenous drug users in New York City, *Science* 242:916 (1988).
18. R. A. Kaslow, W. C. Blackwelder, D. G. Ostrow, D. Yerg, J. Palenicek, A. H. Coulson, and R. O. Valdiserri, No evidence for a role of alcohol or other psychoactive drugs in accelerating immunodeficiency in HIV-1-positive individuals. *J.A.M.A.* 261:3424 (1989).
19. K. M. Farizo, J. W.Buehler, M. E. Chamberland, B. M. Whyte, E. S. Froelicher, S. G. Hopkins, C. M.Reed, E. D. Makotoff, D. L. Cohn, S. Troxler, A. F. Phelps, and R. L. Berkelman, Spectrum of disease in persons with human immunodeficiency virus infection in the United States, *J.A.M.A.* 267:1798 (1992).
20. J. M. Zenilman, B. Erickson, R. Fox, C. A. Reichart, and E. W. Hook, III. Effect of HIV posttest counseling on STD incidence, *J.A.M.A.* 267:843 (1992).
21. Letters to Editor, Psychoactive drug use and AIDS, *J.A.M.A.* 263:371 (1990).
22. P. N. Fultz, A. M. McClure, D. C. Anderson, R. B. Swenson, R. Anand, and A. Srinivasan, Isolation of a T-lymphotropic retrovirus from naturally infected sooty managabey monkeys (Cercocebus atys). *Proc. Natl. Acad., Sci.*, U.S.A. 83:5286 (1986).
23. H. M. McClure, D. C. Anderson, P. N. Fultz, A. A. Ansari, E. Lockwood, and A. Brodie, Spectrum of disease in macaque monkeys chronically infected with SIV/SMM. *Vet. Immunol. Immunopathol.* 21:13 (1989).
24. J. H. Woods, G. D. Winger, F. Medzihradsky, C. B. Smith, D. Gemerek, M. D. Aceto, L. S. Harris, E. L. May, R. L. Balster, and B. L. Slifer, Evaluation of new compounds for opioid activity in rhesus monkey, rat and mouse, *NIDA Res. Monograph Ser.* 55:309 (1984).

25. R. M. Donahoe, and A. Falek, Neuroimmunomodulation by opiates and other drugs of abuse: Relationship to HIV infection and AIDS, *Adv. Bioch. Psychopharmacol.* 44:145 (1988).

26. P. N. Fultz, H. M. McClure, D. C. Anderson, and W. M. Switzer, Identification and biologic characterization of an acutely lethal variant of simian immunodeficiency virus from sooty mangabeys (SIV/SMM). *AIDS Res. Hu. Retrovirol.* 5:397 (1989).

27. M. I. Bukrinsky, T. L. Stanwick, M. P. Dempsey, and M. Stevenson, Quiescent T lymphocytes as an inducible virus reservoir in HIV-1 infection. *Science* 254:423 (1991).

28. V. Riley, Psychoneurocendocrine influences on immunocompetence and neoplasia, *Science* 212: 1100 (1981).

29. D. D. Ho, T. Moudgil, and M. Alam, Quantitation of human immunodeficiency virus type 1 in the blood of infected persons, *N.E.J.M.* 321:1622 (1989).

30. A. S. Fauci, S. M. Schnittman, G. Poli, S. Koenig, and G. Pantaleo, NIH Conference. Immunopathogenic mechanisms in human immunodeficiency virus infection, *Ann. Inem. Med.* 114:678 (1991).

31. Y. Shavit, G. W. Terman, J. W. Lewis, C. J. Zane, R. P. Gale, and J. C. Liebeskind, Effects of footshock stress and morphine on natural killer lymphocytes in rats: studies of tolerance and cross-tolerance, *Brain Res.* 372:382 (1986).

32. S. Tross, and D. A. Hirsch, Psychological distress and neuropsychological complications of HIV infection and AIDS, *Am. Psychologist* 43:919 (1988).

33. J. M. Risdahl, P. K. Peterson, C. Pijoan, and T. W. Molitor, Effects of morphine dependence upon the pathogenesis of swine herpesvirus infection, *J. Infec. Dis.* Submitted, (1992).

34. E. Tubaro, G. Borelli, C. Croc, G. Cavallo, and G. Santiangeli, Effect of morphine on resistance to infection. *J. Infect. Dis.* 148:656 (1983).

35. E. Tubaro, U. Avico, G. Santiangeli, P. Zucarro, G. Cavallo, R. Pacifici, C. Croce, and G. Vorelli, Morphine and methadone impact on human phagocytic physiology, *Int. J. Immunopharmacol.* 7:865 (1985).

36. R. Ader, D. L. Felton, and N. Cohen, *Psychoneuroimmunol.* (2nd edition), Academic Press, New York, (1991).

EFFECTS OF OPIOIDS ON PROLIFERATION OF MATURE AND IMMATURE IMMUNE CELLS

Horace H. Loh, Andrew P. Smith and Nancy M. Lee

Department of Pharmacology
University of Minnesota Medical School
Minneapolis, MN 55414

INTRODUCTION

A large and growing body of evidence indicates that the use of opioid drugs can alter immune system functioning. It has long been known that opioid addicts suffer from an increased incidence of a variety of infectious diseases (1), as well as alterations in a number of immune parameters. A variety of changes in the immune system has also been observed following administration of opioids to laboratory animals (for review, see (2). However, almost all work on opioid-immune associations to date has focussed on mature immune cells. All circulating cells arise from pluripotent stem cells in the bone marrow, which proliferate and differentiate, by means of a complex process involving several specific lymphokines, into mature immune cells and erythrocytes. Any drug of abuse acting on stem cells therefore might have potent, wide ranging effects on the immune system. As an approach to this question, we treated mice chronically with morphine, then isolated their bone marrow cells and tested their sensitivity to several cytokines that normally induce proliferation and/or differentiation of subpopulations of these cells (3).

EFFECT OF MORPHINE ON BONE MARROW CELL PROLIFERATION

Mice were implanted with a 75 mg morphine pellet for 72 hours, or as controls, with two placebo pellets or with morphine and naloxone pellets together (so that all animals had 2 pellets, morphine-treated animals were given 1 morphine pellet and 1 placebo pellet). After 72 hours, the animals were killed, and bone marrow cells isolated and assayed for colony formation by incubating in culture for 5 days with recombinant macrophage-colony stimulating factor (MCSF) or granulocyte/macrophage-colony stimulating factor (GM-CSF). We found that mice treated with morphine for 72 hrs showed a dramatic decrease (70%) in the number of colonies induced by (M-CSF), relative to control or placebo-implanted animals. In contrast, there was no effect on proliferation induced by GM-CSF. The effect of morphine on M-CSF-induced colonies

Drugs of Abuse, Immunity, and AIDS, Edited by
H. Friedman *et al.*, Plenum Press, New York, 1993

was not observed in animals implanted with both morphine and naloxone pellets, indicating that the morphine effect could be blocked by a classical opioid antagonist (3). Further studies demonstrated that the morphine effect on M-CSF-induced colonies was observed as early as 36 hrs after pellet implantation. However, an acute injection of morphine (20 mg/kg body weight) had no suppressive effect. Furthermore, when pellets were removed after 72 hrs, and bone marrow collected and assayed at various times later, there was a time dependent recovery in the colony formation. Five days after removal of the pellet, total recovery of the colony-forming ability of the cells was observed (3). In theory, the effect of chronic morphine on M-CSF-induced proliferation could result from either a direct effect of opioid on the cells, or an indirect effect mediated through the brain or other organ containing opioid receptors. To distinguish between these possibilities, bone marrow cells from untreated animals were incubated with morphine *in vitro* for 7 days in culture. We found that morphine concentrations as low as 25 μM significantly inhibited M-CSF colony formation; moreover, the opioid peptide, β-endorphin, was even more potent, being effective at 0.25 μM. In further agreement with the *in vivo* results, chronic treatment of bone marrow cells *in vitro* with morphine or β-endorphin had no effect on GM-CSF-induced proliferation. Surprisingly, however, naloxone did not antagonize morphine's inhibitory effects in this case; that is, *in vitro* incubation of bone marrow cells with a combination of naloxone (up to 1 mM) and morphine resulted in an inhibition of M-CSF-induced proliferation as great as that seen with cells given morphine alone (3). Thus while morphine inhibits stem cell proliferation both *in vivo* and *in vitro*, our results suggest that different receptors may be involved in the two cases, and the question of whether the *in vivo* effects are mediated by direct action of morphine on bone marrow cells, or indirectly via morphine action in the central nervous system remains open.

EFFECT OF DYNORPHIN ON MORPHINE-INHIBITION OF BONE MARROW CELL PROLIFERATION

Further studies of this effect were carried out using the opioid peptide dynorphin-A(1-13). Some years ago, we reported that dynorphin, though having no antincocice-ptive activity in the brain, is able to modulate morphine antinociception. Specifically, it antagonizes morphine antinociception in naive animals, while enhancing it in morphine-dependent animals (4, 5). In addition, it suppresses morphine withdrawal symptoms (6). These results, which have been replicated to some extent in humans (7), suggest that dynorphin might be useful in treating opioid addiction. For this reason, it was of interest to determine whether dynorphin modulates morphine's effect on M-CSF-induced proliferation of stem cells (8). When mice implanted with morphine pellets were simultaneously administered dynorphin A(1-13) (2 or 4 mg/kg s.c., three times daily), the inhibition of colony formation was partially blocked, with cells from the morphine + dynorphin treated animals exhibiting only slightly depressed levels of proliferation, relative to stem cells from animals not given either drug. This effect appeared to be dose-dependent, in that stem cells from animals given the higher dose of dynorphin exhibited a response to M-CSF that was virtually identical to that of cells from untreated animals. Dynorphin also antagonized morphine inhibition of stem cell proliferation when both drugs were administered *in vitro* to stem cells isolated from untreated mice, with complete antagonism of morphine by dynorphin when the latter was 0.01-0.1 mM. Interestingly, however, the effect of dynorphin was biphasic, with doses of peptide greater than 0.1 mM only partially effective in reversing morphine inhibition of stem cell proliferation. Finally, when stem cells were incubated with dynorphin (up to 0.1 mM) only, there was no effect on M-CSF-induced proliferation. Thus dynorphin's action on stem cells parallels its effect on antinociception, in that it antagonizes morphine, while having no effect of its own. To determine whether morphine inhibition of bone marrow cell proliferation is shared by other opioid alkaloids, two other agonists often used clinically, methadone and pentazocine, were tested *in vitro*. Both were capable of inhibiting M-CSF-stimulated bone marrow proliferation in a dose-dependent manner, although their potencies were somewhat lower than that of morphine. Moreover, dynorphin was able to antagonize the inhibition of these drugs also, and as with its effect on morphine, dynorphin's action was biphasic.

MORPHINE BINDING SITES ARE PRESENT ON BONE MARROW CELLS

These results imply that there are morphine receptors on bone marrow stem cells, which mediate the inhibitory effects of this opioid on proliferation. To obtain direct evidence for this, we prepared a crude membrane fraction from these cells by differential centrifugation, incubated it with ^{3}H-morphine, then determined binding after removal of free tritiated ligand by filtration. A Kd of about 100 nM and a BmaX of 2 pmoles/mg protein was obtained. This binding was potently inhibited by chloride ion and calcium ion, while manganese, surprisingly, increased binding 6-fold. Competition studies revealed that opioid alkaloids were more potent than opioid peptides. However, unlike classical opioid receptors in the brain, the ^{3}H-morphine binding sites present on stem cells were not stereoselective, and had relatively low affinity for the antagonist naloxone. Thus the morphine receptors present on bone marrow cells are clearly different from those mediating antinociception in the brain.

These binding studies were initiated in order to identify receptors that mediate morphine inhibition of bone marrow cell proliferation by M-CSF. The characteristics of this response and of ^{3}H-morphine binding correlate fairly well. Thus the Kd for morphine binding to the cells, 200-300 nM, is consistent with the IC_{50} for morphine inhibition of proliferation, 250 nM, and other opioid alkaloids, such as etorphine, EKC and pentazocine, are much less potent in both inhibition of proliferation and in binding. An exception to the correlation between binding and inhibition of proliferation is provided by β-endorphin, which we have shown is as potent as morphine in inhibition of proliferation, yet has much lower affinity for the ^{3}H-morphine binding sites. However, one would perhaps not expect a perfect correlation, given that binding is carried out with isolated bone marrow cell membranes in buffer, while the proliferation assay is carried out with whole cells in culture medium. Factors in the latter may affect interaction of opioids with their binding sites. In fact, we found that the cytokines IL-l and M-CSF, which are present to some extent endogenously in bone marrow, both affected ^{3}H-morphine binding, though in opposite ways. Thus treatment of the bone marrow cell membranes with interleukin-1 at a concentration of 10 ng/ml resulted in a nearly 50% inhibition of ^{3}H-morphine binding, while treatement with M-CSF increased binding up to 4-fold.

If these ^{3}H-morphine binding sites do mediate morphine inhibition of M-CSF-induced bone marrow cell proliferation, the question remains as to the functional relevance of this phenomenon. We suggest that it may act as a negative feedback system to regulate M-CSF-induced proliferation. In this scheme, proliferation would be controlled by a balance between activation by M-CSF and inhibition mediated through opioid binding sites. Our finding that M-CSF stimulates ^{3}H-morphine binding further establishes the existence of a close relationship between these two processes. This cytokine appears to trigger both proliferation (by interaction with its own receptors) and inhibition of proliferation (by upregulation of inhibitory morphine receptors).

The existence of opposing regulatory forces is well established in the immune system. For example, interferon-γ (IFN-γ) inhibits bone marrow cell proliferation induced by interleukin 3 (IL-3), interleukin-4 (IL-4) or granulocyte/macrophage-colony stimulating factor (GM-CSF) (9, 10, 11), as well as IL-4-induced proliferation of CD4+ thymocytes (12, 13). In the case of the bone marrow system, the effect of (IFN-γ) appears to be mediated indirectly, via secretion of tumor necrosis factor (TNF) from stromal cells. Thus either TNF or IFN-γ can counter the proliferative actions of several other cytokines.

Like IFN-γ, morphine also inhibits thymocyte proliferation (14), and it appears to act through binding sites that are quite similar in their properties to those described here. In fact, we have found that IL-1 treatment of thymocytes greatly enhances their ^{3}H-morphine binding (14). Both proliferation of the thymocytes and the increase in morphine binding sites was increased in a dose-dependent fashion by IL-1, with a maximum of about a 5-fold increase in binding sites. The sites were not stereoselective, again indicating a significant difference from classical opioid receptors in the brain.

Thus opioid binding sites may play an important role in regulating proliferation of several types of immune cells. In fact, given the relatively low affinity of morphine and other opioids for bone marrow cells, we can't rule out the possibility that their binding sites actually represent receptors for IFN-γ, or some other cytokine, with which morphine competes. Our observation that these sites are sensitive to both M-CSF and IL-1 is consistent with this, and further strengthens the conclusion that these binding sites are functionally relevant, and not simply a curiosity.

CONCLUSIONS

Our results indicate that morphine and other often-used opioids can have profound effects on the proliferation of immature as well as mature immune cells. Though the μM concentrations at which morphine and other opioids are effective in these systems are quite high relative to the affinity of opioid ligands for their brain receptors, they are in the range of serum concentrations of opioids in heavy users. Clearly, such effects need to be taken into account when opioids are used chronically in clinical settings. If opioids are suppressing the development of certain types of immune cells, as well as compromising the functions of fully mature cells, then it becomes particularly urgent to seek other means of alleviating pain. At the same time, our findings that dynorphin can antagonize the opioid effects on bone marrow cell proliferation, together with our previously documented effects of this endogenous opioid peptide on morphine antinociception, suggest that this peptide may be extremely useful for treating opioid addicts.

Acknowledgments

The work in our laboratory cited here was supported by NIDA Research Grants DA06011 and DA00564, and by Research Scientist Awards DA-00020 and DA-70554.

REFERENCES

1. D. B. Louria, T. Hensle, and J. Rose, The major medical complications of heroin addiction, *Ann. Int. Med.* 67:1 (1967).
2. N. E. S. Sibinga and A. Goldstein, Opioid peptides and opioid receptors in cells of the immune system, *Ann. Rev. Immunol.* 6:219 (1988).
3. S. Roy, S. Ramakrishnan, H. H. Loh, and N. M. Lee, Chronic morphine treatment selectively suppresses macrophage colony formation in bone marrow, *Eur. J. Pharmacol.* 195:359 (1991).

4. H. J Friedman, M. F. Jen, J. K. Chang, N. M. Lee, and H. H.Loh, Dynorphin: A possible modulatory peptide on morphine or beta-endorphin analgesia in mouse, *Eur. J. Pharmacol.* 69:351 (1981).
5. F. C. Tulunay, M. F. Jen, J. K. Chang, H. H. Loh, and N. M. Lee, Possible regulatory role of dynorphin on morphine- and endorphin-dependent analgesia, *J. Pharmacol. Exp. Ther.* 219:296 (1981).
6. M. D. Aceto, W. L. Dewey, J. K. Chang, and N. M. Lee, Dynorphin-1-13 substitutes for morphine in addicted Rhesus monkeys., *Eur. J. Pharmacol.* 83:139 (1982).
7. H. L. Wen, and W. K. K. Ho, Suppression of withdrawal symptoms by dynorphin in heroin addicts, *Eur. J. Pharmacol.* 82:183 (1982).
8. S. Roy, H. H. Loh, and N. M. Lee, Dynorphin blocks opioid inhibition of M-CSF-induced Proliferation of bone marrow cells, *Eur. J. Pharmacol.* (1992).
9. B. D. Chen, T. H. Chou, and V. Ratanatharathorn, Expression of gamma-interferon receptor in murine bone marrow-derived macrophages associated with macrophage differentiation: Evidence of gamma-interferon receptors in the regulation of macrophage proliferation, *J. Cell Physiol.* 133:313 (1987).
10. S. A. Cannistra, P. Groshek, and J. D. Griffin, Monocytes enhance gamma-interferon induced inhibition of myeloid progenitor cell growth through secretion of tumor necrosis factor, *Exp. Hematol.* 16:865 (1988).
11. T. F. Gajewski, E. Goldwasser, and F. W. Fitch, Anti-proliferative effect of IFN-gamma inhibits the proliferation of murine bone marrow cells stimulated with IL-3, IL-4, or granulocyte-macrophage colony stimulating factor, *J. Immunol.* 141:2635 (1988).
12. P. D. Hodgkin, J. Cupp, A. Zlotnik, and M. Howard, IL-2, IL-6 and IFN-gamma have distinct effects on the IL-4-induced proliferation of thymocyte subpopulations, *Cell Immunol.* 126:57 (1990).
13. J. Ransom, M. Fischer, T. Mosmann, T. Yokota, D. DeLuca, J. Schumacher, and A. Zlotnik, Interferon-gamma is produced by activated immature mouse thymocytes and inhibits the interleukin-4-induced proliferation of immature thymocytes, *J. Immunol.* 139:4102 (1987).
14. S. Roy, B.-L. Ge, S. Ramakrishnan, N. M. Lee, and H. H. Loh, ^{3}H-morphine binding is enhanced by IL-1 stimulated thymocyte proliferation, *FEBS Letters* 287:93 (1991).

IMMUNE ALTERATIONS IN CHRONIC MORPHINE-TREATED RHESUS MONKEYS

Daniel J.J. Carr[1,3] and Charles P. France[2,3]

[1]Departments of Microbiology, Immunology, Parasitology and [2]Pharmacology, [3]Alcohol and Drug Abuse Center and Neuroscience Center of Excellence, LSU Medical Center, New Orleans, LA 70112-1393

ABSTRACT

Both immune and neuroendocrine abnormalities have been documented in heroin abusers. We investigated immunocompetence of peripheral blood mononuclear cells (PBMs) among separate groups of rhesus monkeys that were drug naive or received morphine either infrequently (twice/week) or daily (3.2 mg/kg). Both infrequent and daily morphine-exposed monkeys showed a decrease (10%) in the percentage of $CD4^+$ circulating lymphocytes and an increase (19%) in the percentage of $CD8^+$ cells. However, monkeys exposed daily to morphine showed a 30% increase in the helper-inducer $CD4^+$ lymphocytes, $CD4^+CD29^+$, compared to untreated controls. PBMs taken from animals exposed daily to morphine responded poorly to forskolin in the production of cAMP compared with cells obtained from untreated animals. However, cells from monkeys that received morphine infrequently had elevated levels of cAMP in response to forskolin. These results suggest relatively low doses of morphine have a significant effect on immunocompetence in rhesus monkeys which parallels the effects observed in the opioid-dependent human population. Therefore, rhesus monkeys will provide a beneficial animal model to study the effects of opioid compounds on immunocompetence during exposure, withdrawal and substitution drug therapy in opioid-dependent animals.

INTRODUCTION

Opioids affect a wide spectrum of immune parameters including natural killer (NK) activity, antibody production, mitogen-induced proliferation, generation of cytotoxic T lymphocytes, and cytokine production (1). Human and nonhuman primate studies on opioid dependence and immune responsiveness have also been reported: modulation of CD2 expression (5), reduction in NK activity (9) and a diminution in the CD4/CD8 ratio (4). Drug-induced alterations in immune homeostasis are likely to have serious consequences in opioid abusers in mounting an immune response to infectious agents (6,7). The present study was undertaken to characterize the PBM profile in rhesus monkeys exposed infrequently or daily to relatively low doses of morphine.

Drugs of Abuse, Immunity, and AIDS, Edited by
H. Friedman *et al.*, Plenum Press, New York, 1993

MATERIALS & METHODS

PBM Preparation

Monkeys were administered opioid drug or saline (s.c.) 3-hr prior to collecting blood samples. Whole blood was obtained from the saphenous vein of rhesus monkeys (male & female, 5-7 kg) sitting in primate restraining chairs. The sample was centrifuged (250 x g, 10 min) to separate the plasma from the buffy coat. The plasma was removed and the buffy coat was diluted 1:3 in RPMI-1640 and placed over ficoll-hypaque. The PBMs were collected from the ficoll hypaque following centrifugation (220 x g, 30 min, at room temp.) and subsequently washed and counted with trypan blue dye.

Fluorescence Activated Cell Sorter (FACS) Analysis

PBMs from both treated and untreated monkeys were collected and washed in 1.0 ml of phosphate buffered saline (PBS) containing 0.1 % bovine serum albumin (BSA) and 0.05 M NaN_3 (azide). PBMs were resuspended in 0.1 ml PBS-BSA plus azide containing anti-Leu-2a (CD8) conjugated with phycoerythrin, OKT4 (CD4) conjugated with fluorescein, or OKT4 conjugated with fluorescein and anti-4B4 (CD29) conjugated with RD1 and allowed to incubate for 30 min on ice in the dark. Cells were subsequently washed with ice-cold PBS-BSA plus azide, fixed in 1% paraformaldehyde solution, and analyzed by FACS for the percentage of stained cells in the total cell population. Unstained cells were used to determine the degree of autofluorescence. Light scatter was collected at 488 nm and the emitted light was passed through a long pass filter and analyzed at 525 nm (fluorescein) or 575 nm (phycoerythrin or RD1) on a Coulter Elite (Hialeah, FL). Ten thousand gated events were analyzed per sample.

Determination of cAMP Production by PBMs

PBMs (1×10^6 cells/condition) obtained from the treated and untreated monkeys were stimulated with or without forskolin (10^{-5} M) in the presence or absence of morphine (10^{-6} M) for 30 min in 1.0 ml RPMI-1640 at 37° C. Following the incubation period, 0.5 ml of 10% perchlorate was added to each tube, and the tubes were placed on ice for 5 min. The tubes were subsequently vortexed and 0.5 ml of supernate was removed and added to microcentrifuge tubes containing 0.5 ml of ice-cold 1.5 N KOH. Following a 10 min incubation period on ice, the tubes were centrifuged (10,000 x g, 1 min) and 100 µl of supernate was removed, acetylated, and assayed for cAMP content using a radioimmunoassay kit (Advanced Magnetics Inc., Cambridge, MA).

RESULTS

A study was undertaken to determine the percentage of $CD4^+$ and $CD8^+$ cells in the peripheral blood of monkeys exposed to morphine either daily or infrequently. Monkeys treated either infrequently or daily with morphine showed a 10-12% decrease in the number of $CD4^+$ cells (Fig. 1A). Conversely, their was a 20-22% increase in the number of $CD8^+$ cells in the peripheral blood of morphine-exposed animals (Fig. 1A). Within the $CD4^+$ population, a 30% increase in the percentage of $CD4^+CD29^+$ was observed in the daily morphine-exposed animals compared to untreated controls (Fig. 1B).

Previous studies show that variations in intracellular concentrations of cAMP can modify immune responsiveness (8). Moreover, the endogenous opioid ß-endorphin has been shown to suppress cAMP production in murine splenic lymphocytes in a naloxone-reversible manner (2). Therefore, PBMs obtained from morphine-treated and untreated monkeys were assayed for cAMP in the presence or absence of morphine, forskolin or morphine in combination with forskolin. The results indicate PBMs taken from daily morphine-exposed animals have a diminished response to forskolin while PBMs obtained from infrequent morphine-exposed monkeys have an elevated response to forskolin compared with PBMs from untreated control monkeys (Table 1).

DISCUSSION

The present study suggests that relatively low doses of morphine affect the immune response in rhesus monkeys as measured by (i) changes in the percent of $CD4^+$ and $CD8^+$ cells (Fig. 1a) (ii) increases in the $CD4^+CD29^+$ cells (Fig. 1b) and (iii) altered responses to forskolin-stimulated cAMP production (Table 1). Daily exposure of rhesus monkeys to morphine (3.2 mg/kg) has also been shown to suppress PBM NK activity, reduce the $CD8^+/CD16^+$ population of PBMs, and augment polyclonal IgG and

Table 1. Morphine-induced alteration of forskolin-elicited cAMP production by peripheral blood mononuclear cells[a].

Expt no.	Morphine treatment[b]	cAMP (fmols/10^6 cells) const[c]	(M)[d]	(F)[e]	M+F
1.	none	431	402	4195	3776
2.	none	371	433	2259	2263
3.	none	680	533	3636	3377
4.	none	717	615	14344	15686
1.	infreq.	568	709	20896	18244
2.	infreq.	513	448	28853	28977
3.	infreq.	645	429		34512
26908					
4.	infreq.	456	384	28314	32956
1.	daily	539	530	2509	2440
2.	daily	550	407	969	2065
3.	daily	447	367	1611	640
4.	daily	720	638	691	981

[a]cAMP production was determined by radioimmunoassay. The standards used in the kit consistently gave correlation coefficients of -.9900. Each experiment represents the average of the cAMP generated by PBMs obtained from two animals/group with each measurement in duplicate.

[b]None = animals not treated with opioid; infreq. = animals treated twice/week with an opioid; daily = animals treated daily with 3.2 mg/kg morphine.

[c]Const. = constitutive levels

[d]M = morphine (10^{-6} M)-treated PBMs.

[e]F = forskolin (10^{-5} M)-treated PBMs.

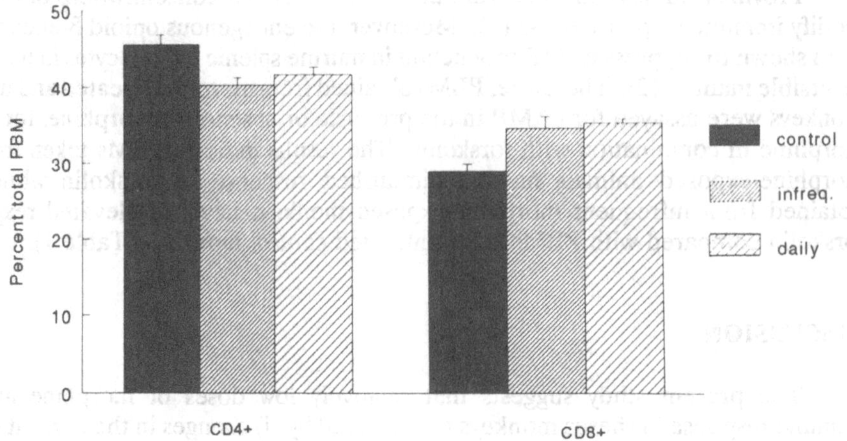

Fig. 1a. Morphine-exposed rhesus monkeys have altered percentages of CD4⁺ and CD8⁺ cells.

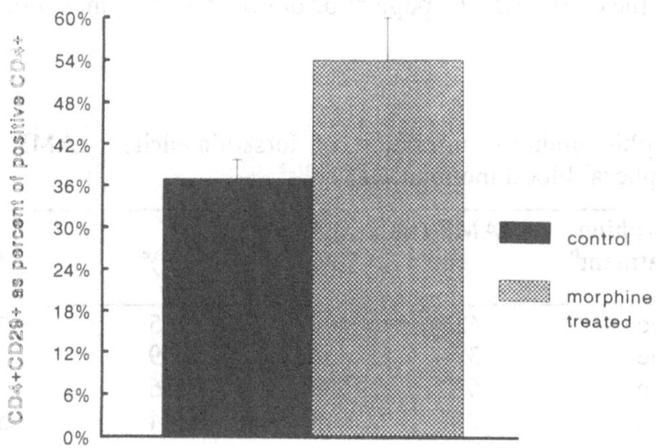

Fig. 1b. Daily morphine-exposed monkeys have elevated levels of peripheral blood $CD4^+CD29^+$ lymphocytes. The percentage of dual stained $CD4^+$ cells was calculated as the percentage of $CD4^+CD29^+$ cells/percentage of total $CD4^+$ cells X 100.
[a]Error bars represent standard error of the mean, n=4.

IgM production as well as enhance interleukin-2 production by PBMs following pokeweed mitogen stimulation (3). It is tempting to speculate that the changes in the production of cAMP by PBMs from morphine-exposed monkeys in response to a stimulator such as forskolin may be responsible for some of the immunoregulatory events (e.g., the suppression of NK activity) similar to cAMP modulation of cytotoxic T lymphocyte activity (10). The data indicating that rhesus monkeys exposed daily to morphine also have a larger percentage of $CD4^+CD29^+$ helper-inducer T lymphocytes supports the results of the interleukin-2 data. Similarly, the results obtained with the daily morphine-exposed rhesus monkeys parallel the observations reported in the human population of opioid abusers (4,9). Future work will address the effects of other opioids on immunocompetence in rhesus monkeys in the hopes of identifying drugs which may be beneficial therapeutically as substitution agents in opioid-dependent patients.

ACKNOWLEDGEMENTS

The authors would like to acknowledge the excellent technical help of Sylvia Mayo, Sandy Wegert and Bob Gump. This work was in part supported by grants from the LSU Cancer Center, The LSU Neuroscience Center of Excellence, and USPHS Grant DA-05018.

REFERENCES

1. D. J.J.Carr, The role of endogenous opioids and their receptors in the immune system, *Proc. Soc. Exp. Biol. Med.* 198: 710 (1991).
2. D. J.J. Carr, K.L. Bost and J.E. Blalock, The production of antibodies which recognize opiate receptors on murine leukocytes, *Life Sci.* 42: 2615.(1988).
3. D. J.J. Carr, and C.P. France, Immune alterations in morphine-treated rhesus monkeys, *J. Pharmacol. Exp. Ther.* in press, (1993).
4. R. M. Donahoe, C. Bueso-Ramos, F. Donahoe, J.J Madden and A. Falek, Mechanistic implications of the findings that opiates and other drugs of abuse moderate T-cell surface receptors and antigenic markers, *Ann. N.Y. Acad. Sci.* 496: 711.(1987).
5. R. M. Donahoe, J.K.A. Nicholson, J.J. Madden, F. Donahoe, D.A. Shafer, D. Gordon, P. Bokos and A. Falek, Coordinate and independent effects of heroin, cocaine, and alcohol abuse on T-cell E-rosette formation and antigenic marker expression, *Clin. Immunol. Immunopath.* 41: 254 (1986).
6. R. L. Hubbard, N.E. Marsden, E. Cavanaugh, J.V. Rachal and H.M. Ginzburg, The role of drug abuse treatment in limiting the spread of AIDS. *Rev. Infect. Dis.* 10:377 (1988).
7. P. A. Lorenzo, Portoles, J.V. Beneit, E. Ronda and A. Portoles, Physical dependence to morphine diminishes the interferon response in mice, *Immunopharmacol.* 14:93. (1987).
8. A. A. Marhazachi, Cholera toxin inhibits interleukin-2-induced, but enhances pertussis toxin-induced T-cell proliferation: regulation by cyclic nucleotides, *Immunol.* 75: 103 (1992).
9. D. M Novick, M. Ochshorn, V. Ghali, T.S. Croxson, W.D. Mercer, N. Chiorazzi and M.J. Kreek, Natural killer cell activity and lymphocyte subsets in parenteral heroin abusers and nd long-term methadone maintenance patients, *J. Pharmacol. Exp. Ther.* 250: 606. (1989).
10. M. G. Plaut, Marone and E. Gillespie, The role of cyclic AMP in modulating cytotoxic T lymphocytes. *J. Immunol.* 131: 2945. (1983).

IMMUNOSUPPRESSIVE EFFECTS OF MORPHINE ON IMMUNE RESPONSES IN MICE

Toby K. Eisenstein[1], Jeanine L. Bussiere,[1,2] Thomas J. Rogers[1], and Martin W. Adler[2]

Department of Microbiology and Immunology[1]
Department of Pharmacology[2], Temple University School of Medicine, Philadelphia, PA 19140

INTRODUCTION

The establishment of a firm connection between the immune and neural systems has led to considerable interest in the mediators of the interactions (1-4). In particular, endogenous opioids have been shown to have significant immunomodulatory effects (5-8). There is evidence that immune cells have opioid receptors (9-12) and can secrete opioids and other hormones that are part of the hypothalamic pituitary-adrenal axis (12-15). The studies presented in this paper focus on the immunomodulatory activities of the exogenous opioid, morphine. Although endogenous opioids have been reported to be both immunostimulatory and immunosuppressive (3, 12, 16-23), morphine tends to be only immunosuppressive. Morphine addicts are reported to have decreased numbers of T cells that can rosette with sheep red blood cells (24) and decreased mitogen responses (25). Morphine given *in vivo* has been shown to sensitize mice to bacterial, fungal, and protozoal infection (26, 27), to inhibit antibody formation to tetanus toxoid (28), to inhibit mitogen responses of spleen cells *in vitro* (29), and to suppress macrophage colony formation (30). In rats, morphine injected into the lateral ventricle or the periaqueductal gray matter in the brain decreased natural killer cell activity in the spleen (31, 32). Further, morphine decreased delayed-type hypersensitivity responses in rats (33).

In vitro, morphine has been reported to inhibit human T cell rosettes (9), alter human and monkey T cell antigenic markers (34), inhibit human granulocyte aggregation and mediator secretion (35), and inhibit phagocytosis of sheep red blood cells by mouse peritoneal macrophages (36). Our laboratories have shown that morphine suppresses the secondary *in vitro* antibody response to sheep red blood cells (37). Of relevance to the societal implications of addiction, morphine has been shown to promote growth of HIV-1 in human mononuclear cells cocultured with antigen-activated cells (38). We have demonstrated that heroin increases syncytia formation in human T cells infected with HIV-1 (unpublished observations).

This paper summarizes studies we have carried out to investigate in greater depth the effects of *in vivo* administration of morphine on the primary *in vitro* response to sheep red blood cells. The effects of mouse strain and sex on immunomodulation

Drugs of Abuse, Immunity, and AIDS, Edited by
H. Friedman *et al.*, Plenum Press, New York, 1993

induced by morphine and by its antagonist naltrexone were studied. Further, the mechanism of morphine-induced immunosuppression was investigated. The macrophage was found to be a key cellular target for the suppressive effects of the drug.

METHODS

Animals

Specific pathogen-free mice of the following strains were purchased from the Jackson Laboratories, Bar Harbor, ME: C3HeB/FeJ, C3H/HeJ, CXBK/ByJ, C57BL/6J, C57BL/6Jbg^J/bg^J (beige), and C57BL/6Jbg^J/+ (beige+). C3H/HeJ mice have a genetically determined defect that maps to chromosome 4, in the capacity of their macrophages to be activated (39), and also in responsiveness of many cell types, including macrophages, to the lipid A portion of gram-negative lipopolysaccharides (40). Beige mice have a genetically determined defect that mimics Chediak-Higashi syndrome, with defective formation of lysosomes in the polymorphonuclear leukocytes, defective phagolysosome fusion, and decreased responsiveness to intracerebroventricular morphine (41, 42). CXBK mice have a decreased number of μ receptors in the brain (43).

Drug Administration and Experimental Design

Under methoxyflurane anesthesia, 75-mg morphine pellets, 30-mg naltrexone pellets or placebo pellets (from the National Institute on Drug Abuse) were implanted subcutaneously. Sham animals were operated on similarly, but no pellet was implanted. Mice were sacrificed 48 or 72 hrs after pellet implantation.

Assay for Antibody Formation

To assess the effect of morphine on the capacity for *in vitro* antibody formation, spleens were removed from mice and single-cell suspensions were obtained by pushing the spleens through nylon mesh bags. Cells were placed into Mishell-Dutton cultures in 24-well plates at 1.0 x 10^7 cells per ml. Sheep red blood cells (3.5 x 10^6 cells) were added to each well. Plates were incubated for five days under conditions previously described (44). The number of plaque forming cells (PFCs) was assessed using the Cunningham modification of the Jerne hemolytic plaque assay (45).

Coculture Experiments

In some experiments spleen cells of normal mice were added to the cells of morphine-treated mice in culture. Normal spleen cells were added either unfractionated, or fractionated into adherent and nonadherent cell populations. For cocultures, 2.5 x 10^6 normal cells were added to wells containing 1 x 10^7 unfractionated cells from morphine-treated animals. Incubations were carried out as described above for Mishell-Dutton cultures.

Cytokines

Interleukins (IL) were obtained as follows: IL-1β, IL-2, IL-5, and IL-6 and Interferon-γ (IFN-γ) were purchased from Genzyme (Cambridge, MA), and recombinant IL-4 was obtained from Biosource International (Camarillo, CA).

RESULTS

The effect of subcutaneously implanted morphine pellets on the *in vitro* PFC response was examined in a variety of mouse strains and in mice of different sexes. The results are summarized in Table 1. Subcutaneous implantation of a morphine pellet 48 hours previous to harvest of spleen cells suppressed the primary *in vitro* PFC response to sheep red blood cells by 70% to 90%, as compared with spleen cells from placebo-pelleted mice. Morphine-induced suppression occurred in male or female mice, as well as in two mouse strains with genetically determined defects in immune responses, C3H/HeJ and C57Bl/6J bg^J/bg^J. CXBK mice, which have decreased μ receptors in the brain, were not responsive to morphine-induced suppression. Simultaneous implantation of a naltrexone pellet with the morphine pellet prevented the morphine-induced suppression of PFC responses in mice in the C3H lineage, the C3H/HeJ and the C3HeB/FeJ strains (44). For three mouse strains in the C57BL/6J lineage-the parent strain, the beige mice and the heterozygous beige litter mates-naltrexone failed to block morphine-induced suppression, and naltrexone itself was found to be immunosuppressive (44, 46). In the beige mice, not only did naltrexone not block the effect of morphine, but placebo pellet implantation also markedly suppressed PFC responses. Because the placebo levels were suppressed, when the number of PFCs was compared in morphine- and placebo-pelleted beige mice on the basis of 10^7 cells, the differences were not statistically significant. However, when the comparison was made on the basis of PFCs per spleen, morphine did induce a significantly greater suppression of the PFC response in beige mice (46).

Implantation of morphine pellets caused significant splenic atrophy. Table 2 examines the effect of pellet implantation on the ratio of spleen weight to body weight in the various mouse strains examined. Morphine resulted in significant reduction in spleen weights as a percent of body weight in all the strains tested, including the beige and the CXBK mice. In C3H lineage mice the spleen/body weight ratio averaged .60 in placebo-pelleted mice and was decreased about 50% by morphine. In C57Bl/6J lineage mice, the placebo ratio averaged .34 and was decreased about 40% by morphine. The naltrexone pellet alone also caused decreases in the spleen/body weight ratio compared with placebo in all strains tested, but the effect was only about half that seen with morphine. Simultaneous implantation of a naltrexone and a morphine pellet gave spleen sizes comparable to those observed with naltrexone alone in C3H lineage mice, but in C57BL/6J lineage animals, naltrexone did not block the morphine-induced spleen size decrease.

Our next studies focused on trying to determine the mechanism of action of the morphine-induced immunosuppression. As shown in Fig. 1, immune suppression can occur by two basic mechanisms. The first is failure of some aspect of responsiveness of the immune system, such as tolerance induced by pneumococcal polysaccharide or failure to process antigen because of lack of induction of class II histocompatibility determinants. The second type of mechanism involves active suppression, in which either T suppressor cells or suppressor macrophages produce factors which down-regulate the immune system. To distinguish between these two mechanisms, coculture experiments were carried out. In these experiments, cells from placebo-treated C3HeB/FeJ mice were mixed with cells from morphine-pelleted animals. It was found that the cells from the morphine-pelleted animals did not induce suppression in the normal spleen cell cultures over and above what would be expected by dilution alone (data not shown). These results suggest that morphine is acting by a refractory mechanism, namely, a lack of some factor required for immune response, rather than by active suppression. Experiments were carried out to try to determine what cells or cytokines might be deficient in the morphine-treated spleens. In the first set of

Table 1. Effects of *in vivo* administered morphine and naltrexone on the *in vitro* PFC response per spleen in various mouse strains.

		In vivo treatment[a]			
Mouse strain	Sex	Placebo[b]	Morphine[c]	Morphine + Naltrexone[c]	Naltrexone[c]
C3H/HeJ	F	-	↓	-	-
C3HeB/FeJ	F	-	↓	-	-
C3HeB/FeJ	M	-	↓	-	-
C57BL/6J	M	-	↓	↓	↓
C57BL/6J bg^J/bg^J	M	↓	↓	↓	↓
C57BL/6J $bg^J/+$	M	-	↓	↓	↓
CXBK/ByJ	F	-	-	ND	ND

[a]Animals received an implantation of a placebo pellet, a 75-mg morphine pellet, a 30-mg naltrexone pellet, or a morphine plus a naltrexone pellet. - = no effect; ↓ = decreased response; ND = not determined.
[b]Compared to untreated control or sham-operated animals.
[c]Compared with placebo treatment.

Table 2. Effects of *in vivo* administered morphine and naltrexone on the ratio of spleen weight to body weight in various mouse strains.

Mouse strain	Sex	*In vivo* treatment[a]			
		Placebo[b]	Morphine[c]	Morphine + Naltrexone[c]	Naltrexone[c]
C3H/HeJ	F	↑	↓↓	↓	↓
C3HeB/FeJ	F	↑	↓↓	↓	↓
C3HeB/FeJ	M	↑	↓↓	↓	↓
C57BL/6J	M	-	↓↓	↓↓	↓
C57BL/6J bg^J/bg^J	M	-	↓↓	↓↓	↓↓
C57BL/6J $bg^J/+$	M	-	↓↓	↓↓	↓
CXBK/By^J	F	-	↓	ND	ND

[a]Animals received an implantation of a placebo pellet, a 75-mg morphine pellet, a 30-mg naltrexone pellet, or a morphine plus a naltrexone pellet. - = no effect; ↑ = increased; ↓↓ ~ 50% decreased response; ↓ ~ 25% decreased response; ND = not determined.

[b]Compared to untreated control or sham-operated animals.

[c] Compared with placebo treatment or sham control.

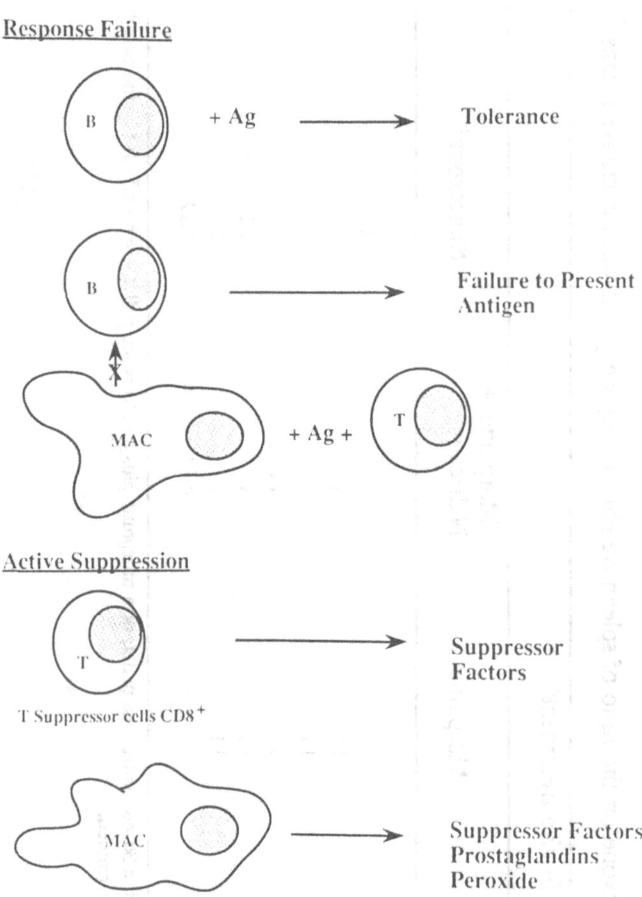

Fig. 1. Mechanisms of immunosuppression

Table 3. Addition of normal adherent spleen cells to spleen cell cultures of morphine-treated animals restores immune responses.

Cells added[a]	Response of spleen cells from morphine-treated mice (% of response of cells from sham mice)
None	16%
Whole cells	40%
Nonadherent cells	27%
Adherent cells	117%

[a] 2.5×10^6 cells from sham-treated mice, of the type indicated, were added to cultures of 1×10^7 cells from morphine-treated mice.

experiments, either normal spleen cells or cell fractions were added to cells taken from morphine-pelleted animals. The results show (Table 3) that addition of normal, unfractionated spleen cells to morphine-suppressed cultures partially alleviated suppression; the addition of nonadherent cells was without effect; and addition of adherent cells completely reversed the suppression (47). Thus, there is a deficiency in the number of macrophages or in macrophage function in the spleens from morphine-treated animals. To further explore deficiencies in the morphine spleen cell cultures, various cytokines were added back to *in vitro* cultures, as shown in Table 4. Addition of IL-1β, IL-6, or IFN-γ restored responsiveness, whereas IL-2, IL-4, or IL-5 did not (47).

DISCUSSION

These studies show that implantation of a morphine pellet causes marked suppression in the capacity of spleen cells taken 48 hrs later to form a primary *in vitro* PFC response to sheep red blood cells in various mouse strains. No differences were observed between the sexes in the effects of the morphine pellet. Of the strains tested, only the CXBK, which are known to have reduced numbers of μ receptors, did not have a suppressed antibody response. These strain differences were mirrored by the changes in spleen/weight ratios, with the exception that morphine decreased spleen size in CXBK mice, but did not suppress. On the other hand, there were marked differences between the strains in the way they responded to naltrexone. In mice in the C57BL/6J lineage, which includes the parent strain, mice with the beige defect, and their heterozygous beige littermates, co-implantation of a morphine and a naltrexone pellet failed to reverse the immunosuppressive effects of morphine or naltrexone. The reason for the difference between mice in the C3H lineage and mice in the C57BL/6J lineage in their responses to naltrexone is not known at present.

In the case of the C3HeB/FeJ mice, the mechanism of morphine-induced suppression was further investigated and found to be due to a deficit in macrophage numbers or function. It was shown that adding back normal macrophages to cultures taken from morphine-treated animals restored PFC responses. Furthermore, two cytokines produced by macrophages, IL-1β, and IL-6, were able to restore responses. Additionally, a cytokine which is known to activate macrophages, IFN-γ, also restored *in vitro* antibody responses. Cytokines whose primary effect is on T cells or B cells were not effective in overcoming the refractoriness of spleen cells taken from morphine-treated animals (IL-2, IL-4, and IL-5). IL-2 and IL-4 suppressed normal cell cultures at 100 U. At lower doses IL-2 was less suppressive of normal cell cultures, but did not reverse inhibition in cultures from morphine-treated mice (data not shown). These studies indicate that morphine pellet implantation causes immunosuppression by impairing macrophage activity, as normal macrophages, macrophage cytokines, and a cytokine which activates macrophages all restore immune function.

There is a relative paucity of published studies on the effect of morphine and other opioids on macrophage function. Our results, suggesting an effect of morphine on macrophages, are in agreement with the findings of Tubaro et al. (26), who reported that morphine administered by injection decreased the number of peritoneal macrophages elicited by thioglycolate, slightly inhibited the phagocytic capacity of sodium caseinate-elicited peritoneal macrophages for *Candida albicans,* and partially

Table 4. Effects of cytokine addition on morphine-induced suppression of the antibody response.

Cytokine	PFC response of spleen cells			
	Sham[a]	Morphine[b]	Sham + cytokine[c]	Morphine + cytokine[c]
IL-1β	173 ± 167	345 ± 62	1883 ± 43	1453 ± 214[d]
IL-2	1053 ± 71	356 ± 45	267 ± 103	417 ± 69
IL-4	1112 ± 74	257 ± 23	238 ± 57	87 ± 36
IL-5	1251 ± 174	391 ± 56	1171 ± 212	719 ± 167
IL-6	984 ± 66	289 ± 43	804 ± 69	729 ± 60[d]
IFN-γ	1904 ± 153	362 ± 37	1973 ± 155	1838 ± 70[d]

[a] Sham-operated mice.
[b] Mice implanted with a morphine pellet 48 hrs prior to sacrifice for spleen cells.
[c] Cytokines added *in vitro* at 100 U/ml.
[d] $p < .05$ when compared to morphine.

inhibited the phagocytic and killing capacities of bone marrow macrophages against *C. albicans.* Morphine given *in vivo* also suppressed superoxide induction by phorbol myristate in elicited murine peritoneal macrophages (26). Casellas et al., (36) reported that morphine, as well as met- and leu-enkephalin, added *in vitro* to thioglycolate-eli cited murine macrophages, slightly decreased phagocytosis of antibody-coated sheep red blood cells, pointing to a direct effect of the drug on phagocytic cells. Similarly, the endogenous opioids met- and leu-enkephalin and β-endorphin depressed human peripheral blood monocyte phagocytosis of *C. albicans,* expression of vimentin, and induction of class II histocompatibility antigens (43). Others have reported that morphine is without effect on human monocyte chemotaxis but endogenous opioid peptides are stimulatory (48, 49). Endogenous opioid peptides added *in vitro* have been shown to enhance secretion of IL-1 by murine bone marrow macrophages already activated by other agents (50). Similarly, dynorphin and leu-enkephalin are reported to enhance tumoricidal activity of activated murine macrophages (51). In another study, morphine and β-endorphin were reported to suppress the respiratory burst of human peripheral blood mammalian cells (52). Investigation of this phenomenon in pigs led to the conclusion that this suppression was caused by an effect of the opioids on lymphocytes, causing them to release transforming growth factor-β, which suppressed the macrophages (53). Thus, the effects of morphine on macrophage function appear to be uniformly depressive, whereas the endogenous opioids have both enhancing and depressing activity, depending on the functional assay.

Our studies did not address the question of whether the effect of morphine given *in vivo* was direct or indirect. The fact that depressive effects of morphine have been observed on macrophages when the drug is added *in vitro* (36, 43, 52) supports the possibility that the immunomodulatory effects of the drug *in vivo* could be direct. We have also shown that morphine added *in vitro* inhibits the secondary PFC response (37). Our observation of the capacity of naltrexone to block immunosuppression induced by *in vivo* administered morphine argues in favor of an opioid receptor-mediated mechanism. Work from other laboratories supports this observation and conclusion (29, 54). Further, Carr et al., (55) have evidence for delta and kappa opioid receptors in P388d$_1$, a macrophage cell line, and others have reported the presence of opioid receptors on human monocytes (56). These observations provide a mechanism by which macrophage functional capacity could be directly down-regulated by administration of morphine.

The role of exogenous opioids, such as morphine, in sensitizing to infection with HIV-1 or in exacerbating the course of AIDS is still to be definitely determined. The observations presented in this paper are consistent with compromised immune function in drug abusers.

SUMMARY

Implantation of a 75-mg morphine sulfate pellet subcutaneously into mice of different strains and sexes caused profound immunosuppression of their spleen cell primary *in vitro* antibody responses to sheep red blood cells. No sex differences were observed. In mice of the C3H lineage, naltrexone blocked the immunosuppression. In mice in the C57BL/6J lineage, naltrexone was ineffective in blocking the effects of morphine and was itself suppressive. In beige C57BL/6J bg^J/bg^J mice, placebo pellets were also suppressive. The mechanism of the morphine-induced immunosuppression was investigated in C3HeB/FeJ mice. Addition of normal splenic macrophages to *in vitro* cultures restored immune responses, as did IL-1, IL-6 and IFN-γ, suggesting that morphine-induced immunosuppression is due to a deficit in macrophage function. Morphine pellet implantation induced splenic atrophy. Whether suppression is attributable to decreased macrophage numbers or to decreased functional capacity of individual macrophages is currently under investigation.

ACKNOWLEDGMENT

This work was supported by NIDA grants DA-06650 and T32-07237.

REFERENCES

1. J. E. Blalock, D. Harbour-McMenamin, and E. M. Smith, Peptide hormones shared by the neuroendocrine and immunologic systems, *J. Immunol.* 135:858s (1985).
2. A. Bateman, A. Singh, T. Kral, and S. Solomon, The immune-hypothalamic-pituitary-adrenal axis, *Endocrin. Rev.* 10:92 (1989).
3. E. J. Goetzl, S. P. Sreedharan, and W. S. Harkonen, Pathogenetic roles of neuroimmunologic mediators, *in:* "Immunology and Allergy Clinics of North America", R. A. Goldstein, ed., W. B. Saunders Co., Philadelphia (1988).
4. Y. Shavit, R. Yirmiya, and B. Beilin, Stress neuropeptides, immunity, and neoplasia, *in:* "Neuroendocrine Network," S. Freier, ed., CRC Press, Boca Raton (1990).
5. D. V. Harbour and E. M. Smith, Immunoregulatory activity of endogenous opioids, *in:* "Neuroendocrine Network," S. Freier, ed., CRC Press, Boca Raton (1990).
6. N. P. Plotnikoff, A. J. Murgo, G. C. Miller, C. N. Corder, and R. E. Faith, Enkephalins: immunomodulators, *Fed Proc.* 44:118 (1985).
7. L. Schadené and J. Wybran, Evaluation of the immunological functions of opioid peptides, *Mod. Methods Pharmacol.* 6:235 (1990).
8. H. M. Johnson, E. M. Smith, B. A. Torres, and J. E. Blalock, Regulation of the *in vitro* antibody response by neuroendocrine hormones, *Proc. Natl. Acad. Sci. USA* 79:4171(1982).
9. J. Wybran, T. Appelboom, J.-P. Famaey, and A. Govaerts, Suggestive evidence for receptors for morphine and methionine-enkephalin on normal human blood T lymphocytes, *J. Immunol.* 123:1068 (1979).
10. D. J. J. Carr, B. R. DeCosta, C.-H. Kim, A. E. Jacobson, K. L. Bost, K. C. Rice, and J.E. Blalock, Anti-opioid receptor antibody recognition of a binding site on brain and leukocyte opioid receptors, *Neuroendocrinol.* 51:552 (1990).
11. H. Ovadia, P. Nitsan, and O. Abramsky, Characterization of opiate binding sites on membranes of rat lymphocytes, *J. Neuroimmunol.* 21:93 (1989).
12. N. E. S. Sibinga, and A. Goldstein, Opioid peptides and opioid receptors in cells of the immune system, *Ann. Rev. Immunol.* 6:219 (1988).
13. J. E. Blalock, Production of neuroendocrine peptide hormones by the immune system, *Prog. Allergy* 43:1 (1988).
14. S. J. Lolait, A. T. W. Lim, B. H. Toh, and J. W. Funder, Immunoreactive β-endorphin in a subpopulation of mouse spleen macrophages, *J. Clin. Invest.* 73:277 (1984).
15. R. T. Radulescu, B. R. DeCosta, A. E. Jacobson, K. C. Rice, J. E. Blalock, and D. J. J. Carr, Biochemical and functional characterization of a μ-opioid receptor binding site on cells of the immune system, *Prog. NeuroEndocrin. Immunol.* 4:166 (1991).
16. D. J. J. Carr, The role of endogenous opioids and their receptors in the immune system (43309B), *Proc. Soc. Exp. Biol. Med.* 198:710 (1991).
17. S. C. Gilman, J. M. Schwartz, R. J. Milner, F. E. Bloom, and J. D. Feldman, β-endorphin enhances lymphocyte proliferative responses, *Proc. Natl. Acad. Sci. USA* 79:4226 (1982).
18. W. Heagy, M. Laurance, E. Cohen, and R. Finberg, Neurohormones regulate T cell function, *J. Exp. Med.* 171:1625 (1990).
19. G. C. Miller, A. J. Murgo, and N. P. Plotnikoff, Enkephalins enhancement of active T-cell rosettes from normal volunteers, *Clin. Immunol. Immunopathol.* 31:132 (1984).
20. F. H. Hucklebridge, B. N. Hudspith, P. M. Lydyard, and J. Brostoff, Stimulation of human peripheral lymphocytes by methionine enkephalin and δ-selective opioid analogues, *Immunopharmacol.* 19:87 (1990).
21. R. N. Mandler, W. E. Biddison, R. Mandler, and S. A. Serrate, β-endorphin augments the cytolytic activity and interferon production of natural killer cells, *J. Immunol.* 136:934 (1986).
22. N. E. Kay, J. E. Morley, and J. I. Allen, Interaction between endogenous opioids and IL-2 on PHA-stimulated human lymphocytes, *Immunol.* 70:485 (1990).

23. H. Bessler, M. B. Sztein, and S A. Serrate, β-endorphin modulation of IL-1-induced IL-2 production, *Immunopharmacol.* 19:5 (1990).
24. R. J. McDonough, J. J. Madden, A. Falek, D. A. Shafer, M. Cline, D. Gordon, P. Bokos, J. C. Kuehnle, and J. Mendelson, Alteration of T and null lymphocyte frequencies in the peripheral blood of human opiate addicts: *in vivo* evidence for opiate receptor sites on T lymphocytes, *J. Immunol.* 125:2539 (1980).
25. S. M. Brown, B. Stimmel, R. N. Taub, S. Kochwa, and R. E. Rosenfield, Immunologic dysfunction in heroin addicts, *Arch. Intern. Med.* 134:1001 (1974).
26. E. Tubaro, G. Borelli, C. Croce, G. Cavallo, and C. Santiangeli, Effect of morphine on resistance to infection, *J. Inf. Dis.* 148:656 (1983).
27. C. C. Chao, B. M. Sharp, C. Pomeroy, G. A. Filice, and P. K. Peterson, Lethality of morphine in mice infected with *Toxoplasma gondii*, *J. Pharmacol. Exp. Ther.* 252:605 (1990).
28. T. K. Eisenstein, J. J. Meissler, Jr., E. B. Geller, and M. W. Adler, Immunosuppression to tetanus toxoid induced by implanted morphine pellets, *Ann. N.Y. Acad. Sci.* 594:377 (1990).
29. H. U. Bryant, E. W. Bernton, and J. W. Holaday, Morphine pellet-induced immunomodulation in mice: temporal relationships, *J. Pharmacol. Exp. Ther.* 245:913 (1988).
30. S. R. S. Ramakrishnan, H. H. Loh, and N. M. Lee, Chronic morphine treatment selectively suppresses macrophage colony formation in bone marrow, *Eur. J. Pharmacol.* 195:359 (1991).
31. Y. Shavit, A. Depaulis, F. C. Martin, G. W. Terman, R. N. Pechnick, C. J. Zane, R. P. Gale, and J. C. Liebeskind, Involvement of brain opiate receptors in the immune-suppressive effect of morphine, *Proc. Natl. Acad. Sci. USA* 83:7114 (1986).
32. R. J. Weber, and A. Pert, The periaqueductal gray matter mediates opiate-induced immunosuppression, *Science* 245:188 (1989).
33. N. R. Pellis, C. Harper, and N. Dafny, Suppression of the induction of delayed hypersensitivity in rats by repetitive morphine treatments, *Exp. Neurol.* 93:92 (1986).
34. R. M. Donahoe, C. Buesco-Ramos, A. Falek, H. McClure, and J. K. A. Nicholson, Comparative effects of morphine on leukocytic antigenic markers of monkeys and humans, *J. Neurosci. Res.* 19:157 (1988).
35. A. Mazzone, G. Ricevuti, D. Pasotti, A. Fioravanti, M. Marcoli, S. Lecchini, A. Notario, and G. M. Frigo, Peptide opioids and morphine effects on inflammatory process, *Inflammation* 14:717 (1990).
36. A. M. Casellas, H. Guardiola, and F. L. Renaud, Inhibition by opioids of phagocytosis in peritoneal macrophages, *Neuropeptides* 18:35 (1991).
37. D. D. Taub, T. K. Eisenstein, E. B. Geller, M. W. Adler, and T. J. Rogers, Immunomodulatory activity of μ- and κ-selective opioid agonists, *Proc. Natl. Acad. Sci. USA* 88:360 (1991).
38. P. K. Peterson, B. M. Sharp, G. Gekker, P. S. Portoghese, K. Sannerud, and H. H. Balfour, Jr., Morphine promotes the growth of HIV-1 in human peripheral blood mononuclear cell cocultures, *AIDS* 4:869 (1990).
39. L. P. Ruco, and M. S. Meltzer, Defective tumoricidal capacity of macrophages from C3H/HeJ mice, *J. Immunol.* 120:329 (1978).
40. B. M. Sultzer, Genetic control of leucocyte responses to endotoxin, *Nature (London)* 219:1253 (1968).
41. A. Sato, Chediak and Higashi's disease. Probable identity of "A new leucocytal anomaly (Chediak) and "Congenital gigantism of peroxidase granules (Higashi)," *Tokyo J. Exp. Med.* 61:201 (1955).
42. J. R. Mathiasen, R. B. Raffa, and J. L. Vaught, C57BL/6J-bg^{J} (beige) mice: differential sensitivity in the tail flick test to centrally administered mu- and delta-opioid receptor agonists, *Life Sci.* 40:1989 (1987).
43. J. Prieto, M. L. Subirá, A. Castilla, J. L. Arroyo, and M. Serrano, Opioid peptides modulate the organization of vimentin filaments, phagocytic activity, and expression of surface molecules in monocytes, *Scand. J. Immunol.* 29:391 (1989).
44. J. L. Bussiere, M. W. Adler, T. J. Rogers, and T. K. Eisenstein, Differential effects of morphine and naltrexone on the antibody response in various mouse strains, *Immunopharmacol. Immunotoxicol.* 14:657 (1992).
45. A. Cunningham and A. Szenberg, Further improvements in the plaque technique for detecting single antibody producing cells, *Immunology* 14:599 (1968).
46. J. L. Bussiere, M. W. Adler, T. J. Rogers, and T. K. Eisenstein, Effects of *in vivo* morphine treatment on antibody responses in C57BL/6 bg^{J}/bg^{J} (beige) mice, *Life Sci.* 52:43 (1993).
47. J. L. Bussiere, M. W. Adler, T. J. Rogers, and T. K. Eisenstein, Cytokine reversal of morphine-induced suppression of the antibody response, *J. Pharmacol. Exp. Ther.*, in press (1993).
48. M. R. Ruff, S. M. Wahl, S. Mergenhagen, and C. B. Pert, Opiate receptor-mediated chemotaxis of human monocytes, *Neuropeptides* 5:363 (1985).
49. D. E. van Epps and L. Saland, β-endorphin and met-enkephalin stimulate human peripheral blood mononuclear cell chemotaxis, *J. Immunol.* 132:3046 (1984).

50. R. N. Apte, S. K. Durum, and J. J. Oppenheim, Opioids modulate interleukin-1 production and secretion by bone-marrow macrophages, *Immunol. Lett.* 24:141(1990).
51. J. S. Foster and R. N. Moore, Dynorphin and related opioid peptides enhance tumoricidal activity mediated by murine peritoneal macrophages, *J. Leukocyte Biol.* 42:171(1987).
52. P. K. Peterson, B. Sharp, G. Gekker, C. Brummitt, and W. F. Keane, Opioid-mediated suppression of cultured peripheral blood mononuclear cell respiratory burst activity, *J. Immunol.* 138:3907 (1987).
53. M. P. Murtaugh, Y. Zhou, T. W. Molitor, and P. K. Peterson, Effects of opiates on transforming growth factor beta (TGF-β) expression in porcine peripheral blood leukocytes, *in:* "Molecular and Cellular Biology of Cytokines," Wiley-Liss, Inc., New York (1990).
54. B. M. Bayer, S. Daussin, M. Hernandez, and L. Irvin, Morphine inhibition of lymphocyte activity is mediated by an opioid dependent mechanism, *Neuropharmacol.* 29:369 (1990).
55. D. J. J. Carr, B. R. DeCosta, C.-H. Kim, A. E. Jacobson, V. Guarcello, K. C. Rice, and J. E. Blalock, Opioid receptors on cells of the immune system: evidence for δ- and κ-classes, *J. Endocrinol.* 122:161 (1989).
56. A. Lopker, L. G. Abood, W. Hoos, and F. J. Lionetti, Stereoselective muscarinic acetylcholine and opiate receptors in human phagocytic leukocytes, *Biochem. Pharmacol.* 29:1361 (1980).

MORPHINE-INDUCED MODULATION OF IMMUNE STATUS: EVIDENCE FOR OPIOID RECEPTOR MEDIATION AND COMPARTMENT SPECIFICITY

Donald T. Lysle, Mary E. Coussons, Val J. Watts,
Elizabeth H. Bennett, and Linda A. Dykstra

Department of Psychology, University of North Carolina at Chapel Hill, Chapel Hill, NC 27599-3270

There is considerable evidence that opioid use alters immune status. Studies of chronic opioid users indicate that increased susceptibility to infectious diseases such as hepatitis and endocarditis in this population is related to altered immune status (1, 2). In animals, chronic administration of morphine is associated with a decrease in a number of immune parameters (3). Although these studies suggest that opioids have immunomodulatory effects, it is not clear whether these effects are dose-dependent nor whether they can be attenuated by an opioid antagonist such as naltrexone.

Studies conducted in our laboratory were designed to provide an extensive assessment of the immunomodulatory effects of single administrations of the opioid agonist, morphine, to determine whether morphine's effects are dose-dependent and antagonized by naltrexone in a dose-dependent manner. To determine whether morphine's immunomodulatory effects are dose-dependent, male Lewis rats were assigned to one of 5 groups (n = 6) each of which received either a subcutaneous injection of saline or morphine dissolved in saline at a dose of 5, 10, 15, or 25 mg/kg in a ml/kg volume. One hour following the injection, the rats were rapidly sacrificed, and the spleen and mesenteric lymph nodes were removed. In a subsequent manipulation designed to assess whether the opioid antagonist, naltrexone, would dose-dependently block the immunomodulatory effects of morphine, 5 groups of rats (n = 10) received either a subcutaneous injection of saline or naltrexone at doses of 0.1, 1.0, or 10.0 mg/kg. Fifteen minutes following these injections, half of each of the 5 groups received an injection of saline and the other half an injection of morphine (15 mg/kg). One hour later the rats were sacrificed and the spleen was removed. To assess immune status, a mitogen stimulation assay was performed with leukocytes from the spleen and lymph nodes using the T-cell mitogen, concanavalin-A (Con-A), and the B-cell mitogen, lipopolysaccharide (LPS). Natural killer cell activity of splenic lymphocytes was measured in a standard chromium release assay using YAC-1 murine lymphoma cells as targets. The production of interleukin-2 (IL-2) and γ-interferon (INF) by Con-A stimulated splenic and lymph node lymphocytes was also determined. This battery of immune assays provides a broad assessment of the functional status of lymphocytes across two compartments of the immune system.

Drugs of Abuse, Immunity, and AIDS, Edited by
H. Friedman *et al.*, Plenum Press, New York, 1993

Table 1 shows the results of the manipulation of the dose of morphine on immune status. The results of the assessment of natural-killer cell activity showed that morphine induced a dose-dependent reduction in the cytotoxic response of natural killer cells. The results of the mitogen stimulation assay showed that morphine suppressed the responsiveness of splenocytes to Con-A and LPS in a dose-dependent manner. The results are expressed as the mean DPM for the optimal concentration of Con-A and LPS. Moreover, morphine produced a dose-dependent reduction in the production of IL-2 and INF by Con-A stimulated splenocytes. In contrast, the results of the mitogen stimulation assay for Con-A and LPS stimulated lymphocytes from the mesenteric lymph nodes showed no significant effect of morphine administration. Furthermore, morphine did not alter the capability of lymphocytes in the mesenteric lymph nodes to produce cytokines. Thus, morphine's immunomodulatory effects were evident for splenic lymphocytes, but not for lymphocytes in the mesenteric lymph nodes.

Since morphine's immunomodulatory effects were evident for splenic, but not lymph node lymphocytes, antagonism experiments were only performed on splenic lymphocytes. Table 2 shows that naltrexone antagonized the immunomodulatory effects of morphine in a dose-dependent manner. It should be noted that for the proliferation of splenocytes to LPS, approximately half of the samples were lost from each treatment due to a technical error; nevertheless, there was still a significant dose-dependent antagonism of the suppressive effects of morphine indicating that the effects were quite robust.

The results of our experiments clearly indicate that morphine dose-dependently suppresses immune status, and that this suppression is antagonized by naltrexone in a dose-dependent manner. A single injection of morphine dose-dependently suppressed the mitogenic responsiveness of splenic lymphocytes, production of IL-2 and interferon by splenic lymphocytes, and splenic natural killer cell activity. These immunomodulatory effects are robust and clearly compartment specific, as demonstrated by the failure of any dose of morphine to affect the responsiveness of lymphocytes from the mesenteric lymph nodes. Additionally, the opioid antagonist naltrexone dose-dependently attenuated the immunomodulatory effects of morphine. Taken together, our investigations provide the first clear demonstration of dose-dependent, compartment-specific immunomodulatory effects of a single dose of morphine, and dose-dependent attenuation of these effects by naltrexone, suggesting that opioid receptor activation is involved in the immunomodulatory effects of morphine. Our findings are consistent with those of several other investigators that have found immunomodulatory effects of a single administration of morphine. Those studies showed that either peripheral or central administration of a single dose of morphine reduces natural killer cell cytotoxicity (4,5,6). Bayer and colleagues (7) found that a high dose of morphine reduces the mitogenic response of blood, but not splenic, lymphocytes to Con-A and decreases splenic natural killer cell activity. These findings also suggest that the immunomodulatory effects of opioid administration are not uniform across the compartments of the immune system. Other investigators have also examined the effect of opioid antagonists on morphine's immunomodulatory effects. Morphine-induced suppression of the cytotoxic response of natural killer cells is attenuated by a high dose of naltrexone (4,5,6). Bayer and colleagues[7] also found that morphine-induced suppression of natural killer cell activity is antagonized by a high dose of naltrexone and that the reduction of the mitogenic response of blood lymphocytes is partially attenuated by naltrexone. Ho and Leung (8) found that the reduction of lymphocyte responsiveness to Con-A following chronic morphine administration is partially attenuated by naloxone. Collectively, these studies suggest that the immunomodulatory effects of morphine are mediated by activity at opioid receptors.

Table 1. Effects of morphine dose on immune status.

	MORPHINE (mg/kg)				
	0.0	5.0	10.0	15.0	25.0
NK cell activity* (lytic units ± SE)	53 ± 2.6	42 ± 2.8	41 ± 2.9	37 ± 2.6	37 ± 3.2
Spleen Con-A* (DPM x 10^{-3} ± SE)	421 ± 64	243 ± 57	76 ± 20	41 ± 12	37 ± 7.3
Spleen LPS* (DPM x 10^{-3} ± SE)	75 ± 1.1	68 ± 7.0	55 ± 4.4	49 ± 5.1	60 ± 8.3
Spleen IL-2* (1/2 max units ± SE)	40 ± 5.2	37 ± 4.7	35 ± 2.4	29 ± 2.7	29 ± 3.0
Spleen INF* (units/ml ± SE)	211 ± 47	187 ± 35	101 ± 18	94 ± 21	81 ± 11

Table 1 continued

Lymph node Con-A (DPM x 10^{-3} ± SE)	892 ± 29	938 ± 21.8	950 ± 9.4	871 ± 29.1	948 ± 27
Lymph node LPS (DPM x 10^{-3} ± SE)	60 ± 12.1	66 ± 5.9	62 3.4	51 ± 6.4	56 ± 7.2
Lymph node IL-2 (1/2 max units ± SE)	23 ± 6.1	34 ± 6.8	28 ± 6.7	27 ± 8.2	24 ± 5.9
Lymph node INF (units/ml ± SE)	289 ± 50	300 ± 23.7	324 ± 42	246 ± 28.7	278 ± 35

* significant effect of morphine dose, $p<.05$

Table 2. Effect of the opioid antagonist naltrexone on the immunomodulatory effects of morphine.

		NALTREXONE (mg/kg)			
		0.0	0.1	1.0	10.0
Spleen Con-A* (DPM x $10^{-3}\pm$SE)	morphine	46 ± 23.2	205 ± 26	304 ± 47.8	313 ± 21
	saline	390 ± 42	307 ± 29	338 ± 22.8	336 ± 24
Spleen LPS* (DPM x $10^{-3}\pm$SE)	morphine	23 ± 12	71 ± 31	72_± 49	68 ± 31
	saline	93 ± 5	75 ± 23	68 ± 3.4	80 ± 29
Spleen IL-2* (1/2 max units±SE)	morphine	6 ± 0.8	14 ± 2.1	18 ± 1.8	20 ± 2.8
	saline	15 ± 0.7	15 ± 0.9	17 ± 1.7	17 ± 1.8
NK cell activity* (lytic units±SE)	morphine	14 ± 1.6	18 ± 1.5	23 ± 2	22 ± 1.1
	saline	27 ± 2	25 ± 1.5	23 ± 1.1	26 ± 2.7
Spleen INF* (units/ml±SE)	morphine	109 ± 8.5	178 ± 13	191 ± 16.4	188 ± 12
	saline	198 ± 21	182 ± 10	199 ± 8.1	199 ± 6.0

* significant antagonism of morphine's effects by naltrexone, $p<.05$

Although the results of our experiments clearly demonstrate that opioid receptors are involved in morphine's immunomodulatory effects, the exact mechanism of these alterations is poorly understood. The work indicating the existence of opioid receptors on lymphocytes suggests a direct effect of morphine on immune status (9). However, *in vitro* work has shown that opioid agonists can enhance as well as suppress immune responses, and these effects are not consistently blocked by opioid antagonists. For example, methadone markedly suppresses T-cell proliferation when added to cultures of human peripheral blood mononuclear cells (10). In contrast, when lymphocytes are incubated with morphine, PHA-stimulated T-cell proliferation is enhanced (11). Moreover, naloxone has been shown to enhance the T-cell proliferative response (11). ß-endorphin suppresses PHA-induced blastogenesis of human T-lymphocytes in culture, but enhances other measures of immune function, such as interferon production (12). Similarly, these *in vitro* immunomodulatory effects of ß-endorphin are not always blocked by naloxone, which suggests the involvement of nonopioid mechanisms (12). Taken together, these findings suggest that indirect mechanisms may be responsible for the *in vivo* effects of morphine and other opioids.

There is growing evidence that the *in vivo* effects of morphine may be mediated through the activation of opioid receptors in the central nervous system. Support for central mediation of morphine's immunomodulatory effects is provided by an investigation showing that microinjection of morphine directly into the periaqueductal gray matter suppressed natural killer cell activity, an effect which was blocked by an opioid antagonist (6). It has also been shown that whereas peripheral injection of morphine suppressed immune function, injection of N-methylmorphine, which does not cross the blood-brain barrier, did not alter immune function (4).

Although these results suggest that activation of central opioid receptors by opioid agonists is responsible for morphine-induced alterations of immune status, these findings raise the question of how central opioid activity alters the peripheral immune system. There is no shortage of potential mediators of neuroimmune interactions. The central nervous system can signal the cells of the immune system via hypothalamo-pituitary-neuroendocrine activity and via direct nerve fiber connections with primary and secondary lymphoid compartments (13). There is evidence that morphine and related opioid agonists increase concentrations of catacholamines in plasma (14). Thus, neuroendocrine activation is one of several possible mechanisms through which morphine can regulate immune status. The compartment-specificity of morphine's immunomodulatory effects may be clarified by the examination of different neuroendocrine pathways with respect to the different lymphoid compartments.

Acknowledgement

This work was supported by grants from the National Institute of Mental Health (MH46284) and the National Institute on Drug Abuse (DAO7481). Linda A. Dykstra is the recipient of a Research Scientist Award, DA00033 from the National Institute on Drug Abuse. Mary E. Coussons was supported by National Institute on Drug Abuse training grant (DA07244), and subsequently a National Research Service Award (DAO5522). A more complete version of this work is published in the Journal of Pharmacology and Experimental Therapeutics. Address correspondence to either Donald T. Lysle or Linda A Dykstra, Department of Psychology, Davie Hall, CB # 3270, University of North Carolina, at Chapel Hill, Chapel Hill, NC 27599-3270.

REFERENCES

1. H. H. Hussey and S. Katz, Infections resulting from narcotic addiction: Report of 102 cases, *Am. J. Med.* 9:186 (1950).
2. D. M. Novick, M. Ochshorn, V. Ghali, T.S. Croxson, W.D. Mercer, N. Chiorazzi, and M.J. Kreek, Natural killer cell activity and lymphocyte subsets in parenteral heroin abusers and long-term methadone maintenance patients, *J. Pharmacol. Exp. Ther.* 250:606 (1989).
3. H. U. Bryant, E.W. Bernton, and J.W. Holaday, Immunosuppressive effects of chronic morphine treatment in mice, *Life Sci.* 41:1731 (1987).
4. Y. Shavit, A. DePaulis, F.C. Martin, G.W. Terman, R.N. Pechnick, C.J. Zane, R.P. Gale and J.C. Liebeskind, Involvement of brain opiate receptors in the immune-suppressive effect of morphine, *PNAS* 83:7114 (1986).
5. Y. Shavit, F.C. Martin, R. Yirmiya, S. Ben-Eliyahu, G.W. Terman, H. Weiner, R.P. Gale, J.C. Liebeskind, Effects of a single administration of morphine or foot shock stress on natural killer cell cytotoxicity, *Brain, Behav. and Immun.* 1:318 (1987).
6. R. J. Weber and A. Pert, The periaqueductal grey matter mediates opiate-induced immunosuppression, *Behav. Neurosci.* 102:534 (1989).
7. B. M. Bayer, S. Daussin, M. Hernandez, and L. Irvin, Morphine inhibition of lymphocyte activity is mediated by and opioid-dependent mechanism, *Neuropharmacol.* 29:369 (1990).
8. W. K. K. Ho and A. Leung, The effect of morphine addiction on concanavalin A-mediated blastogenesis, *Pharmac. Res. Commun.* 11:413 (1979).
9. D. J.J. Carr, B.R. DeCosta, C.H. Kim, A.E. Jacoben, K.C. Rice and J.E. Blalock, Opioid receptors on cells of the immune system: Evidence for delta and kappa classes, *J. Endocrinol.* 122:161 (1989).
10. V. K. Singh, A. Jakubovic and D.A. Thomas, Suppressive effects of methadone on human blood lymphocytes, *Immunol. Let.* 2:177 (1980).
11. G. Bocchini, G. Bonanno and A. Canevari, Influence of morphine and naloxone on human peripheral blood T-lymphocytes, *Drug Alcohol Dependence*, 11:233 (1983).
12. H. W. McCain, I.B. Lamster, J.M. Bozzone and J.T. Grbic, ß-endorphin modulates human immune activity via non-opiate receptor mechanisms, *Life Sci.* 31:1619 (1982).
13. D. L. Felten, S.Y. Felten, K.D. Ackerman, D.L. Bellinger, K.S. Madden, S.L. Carlson and S. Livnat, Peripheral innervation of lymphoid tissue, *in*: "The Neuroendocrine-Immune Network", S. Freier ed., pp. 9-18, Boca Raton, Florida: CRC Press, (1990).
14. G. R. Van Loon, N.M. Appel and D. Ho. ß-endorphin-induced stimulation of central sympathetic outflow: B-endorphin increases plasma concentrations of epinephrine, norepinephrine, and dopamine in rats, *Endocrinol.* 109:49 (1981).

MORPHINE BINDING SITES ON HUMAN T LYMPHOCYTES

John J. Madden, David Ketelsen and William L. Whaley

Department of Psychiatry, Emory University, Atlanta, GA 30322 and Human and Behavioral Genetics Laboratory, Georgia Mental Health Institute, 1256 Briarcliff Road, NE, Atlanta, GA 30306

INTRODUCTION

The search for classic opiate receptors on cells of the human immune system has been essentially futile (1,2). However, a large block of replicable data have suggested that opiates are potent modulators of immune status or function. This quandary has been partially resolved by the demonstration of non-classic opiate binding sites or situational binding sites on cellular elements of the immune system. These sites appear to be highly ligand specific; but their pattern of specificity does not mirror those of the opiate receptors of the central nervous system (CNS).

In attempting to define a lymphocyte mu-like binding site, the binding of B-endorphin to human lymphocytes was studied by several groups (3,4). While saturable specific binding was found, the binding was not displaceable by any of the expected ligands, with the exception of alpha-endorphin and various C-terminal peptides from B-endorphin. Since it had already been shown that the binding of B-endorphin in the CNS was via the N-terminal end, this binding site on the lymphocyte fails to mimic any of the known opiate receptors formerly described and thus has been called a "non-opiate" binding site. Further confusing the issue, it has been reported that a 72 kD protein is involved in the active transport of B-endorphin into the lymphocyte (5). Thus, while B-endorphin is undeniably potent in the modulation of the immune system *in vitro*, the binding site for B-endorphin is quite dissimilar from known CNS sites. Quite possibly, the mechanisms by which B-endorphin affects lymphocyte function are different from those found in the CNS, e.g., in the generation of secondary messengers. The role of uptake in those mechanisms has yet to be determined.

A second ligand which has been used to assess the presence of opiate binding sites on lymphocytes is (-)-naloxone. A low affinity site (K_d 40-50 nM) has been reported for G_o human lymphocytes with some displacement by various mu and delta ligands (6). On mouse splenocytes at least 2 binding sites are apparent - one corresponding to the low affinity site reported for human lymphocytes and a high affinity site (K_d approx. 1 nM)(7). Ligand displacement properties at these sites are not yet known.

Using an irreversible mu binding ligand (BIT), Radulescu et al. (8) labeled a 58 kD protein from mouse splenocytes. Binding could be prevented by competition with

Drugs of Abuse, Immunity, and AIDS, Edited by
H. Friedman *et al.*, Plenum Press, New York, 1993

another mu selective ligand (DAGO) further suggesting mu-like characteristics for this protein. Binding of BIT to mouse T splenocytes altered calcium uptake while the uptake in B splenocytes was unaffected by BIT. Surprisingly, the protein labeled is present at 3,000-30,000 sites per cell. At that level, it is not clear why the site cannot be seen by standard saturation binding techniques using compounds like morphine as the labeling compound. To date, all reports of specific binding of morphine to G_o lymphocytes, including mouse splenocytes, have been negative (1,9). The only way of reconciling these results is to assume that morphine has a very low affinity and occupancy for the site bound by the BIT which is not what is measured for the CNS mu receptor. Thus it is not yet certain that the protein bound by BIT in the mouse splenocyte is in fact the same protein bound by BIT in the CNS.

A recent report from Minnesota (9) has provided the first clear evidence for a high affinity (-)-morphine binding site of mouse thymocytes - albeit cells that had first been stimulated to division by a mitogen (phytohemagglutin [PHA]). This binding is competitive with (-)-naloxone and, interestingly with the pharmacologically inactive enantiomers (+)-morphine and (+)-naloxone. Again, this is diametrically opposed to what is seen in the CNS where the inactive enantiomers do not affect binding at the mu receptor. Also, at least some of the biological activities of morphine in the mouse lymphocyte are stereospecific suggesting that this site is probably not involved in those biological activities (10). Its role in immunomodulation therefore has yet to be determined.

Thus, while much progress has been made in the analysis of opiate binding to mouse lymphocytes, very little has been published concerning the human peripheral lymphocyte. This report will present some preliminary observations concerning morphine binding to human peripheral lymphocytes.

RESULTS

In evaluating morphine binding to lymphocytes, several pharmacological criteria were employed to determine whether the binding observed might be significant. The primary criteria included specificity, saturability, high affinity (K_d < 10 nM), stereospecificity, (-)-naloxone reversibility and competition with appropriate opiate ligands. In particular, reversibility by B-endorphin was investigated because of its physiological importance. The radioactive ligands used were ^{3}H-(-)-morphine and ^{3}H-(-)-naloxone.

Materials Used

Selection of an appropriate human starting material is difficult because of the continuing need for large numbers of cells for the assays. Thus leukopheresis has been used in these studies as the primary source of cells. Purification and freezing procedures are as previously described as are sonication methods for the production of the cell membrane fractions used in the binding studies reported here (6).

Binding of Morphine to G_o Lymphocytes

With one very unusual exception (an individual who had suffered a severe allergic reaction a few days before donating lymphocytes), morphine does <u>not</u> bind specifically to either intact human peripheral lymphocytes or sonicated lymphocyte membrane at morphine concentrations below 100 nM. There is a high level of non-specific binding compared to that found for comparable concentrations of ligand and CNS derived tissue. None of this binding is displaceable by morphine, (-)-naloxone, morphiceptin, levorphanol or dextrorphan. This lack of competition by various mu opiate agonists is not affected by the sodium chloride concentration or the presence or absence of sulfydryl reagents. Several dozens of cell preparations from over a dozen subjects were tested unsuccessfully. Length of incubation was varied up to 2 hours, although 45 minutes was most frequently used, unsuccessfully. Temperatures of 0, 23 and 37°C were used without apparent effect. Thus, as has been noted by many other groups, human peripheral G_0 lymphocytes lack the ability to competitively bind (-)-morphine above the high level of non-specific binding seen for these preparations.

Binding of Morphine to Activated Lymphocytes

G_0 lymphocytes, which had no demonstrable binding affinity for morphine, were grown for 72 hours with PHA in RPMI 1640 and 10% fetal calf serum (FCS). The PHA was removed by centrifugation and new media, containing 30 units/ml interleuken 2 (IL-2) in place of the PHA added. The cells can then be grown for several weeks with suitable addition of fresh media.

Within 24 hrs of stimulation by mitogen (PHA), the cells begin to express specific binding sites for morphine. The K_d for this saturable binding was approximately 1 nM. Further growth of the cells for 48 to 72 hrs yielded maximal binding 3-10 times greater than that observed at 24 hrs.

Displacement of Morphine from Activated Lymphocytes by Other Ligands

As expected, morphine binding was competitive with a number of other opiate ligands including (-)-naloxone, B-endorphin and the mu specific ligand, morphiceptin. An attempt to assess stereospecificity using competition with levorphanol and dextrorphan failed when both compounds failed to significantly reduce morphine binding.

Effect of Sulfur Compounds on Morphine Binding

Beta-mercaptoethanol and glutathione significantly diminished specific morphine binding suggesting that the specific binding was sensitive to reduced sulfhydryl compounds. Neither of these compounds had an effect on the non-specific binding.

Cleland's reagent (dithiotheitol [DTT]), on the other hand, essentially eliminated specific binding and significantly diminished non-specific binding. One of the great difficulties with measuring specific opiate binding to immune system cells is the high level of nonspecific binding seen compared to that found for CNS membrane preparations. The ability of DTT to greatly reduce lymphocyte non-specific binding suggests that this binding may in fact be to proteins unique to the lymphocyte membrane which contain important disulfide bridges.

Reduction of Morphine Binding by Proteolytic Enzymes

Preincubation for 1 hour of the lymphocyte membrane fraction with trypsin eliminated specific morphine binding and at higher concentrations reduced or eliminated non-specific binding. This again suggests that the both the specific and non-specific binding sites are primarily protein in nature.

Neither neurominidase or phospholipase C had a significant effect on specific, non-specific or total binding.

Effect of Salt Concentration on Morphine Binding

Morphine binding was tested as a function of sodium chloride concentration. Potassium chloride concentration was simultaneous altered to maintain constant molarity. Maximum specific binding was found at 0.15 M sodium chloride falling essentially to zero at concentrations below 0.05 M.

Binding of Opiates to Cell Organelles

Sonication of lymphocytes shatters not only the outer cell membranes, but also much of their internal structures and organelles. Using nitrogen cavitation allows for better recovery of these internal structures using ultracentrifugation methods (11). When G_0 lymphocytes were fractured using nitrogen cavitation, and the cell fractions obtained by centrifugation, it was found that the highest specific activity fractions were the microsomes and the mitochondria. The ligand used in these experiments was ^{3}H-(-)-naloxone at a concentration of 40 nM.

While this binding of opiates to internal cell fraction may seem unexpected, it is in line with some early results that demonstrated that an active process existed for the uptake of these compounds by a variety of cells. In fact, in some preliminary experiments, we could demonstrate that a lymphocyte uptake path existed for morphine. This path could be blocked by 0.1 mM chloroquine.

CONCLUSIONS

After 15 years of concerted efforts by many laboratories, it is now apparent that the control of lymphocyte function by morphine is mediated by processes quite different from those employed by opiates within the CNS. Lack of measurable levels of high affinity, G_0 lymphocyte binding sites make analogy to the known and well described CNS mu receptor somewhat futile. This has not meant however that the pharmacology of the process is totally unknown. Data presented by several laboratories have suggested several novel mechanisms by which morphine might in fact act on the peripheral lymphocyte.

In terms of the non-dividing peripheral lymphocyte at least two mechanisms have presented themselves as viable candidates for lymphocyte modulation - the low affinity receptor reported for both human peripheral lymphocyte and mouse splenocyte and an internalization mechanism followed by interaction of the opiate with a specific subcellular component or organelle. The low affinity receptor, which has a K_d for (-)-naloxone of 40 nM and for morphine somewhere between 300 and 500 nM, may in fact be responsible for the blastogenic modulation seen for mouse splenocyte because of the similarity of the quantitative results of the binding experiments and the growth experiments (10). As is the case with many of the binding studies of the immune system, the applicability of these results must be tempered by the knowledge of the high levels of non-specific binding seen for lymphocyte membrane preparations at these high ligand concentrations (200 - 2,000 nM). At these concentrations and levels of "non-specific" binding, it may well be appropriate to ask how much of the "non-specific" binding is truly non-productive binding and how much represents cellular uptake of ligand. The lymphocyte is after all a much more permeable cell than the brain cell giving it a greater capacity for drug uptake. And if uptake is an significant phenomenon, might morphine play a significant modulating role in the intracellular milieu of the cell?

Earlier studies of the drug uptake by leukocytes (12,13) reported K_m's for such drugs as morphine, codeine and methadone ranging from the micromolar to the millimolar range. The low specific activity of the drugs available precluded studies down to the nanomolar range. Further work is needed to determine whether uptake is a significant component of morphine's action on human lymphocytes and mouse splenocytes. Evidence is starting to accumulate which suggests that once inside the lymphocyte, the opiate binds to the microsomal fraction and possibly the mitochondrial fraction. The effect and specificity of that binding are both unknown.

For the dividing lymphocyte, both the human peripheral lymphocyte (this report) and the mouse thymocyte (9), a receptor mechanism seems more plausible. The binding of morphine to these cells is saturable and naloxone-reversible. For the human lymphocyte, the binding was competitive with B-endorphin and the mu-specific ligand morphiceptin. The salt requirements and sulfhydryl sensitivity of the morphine binding site on the human lymphocytes were significantly different from those requirements for the CNS mu receptor. The actions of trypsin and DTT on the binding indicates the protein nature of the binding site. In the case of the mouse thymocyte, the binding is not stereospecific as judged by competition with either (+)-morphine and (+)-naloxone. Thus in both models, the morphine binding is of high affinity, competitive with a number of biologically important compounds and protein in nature. This binding however is quite dissimilar to that reported for the CNS mu receptor.

The results synopsized in this report affirm the fact that the immune system and central nervous system functionally interact via common intermediates. They further affirm the possibility that the mechanisms used to respond to those stimuli might be site-specific.

Acknowledgements

This work was supported in part by NIDA grants DA-05002 and DA-01451.

REFERENCES

1. N. E. S. Sibinga and A. Goldstein, Opioid peptides and opioid receptors in cells of the immune system, *Ann. Rev. Immunol.* 6:219 (1988).
2. J. J. Madden and R.M. Donahoe, Opiate binding to cells of the immune system, *in*: "Drugs of Abuse and Immune Function" R.R. Watson, ed., CRC Press, Boca Raton (1990).
3. E. Hazum, K.J. Chang and P. Cuartrecases, Specific non-opiate receptors for B-endorphin, *Science* 205:1033 (1979).
4. N. A. Shahabi, P.K. Peterson and B. Sharp, B-endorphin binding to naloxone-insensitive sites on a human mononuclear cell line (U937): effects of cations and guanosine triphosphate, *Endocrinol.* 126:3006 (1990).
5. L. Schweigerer, W. Schmidt, H. Teschmacher and C. Gramsch, B-endorphin surface binding and internalization in thymoma cells, *Proc. Natl. Acad. Sci.*, USA 82:5751 (1985).
6. J. J. Madden, R.M. Donahoe, J. Zwemer-Collins, D.A. Shafer and A. Falek, Binding of naloxone to human T lymphocytes, *Biochem. Pharmacol.* 36:4103 (1987).
7. H. Ovadia, P. Nitsan and O. Abramsky, Characterization of opiate binding sites on membranes of rat lymphocytes, *J. Neuroimmunol.* 21:93 (1989).
8. R. T. Radulescu, B.R. DeCosta, A.E. Jacobson, K.C. Rice, J.E. Blalock and D.J.J. Carr, Biochemical and functional characterization of a u-opioid receptor binding site on cells of the immune system, *Prog. Neuroendocrin. Immnol.* 4:166 (1991).
9. S. Roy, B.-L. Ge, S. Ramakrishnan, N.M. Lee and H.H. Loh, ^{3}H-Morphine binding is enhanced by IL-1-stimulated thymocyte proliferation, *FEBS Lett.* 287:93 (1991).
10. D. D. Taub, T.K. Eisenstein, E.B. Geller, M.W. Adler and T.J. Rogers, Immunomodulatory activity of mu and kappa selective opioid agonists, *Proc. Natl. Acad. Sci.*, USA 88:360 (1991).
11. J. P. Quigley, Association of a protease (plasminogen activator) with a specific membrane fraction isolated from transformed cells, *J. Cell Biol.* 71:472 (1976).
12. M. J. Marks and F. Medzihradsky, Transport and interactions of drugs in leukocytes, *Biochem. Pharmacol.* 23:2951 (1974).

13. F. Medzihradsky, M.J. Marks and J.I. Metcalfe, Cellular transport of CNS drugs, *Adv. Biochem. Psychopharmacol.* 8:537 (1974).

MARIJUANA AND BACTERIAL INFECTIONS

Thomas W. Klein, Catherine Newton, Raymond Widen, and Herman Friedman

Department of Medical Microbiology and Immunology
University of South Florida College of Medicine
Tampa, Florida 33612

INTRODUCTION

Many studies in rodent models have demonstrated that Δ^9 tetrahydrocannabinol (THC) can modulate the function of the immune system (1). Either injecting the drug into rodents or adding the drug to cultures of rodent T lymphocytes, B lymphocytes, natural killer cells or macrophages (1,2,3,4,5) has been consistently reported to be associated with suppressing cellular functions. However, as compelling as these reports are, the question still remains whether these drug-induced immune alterations lead to a heightened state of susceptibility of the animals to bacterial infections. A few reports have attempted to address this question and have examined the influence of cannabinoids on *in vitro* infection models and on resistance to challenge infections with various bacteria. Huber et al., (6) reported that the addition of marijuana smoke to pulmonary alveolar macrophage cultures resulted in the suppression of the bactericidal capacity for *Staphylococcus albus* and recently we reported (7) a similar finding in THC treated peritoneal macrophage cultures infected with *Legionella pneumophila*. Regarding drug effects on challenge infections, Bradley et al., (8) reported an enhanced susceptibility of mice to combination injections of THC and living or killed gram-negative bacteria and Morahan et al., (9) reported similar findings in a murine infection model with *Listeria monocytogenes*. In both of these studies, however, drug doses in excess of 100 mg/kg were found to be most effective therefore frustrating attempts to extrapolate these findings to the human drug abuse situation. Also, although these studies showed that drug treatment suppressed host resistance, little is known concerning the immune cellular and humoral defects involved.

The resistance of humans and experimental animals to infectious diseases can be studied on two levels. The first of these is resistance to primary infection in an immunologically naive animal while the second involves resistance to subsequent infections in an animal previously immunized by either a primary infection or vaccination. The primary response is heavily dependent upon natural immunity and the activation of acute phase proteins and cells (10) while the secondary response involves acquired immunity and a heavy dependence upon lymphocyte activation and function. With these thoughts in mind, we designed a series of studies in mice utilizing THC

Drugs of Abuse, Immunity, and AIDS, Edited by
H. Friedman *et al.*, Plenum Press, New York, 1993

doses of relevance to the human experience and infection paradigms involving susceptibility to primary and secondary infections with *Legionella pneumophila* (Lp). Lp is a gram-negative, facultative, intracellular bacterium which is avirulent for most mouse strains including BALB/c (11). This low virulence is do to the fact that murine macrophages poorly support the intracellular growth of Lp, produce acute phase cytokines in response to Lp infection, and murine lymphocytes respond vigorously to Lp antigens (12). In the present study, we found the injection of relatively low doses of THC at the time of primary infection had no overt effect on the course of infection but did inhibit the acquisition of immunity to a subsequent secondary Lp challenge. Higher THC doses drastically altered the course of the primary infection in that the mice died within a few hours to an otherwise nonlethal inoculum of Lp and this acute mortality coincided with a rise in the blood level of the acute phase cytokine, tumor necrosis factor (TNF). These results suggest THC can modulate host resistance mechanisms during both primary and secondary infections. The primary infection appears to be augmented by the drug with lethal consequences while the secondary immune response is inhibited leaving the animal deficient in the development of immunity and vulnerable to reinfection.

MATERIALS AND METHODS

Animal Infection

Female, BALB/c mice were obtained from Harlan Sprague Dawley, Inc. (Indianapolis, IN) and were used in these studies at 7-10 wk of age. The mice were housed and cared for in our animal facility, which is fully accredited by the American Association for Accreditation of Laboratory Animal Care. A virulent strain of *Legionella pneumophila* (Lp), serogroup 1, was obtained from a case of legionellosis and cultured on buffered charcoal yeast extract medium (BCYE; Becton Dickinson) as previously described (11). The LD_{50} dose of this strain of bacteria in BALB/c mice is 2.5×10^7.

Bacteria were grown on BCYE, suspended in pyrogen-free saline, and injected intravenously into mice. For primary infection studies, a dose of 8×10^6 bacteria was used while 4×10^7 was used for studies involving secondary challenge. These doses are either sublethal or lethal, respectively. Δ^9 tetrahydrocannabinol (THC; NIDA, Research Technology Branch, Rockville, MD) was suspended in DMSO as previously described (4) and further diluted in normal, heat-inactivated mouse serum prior to intravenous injection into mice.

Tumor necrosis factor (TNF) assay

Serum TNF levels were measured in bloods obtained at various times following the second THC injection. Blood was collected by cardiac puncture, allowed to clot, and the serum extracted by centrifugation. TNF was measured using a lytic assay as previously described (14). Briefly, serum samples and recombinant TNF standards (Genzyme, Cambridge, MA) were serially diluted in 96 well culture plates and ^{51}Cr-labelled WEHI-164 cells were added as targets to each well. Supernatants were collected after 18 hrs and counted in a gamma counter. The extent of TNF mediated lysis was estimated from the amount of ^{51}Cr release. The number of lytic units in the serum samples was obtained from comparisons to a recombinant TNF standard curve.

RESULTS AND DISCUSSION

THC Suppresses Acquired or Secondary Immunity

Previous studies designed to examine the effect of THC injection on resistance to bacterial infection found little drug effect at doses below 50 mg/kg (9). Also, in these studies THC was given after infection and not before. Because of this, the first objective in the current study was to examine the influence of relatively low doses of THC given either before or after bacterial infection. Drug doses ranging from 1.0 to 5.0 mg/kg were tried in association with a sublethal Lp primary infection. Figure 1 shows that the injection of 4 mg/kg THC either before or after Lp infection had no effect on the number of surviving animals. Groups given the drug displayed 100% survival as did the DMSO (drug vehicle) and saline injected groups (Figure 1). A subjective evaluation of the clinical course of the illness in these animals suggested that drug treatment also was with out effect on infection associated morbidity.

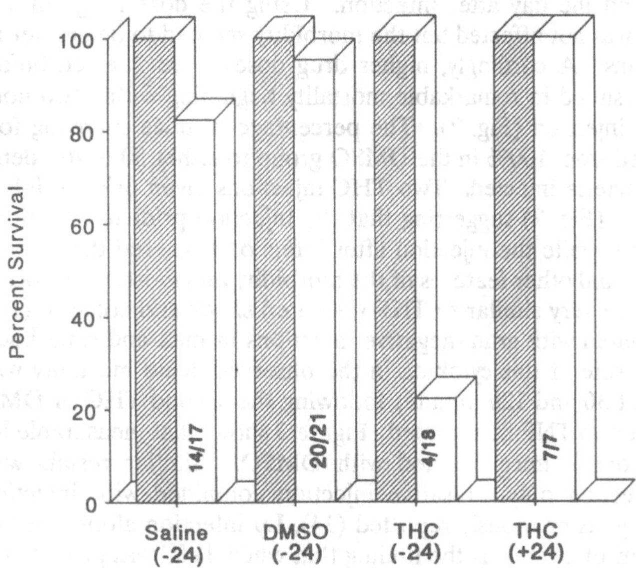

Fig.1. A single injection of THC 24 hr prior to a primary infection has no effect on the course of the primary infection but inhibits acquired immunity to a second infection. For primary infection (striped bars), mice were injected i.v. with 8 x 10^6 *Legionella* 24 hr after (-24) or 24 hr before (+24) a single injection of THC (4 mg/kg), saline or DMSO. For acquired immunity (open bars), the mice from the primary infection studies were given, three weeks after priming, an i.v. infection with a lethal dose (4 x 10^7) of *Legionella*. Note, in the control groups (saline and DMSO), the mice survive the lethal secondary challenge indicating the development of acquired immunity. The numbers on the bars represent the number of animals surviving over the total number tested.

Animals which are exposed to sublethal quantities of bacterial pathogens often develop an acquired resistance or secondary immunity to reinfection with the same pathogen. This secondary immune response can be demonstrated experimentally by priming the animals with a sublethal primary infection and then challenging the animals later with a lethal dose of bacteria. BALB/c mice can be primed for a secondary response to Lp and therefore studies of THC effects on the primary infection phase of the model were conducted. Figure 1 shows that animals given a single THC dose (4 mg/kg) one day prior to primary infection were unable, 3 weeks later, to adequately resist a lethal challenge infection with Lp. In other words, the capacity to develop acquired immunity was compromised by drug treatment during the primary infection. Interestingly, a single drug injection after the primary infection had no effect (Fig. 1) suggesting THC alters the immune response during the very early phases of the primary infection. The results also suggest that the drug effects on the various phases of primary immunity are very subtle in that the effects are not detected until weeks later, and that the secondary immunity model may be a more sensitive indicator of THC effects on host resistance than the primary infection model.

THC increases susceptibility to primary infection

The above studies involved the single injection of THC in association with Lp infection. However, THC is frequently given more than one time in animal studies and so a series of experiments was begun wherein the drug was given on two occasions, i.e. the day before and the day after infection. Using the dose range of 1 to 5 mg/kg, animal mortality was not affected but the morbidity seemed to be greater following the two drug injections. Accordingly, higher drug doses were injected before and after infection. This resulted in remarkable mortality beginning within two hours following the second THC injection (Fig. 2). The percentage of mice surviving following drug treatment dropped from 100% in the DMSO group to either 50 or 0% depending upon the number of bacteria injected. Two THC injections given prior to infection had no effect on mortality (Fig. 2) suggesting that the injection prior to infection primed the animal for collapse while the injection after infection triggered the collapse.

The kinetics and other features of the morbidity and mortality associated with this phenomenon where very similar to TNF mediated shock and collapse (13). This type of shock is associated with gram-negative infections in man and experimental animals and, therefore, a role of this cytokine in the observed acute mortality was examined. Mice were bled at 30 and 120 minutes following the second THC or DMSO injection and the level of serum TNF determined. Figure 3 shows that measurable levels of TNF were found in control mice injected with DMSO. Similar results were obtained following Lp infection only, or saline injection combined with infection (data not shown), suggesting, as previously reported (14), Lp infection alone causes an increase in TNF. However, of interest is the finding that when THC was given before and after infection the TNF level was increased significantly over the DMSO control group (Fig. 3). These results combined with the central role TNF is known to play in septic shock and collapse suggest that THC treatment combined with gram-negative bacterial infection might contribute to host toxicity by exacerbating to a lethal extent the release of inflammatory cytokines normally accompanying the host response to microbial antigens. Additional studies in this area appear warranted which are designed to examine the involvement of other acute phase cytokines in this drug induced phenomenon and determine the mechanism of action of THC on increased cytokine production and mortality.

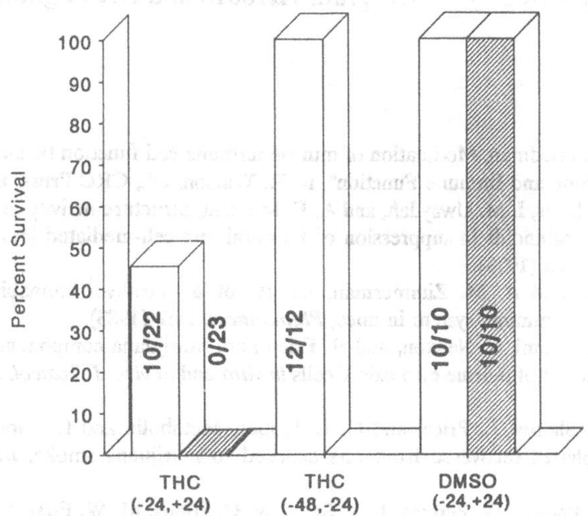

Fig.2. **Two injections of THC, one before and the other after infection, cause an acute mortality. Mice were infected i.v. with either 7 x 10^6 (open bars) or 1 x 10^7 (striped bars) *Legionella* and also were injected with THC (8 mg/kg) or DMSO 24 hr before infection (-24) and 24 hr after (+24). In one experiment, THC was given 48 hr (-48) and 24 hr (-24) before infection. Note, in the control group (DMSO), all mice survived the sublethal infection with *Legionella*. The numbers on the bars represent the number of animals surviving over the total number tested.**

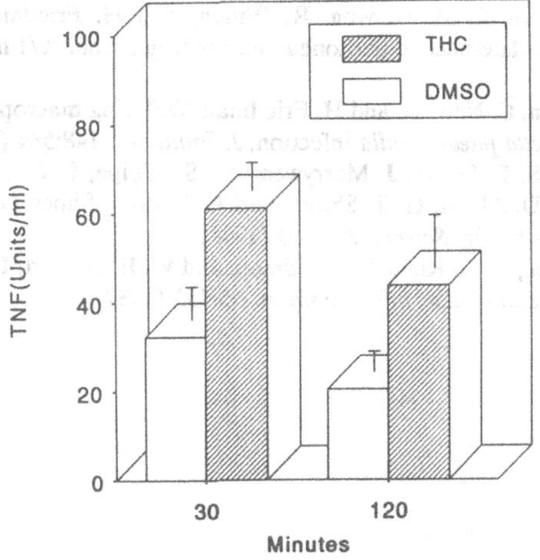

Fig.3. **THC injection increases serum TNF levels in Legionella infected animals. Mice were treated as in Fig. 2 and in addition bled at 30 and 120 min following the second (+24) THC (striped bars) or DMSO (open bars) injection. See Materials and Methods for details.**

Acknowledgements

This work supported by NIAID grant AI16618 and NIDA grant DA03646.

REFERENCES

1. T. W. Klein and H. Friedman, Modulation of murine immune cell function by marijuana components, *in*: "Drugs of Abuse and Immune Function", R. R. Watson, ed., CRC Press, Boca Raton (1990).
2. S. H. Smith, L. S. Harris, I. M. Uwaydah, and A. E. Munson, Structure-activity relationships of natural and synthetic cannabinoids in suppression of humoral and cell-mediated immunity, *J. Pharmacol. Exp. Therap.* 207:165 (1978).
3. W. O. T. Baczynsky and A. M. Zimmerman, Effects of Δ^9-tetrahydrocannabinol, cannabinol and cannabidiol on the immune system in mice, *Pharamacol.* 26:1 (1983).
4. T. W. Klein, Y. Kawakami, C. Newton, and H. Friedman, Marijuana components suppress induction and cytolytic function of murine cytotoxic T cells *in vitro* and *in vivo*, *J. Toxicol. Environ. Hlth.* 32:465 (1991).
5. D. B. Drath, J. M. Shorey, L. Price, and G. L. Huber, Metabolic and functional characteristics of alveolar macrophages recovered from rats exposed to marijuana smoke, *Infect. Immun.* 25:268 (1979).
6. G. L. Huber, V. E. Pochay, W. Pereira, J. W. Shea, W. C. Hinds, M. W. First, and G. C. Sornberger, Marijuana, tetrahydrocannabinol, and pulmonary antibacterial defenses, *Chest* 77:403 (1980).
7. S. Arata, T. W. Klein, C. Newton, and H. Friedman, Tetrahydrocannabinol treatment suppresses growth restriction of *Legionella pneumophila* in murine macrophage cultures, *Life Sci.* 49:473 (1991).
8. S. G. Bradley, A. E. Munson, W. L. Dewey, and L. S. Harris, Enhanced susceptibility of mice to combinations of Δ^9-tetrahydrocannabinol and live or killed gram-negative bacteria, *Infect. Immun.* 17:325 (1977).
9. P. S. Morahan, P. C. Klykken, S. H. Smith, L. S. Harris, and A. E. Munson, Effects of cannabinoids on host resistance to *Listeria monocytogenes* and herpes simplex virus, *Infect. Immun.* 23:670 (1979).
10. P. C. Heinrich, J. V. Castell, and T. Andus, Interleukin-6 and the acute phase response, *Biochem. J.* 265:621 (1990).
11. Y. Yamamoto, T. W. Klein, C. A. Newton, R. Widen, and H. Friedman, Growth of *Legionella pneumophila* in thioglycolate-elicited peritoneal macrophages from A/J mice, *Infect. Immun.* 56:370 (1988).
12. Y. Yamamoto, T. W. Klein, C. Newton, and H. Friedman, Differing macrophage and lymphocyte roles in resistance to *Legionella pneumophila* infection, *J. Immunol.* 148:584 (1992).
13. K. J. Tracey, B. Beutler, S. F. Lowry, J. Merryweather, S. Wolpe, I. W. Milsark, R. J. Mariri, T. J. Fahey, A. Zentella, J. D. Albert, G. T. Shires, and A. Cerami, Shock and tissue injury induced by recombinant human cachectin, *Science* 234:470 (1986).
14. D. K. Blanchard, J. Y. Djeu, T. W. Klein, H. Friedman, and W. E. Stewart, Induction of tumor necrosis factor by *Legionella pneumophila*, *Infect. Immun.* 55:433 (1987).

EFFECTS OF MARIJUANA ON SPLEEN LYMPHOCYTES FROM MICE OF DIFFERENT AGE GROUPS

Susan Pross, Yasunobu Nakano, Sharon Bowen, Ray Widen, and Herman Friedman

Department of Medical Microbiology and Immunology, University of South Florida College of Medicine, Tampa, FL

INTRODUCTION

Marijuana has widespread use, both as a recreational drug and as an anti-emetic obtained by prescription of a synthesized version (Marinol). A number of laboratories, including this one, have been concerned with the effect of marijuana and its components on the immune response. In 1974, Nahas et al., (1) reported a decrease in the ability of lymphocytes obtained from chronic marijuana smokers to proliferate to mitogens or allogeneic antigens in vitro. Since this time, THC (delta-9-tetrahydrocannabinol), the most psychoactive component of marijuana, has been shown to impact on cell proliferation in general (2,3), as well as on specific cell types including effector functions of NK cells (4,5), neutrophils (6) and macrophages (7,8). Further, there is increasing evidence that THC influences production of hormones and cytokines including ß-endorphins, plasma prolactin, and various cytokines including IL-2 and interferon (9,10).

The majority of these studies have used either adult animals for either *in vivo* or *in vitro* analyses. However, limitation of these investigations to this age range may restrict the relevant information obtained since the immune status of individuals strongly correlates with their age. Both very young and elderly individuals have suppressed immune responses (10-12). The suppression has been shown to reside primarily at the T lymphocyte level. The aim of these studies, therefore, is to determine age related differences in the immunomodulatory effects of THC.

MATERIALS AND METHODS

Experimental Animals

Balb/c female mice were purchased from Jackson Laboratories, Bar Harbor, ME. Aged animals were purchased either from Jackson Laboratories or from the National Institute on Aging of the National Institutes of Health. Baby mice were bred in our institution. All mice were kept in our animal facilities and fed Purina mouse pellets and water *ad libitum*.

Drugs of Abuse, Immunity, and AIDS, Edited by
H. Friedman *et al.*, Plenum Press, New York, 1993

Preparation of Marijuana Components

Delta-9 tetrahydrocannabinol was supplied by the Research Technology Branch, National Institute on Drug Abuse, dissolved in ethyl alcohol. The ethanol was evaporated from the cannabinoid stock with a stream of nitrogen gas and suspended in dimethyl sulfoxide (DMSO). Subsequent dilutions of the cannabinoid-DMSO preparation were made with tissue culture medium (RPMI).

Preparation of Lymphoid Cells

Following cervical dislocation, single cell suspensions of individual organs were prepared in a Stomacher 80 Lab-Blender (Tekmar Co., Cincinnati, OH), washed by centrifugation in Hanks' balanced salt solution, and resuspended in RPMI-1640 containing 10% fetal calf serum, antibiotics, and 2-mercaptoethanol (5×10^{-5}M). Cell viability (exceeding 95%) is determined by the trypan blue exclusion technique.

Stimulants

Con A (Sigma Co, St. Louis, MO) and PHA (Burroughs-Welcome, Greenville, NC) were used at final concentrations of 5 μg/ml in media. Anti-CD3 antibody (Pharmingen, Mt. View, CA) was used at a final concentration of 0.5 μg/ml.

Lymphocyte Proliferation Assay

Cells (0.1 ml) were dispensed into individual wells of 96-well flat bottom plates (Costar, Cambridge MA). The mitogens and the marijuana components were each added in 0.05 ml volumes to the wells. The cultures were incubated at 37°C for 48 hr in 5% CO_2 and air. At this time, the plates were pulsed with 0.5 uCi ^{3}H-thymidine for 18 hr. The cells were harvested on glass fiber filters and the incorporated radioactivity determined by liquid scintillation counting. Count/min ± S.E.M. were calculated for triplicate cultures. All experiments were performed at least four times. Results were determined as count/min = [counts/min experimental-counts/min medium alone] x 10^3.

Flow Cytometry

Cells (1×10^6 cell/ml) were incubated for 72 hr in tissue culture flasks with either media alone, mitogens (Con A, PHA, or anti-CD3 antibody), and THC. Cells were then counted and stained with antibodies to either CD3, Ly2, or L3T4 receptors. Four microliters of label were added to 0.1 ml of 1×10^6 cells and incubated at 4°C for 30 min. Following a wash procedure, cells were resuspended in 1% paraformaldehyde and analyzed in the flow cytometer (Becton-Dickinson FACScan).

IL-2

Cell supernatants (0.1 ml) from cells stimulated 48 hrs with mitogens with or without THC were added to 96 well flat bottom culture plates containing 0.1 ml of the IL-2 dependent T cell line CTLL-2 (10^4 cells per well). Following overnight cultivation at 37°C, the wells were pulsed with 1 uCi of ^{3}H-thymidine for 4-6 hr, the cultures were harvested and the amount of incorporated thymidine determined by scintillation spectrometry.

Table 1. Effect of THC on adult spleen cell blastogenic response to Con A, PHA, and anti-CD3 antibody

THC concentration[a] (μg/ml)	Blastogenic Response: Delta cpm (x 10^3)[b] Con A	PHA	anti-CD3
None (control)	111.1 ± 9.0	58.7 ± 5.3	75.6 ± 10.9
1.0	110.0 ± 9.6	53.6 ± 4.3	83.2 ± 7.1
3.0	101.3 ± 7.9	44.1 ± 3.2[c]	123.3 ± 9.4[c]
5.0	69.2 ± 8.1[c]	42.3 ± 5.4[c]	138.4 ± 13.2[c]
7.0	26.5 ± 4.7[d]	21.6 ± 4.3[d]	89.3 ± 6.2

[a]Indicated concentration of THC added to 10^6 mouse spleen cells stimulated with 5.0 μg/ml of mitogen or 1.0 μg/ml of anti-CD3 antibody.
[b]Average delta cpm ± SE determined for cell cultures stimulated with indicated mitogen or antibody; delta cpm calculated as cpm experimental-cpm THC alone.
[c]$p < 0.05$ versus control.
[d]$p < 0.01$ versus control.

RESULTS

THC markedly suppressed the Con A and PHA induced proliferation of adult murine spleen cells. In contrast, THC enhanced the proliferation of adult spleen cells stimulated with anti-CD3 antibody (Table 1). The Con A and PHA induced proliferation of spleen cells obtained from either very young, adult, or very old mice was suppressed by THC. When anti-CD3 antibody was used as the stimulant, the adult cells were up-regulated by THC exposure. Interestingly, there was no enhancement by the drug when murine cells at either age extreme (either very young or old) were used (Table 2).

The responding cells to these THC exposures were subjected to FACS analysis. It was found that in all situations, the numbers of Ly2 and L3T4 cells were increased following stimulation by either the plant mitogens or the anti-CD3 antibody. THC was shown to suppress the proliferation of the Ly2 cells to either Con A or PHA, and to enhance the proliferation to anti-CD3 antibody stimulation (Table 3) in adult cells. When cells from mice of either age extreme were studied, it was found that THC treatment in conjunction with anti-CD3 stimulation, did not enhance the number of Ly2 cells (Table 4). This is in contrast to the findings using adult mice.

It was hypothesized that various cytokine activities may account for the differences seen in these proliferation studies. In order to approach this question, IL-2 activity was assayed in supernatants from these experimental conditions. Table 5 shows that exposure of adult murine cells to plant mitogens resulted in an increase in IL-2 production. This effect was suppressed by THC. In contrast, the increase in IL-2 production following anti-CD3 antibody stimulation was enhanced following THC

Table 2. Effect of THC on spleen cell blastogenic response to Con A, PHA, and anti-CD3 antibody

	2 week mice		
THC concentration	Blastogenic response delta cpm (x 10^3)		
(μg/ml)	Con A	PHA	anti-CD3
None (control)	20.8 ± 1.7[c]	14.0 ± 2.8	44.7 ± 8.2
1.0	19.2 ± 2.3	13.1 ± 2.9	46.3 ± 7.7
3.0	18.9 ± 1.6	14.9 ± 3.3	49.5 ± 8.6
5.0	9.5 ± 1.7[c]	8.9 ± 2.8[c]	41.8 ± 7.7
7.0	2.3 ± .6[d]	2.3 ± .7[d]	17.5 ± 4.4[c]

	15 month mice		
	Blastogenic response delta cpm (x 10^3)		
THC concentration (μg/ml)	Con A	PHA	anti-CD3
None (control)	54.7 ± 5.8	44.6 ± 6.7	91.0 ± 3.9
1.0	57.3 ± 5.0	47.7 ± 7.7	93.3 ± 9.6
3.0	56.3 ± 5.1	49.3 ± 2.7	105.3 ± 7.4
5.0	40.1 ± 6.2	37.8 ± 4.5	83.8 ± 5.5
7.0	12.2 ± 4.6[d]	20.6 ± 5.5[d]	43.7 ± 4.5[d]

(see legend, Table 1).

Table 3. Number of adult splenocytes with the Ly2 marker after culture with THC and stimulant

THC concentrate (μg/ml)	Ly2 cell number (x 10^4)[b] Con A	PHA	anti-CD3
None (control)	85.4 ± 3.2	76.7 ± 4.8	42.6 ± 2.8
1.0	80.3 ± 4.7	68.9 ± 4.3	56.1 ± 3.4
3.0	76.5 ± 2.5	48.5 ± 3.7[c]	73.5 ± 4.3[c]
5.0	42.7 ± 3.9[c]	15.3 ± 2.5[d]	77.6 ± 3.9[c]
7.0	12.3 ± 5.9[d]	2.5 ± 2.5[d]	42.1 ± 4.3

[a]Data expressed as mean ± SE, numbers of splenocytes determined by:

$$\frac{\text{No. of cells after culture}}{\text{ml}} \times \%\ \text{subpopulation}$$

[b]Before stimulation, cell number per culture was 10.5 ± 2.1 (x 10^4)
[c]$P < 0.05$ versus control
[d]$P < 0.01$ versus control

treatment, analogous to the proliferation results. When cells were obtained from either very young or very old mice, this enhancement resulting from THC in combination with anti-CD3 antibody was not seen (Table 6).

DISCUSSION

The results of this study affirm the relationship of aging to the immunomodulation of drugs of abuse. It was found that the effect of THC depended both upon the method of stimulating the cells (plant mitogen or anti-CD3 antibody), as well as the age of the mice. The results presented show that THC can act on an already suboptimal immune system, that of either the young or aged mouse, to further down-regulate the proliferative response as well as the IL-2 activity. Although the pattern of down-regulation in cells obtained from either very young or old mice was similar to that seen in the adult animals, the absolute values both before and after THC exposure were much lower. Down-regulation of an already suppressed system may have relevant biologic consequences. In this regard, decreased levels of this cytokine have been associated with clinical problems (14).

The proliferative enhancement as well as the up-regulation in IL-2 activity found in adult spleen cells following exposure to anti-CD3 antibody and THC was seen in cells from either very young or very old mice. Aging appears, therefore, to be an important factor in terms of considering the immunomodulatory effects of this drug of abuse. The

Table 4. Numbers of splenocytes with the Ly2 marker following culture with THC and stimulant[a]

2 week mice

THC concentration	Ly2 cell numbers (x10^4) Con A	PHA	Anti-CD3
None (control)	12.9 ± 2.5	33.0 ± 10.3	35.0 ± 5.1
3.0	16.3 ± 2.3	34.1 ± 8.3	44.6 ± 7.0
5.0	8.6 ± 1.8	11.7 ± 2.6[c]	37.4 ± 11.6
7.0	4.2 ± 1.8	3.7 ± 1.1[d]	13.1 ± 5.6[c]

Ly2 cells in media alone were 1.3 x 10^4 cells/culture

15 month mice

THC concentration (µg/ml)	Ly2 cell numbers (x 10^4) Con A	PHA	anti-CD3
None (control)	10.0 ± 2.7	15.8 ± 1.6	25.8 ± 5.8
3.0	9.8 ± 1.1	6.5 ± 2.1[c]	32.1 ± 3.4
5.0	6.0 ± 2.7	6.0 ± 0.6	33.9 ± 7.0
7.0	1.0 ± 0.3[d]	1.5 ± 0.4[d]	15.0 ± 2.2

Ly2 cells in media alone were 2.5 x 10^4 cells/culture

Table 5. IL-2 activity following THC in adult splenocytes

THC concentration (µg/ml)	IL 2 activity (units/ml)[a] Con A	PHA	anti-CD3
None (control)	27.9 ± 1.5	12.5 ± 1.2	15.8 ± 1.3
1.0	26.3 ± 1.9	12.1 ± 1.8	20.3 ± 2.1
3.0	23.2 ± 1.7	9.7 ± 1.7[b]	28.8 ± 1.9[b]
5.0	18.9 ± 1.5[b]	8.7 ± 1.3[b]	31.6 ± 1.5[c]
7.0	17.8 ± 1.4[c]	6.7 ± 1.4[c]	18.0 ± 1.5

[a]The concentration of IL-2 in experimental samples was determined by the formula:

$$[\text{IL-2}] = \frac{\text{experimental reciprocal titer}}{\text{standard reciprocal titer}}$$

where a titer is defined as the dilution that yields 50% of maximum CTLL-2 [^{3}H] thymidine incorporation.

[b]$p < 0.05$ versus control
[c]$p < 0.01$ versus control

Table 6. IL-2 activity following THC

THC concentration (µg/ml)	2 week mice IL-2 activity (units/ml) Con A	anti-CD3
None (control)	13.1 ± 1.4	17.0 ± 1.8
1.0	12.0 ± 1.2	16.0 ± 1.5
3.0	10.8 ± 1.1	15.8 ± 1.3
5.0	7.0 ± 0.9	14.5 ± 1.7
7.0	5.8 ± 1.4	8.5 ± 1.5
THC concentration (µg/ml)	**15 month mice IL-2 activity (units/ml) Con A**	**anti-CD3**
None (control)	14.3 ± 1.1	17.9 ± 1.6
1.0	13.1 ± 1.3	16.8 ± 1.4
3.0	11.5 ± 1.5	17.0 ± 1.8
5.0	8.0 ± 0.9	15.9 ± 1.3
7.0	7.2 ± 1.2	10.0 ± 1.5

(see legend Table 5)

precise mechanisms of these age related differences in THC effect require further research. Studies involving the role of accessory cells in these effects as well as investigations into the relationship of these modulations to specific second message signals are currently in progress.

Acknowledgement

These studies were supported by a grant from the U.S. Public Health Service, NIDA #DAO6385.

REFERENCES

1. G. G. Nahas, N. Succiu-Foca, J. Armand, et al., Inhibition of cellular mediated immunity in marihuana smokers, *Science,* 183:419 (1974).
2. T. W. Klein, C. A. Newton, R. Widen, H. Friedman, The Effect of delta-9-tetrahydrocannabinol and 11-hydroxy-delta-9-tetrahydrocannabinol on T-lymphocyte and B-lymphocyte mitogen responses, *J. Immunopharm.*, 7:451 (1985).
3. S. Pross, Y. Nakano, R. Widen, S. McHugh, R. Widen, T. Klein, H. Friedman, Contrasting effects of THC on adult murine lymph node and spleen cell populations stimulated with mitogen or anti-CD3 antibody, *Immunopharmacol. and Immunotoxicol.* 14:675 (1992).

4. S. Specter, M. Rivenbark, C. Newton, Y. Kawakami, G. Lancz, Prevention and reversal of delta-9-tetrahydrocannabinol induced depression of natural killer cell activity by interleukin 2, *Int. J. Immunopharm.*, 11:63 (1989).
5. T. W. Klein, C. Newton, H. Friedman, Inhibition of natural killer cell function by marijuana components, *J. Tox. Environ. Hlth.*, 20:321 (1987).
6. J. Y. Djeu, M. Wang, H. Friedman, Adverse effect of delta 9-tetrahydrocannabinol on human neutrophil function, *Adv. Exp. Med. Biol.*, 288:57 (1991).
7. G. A. Cabral, E. M. Mishkin, Delta-9-tetrahydrocannabinol inhibits macrophage protein expression in response to bacterial immunomodulators, *J. Toxicol. Environ. Hlth.*, 26:175 (1989).
8. S. Specter, G. Lancz, D. Goodfellow, Suppression of human macrophage function *in vitro* by delta 9-tetrahydrocannabinol, *J. Leuk. Biol.*, 50:423 (1991).
9. D. K. Blanchard, C. Newton, T. W. Klein, W. E. Stewart, II, H. Friedman, *In vitro* and *in vivo* suppressive effects of delta-9-tetrahydrocannabinol on interferon production by murine spleen cells, *Int. J. Immunopharmacol.* 8:819 (1986).
10. Y. Nakano, S. H. Pross, H. Friedman, Modulation of IL-2 activity by tetrahydrocannabinol (THC) following stimulation with Con A, PHA, or anti-CD3 antibody, *Proc. Soc. Exp. Biol. Med.*, 201:1165 (1992).
11. D. Segre, R. A. Miller, G. N. Abraham, W. Weigle, H. R. Warner, Workshop report: Aging and the immune system, *Aging: Immunol. and Infect. Dis.* 1:255 (1988).
12. R. A. Miller, Aging and immune function, *Int. Rev. Cytol.* 124:187 (1991).
13. K. Welte, R. Mertersmann, Human interleukin 2: Biochemistry, physiology, and possible pathogenetic role in immunodeficiency syndromes, *Cancer Investigation* 3:35 (1985).

SYPHILIS AND DRUGS OF ABUSE

Lois J. Paradise and Herman Friedman

Department of Medical Microbiology and Immunology
University of South Florida College of Medicine
Tampa, FL 33612

INTRODUCTION

For several decades following the advent of benzathine penicillin chemotherapy for syphilis, its incidence in the United States remained low. However, in 1990, the number of new primary and secondary cases reported reached a new peak of 50,223 and there were 2899 cases of congenital syphilis in this country (1). The rise in syphilis started with increased sexual promiscuity, particularly among the homosexual population, but stabilized for a while after recognition of the severity and source of human immunodeficiency viral infections was accepted. Several published reports relate the most recent increase in syphilis to abuse of recreational drugs (2,3).

Since application of molecular procedures for identification of antigenic epitopes is opening the road to greater understanding of the spirochete of syphilis (4-6), the possibility of vaccine development for protection against this disease becomes less remote. The likelihood is that, once it becomes available, an anti-syphilis vaccine would be applied to populations at risk rather than to all pre-schoolers, as are vaccines for childhood infections and for adult infections that are widespread among the general population. In that case, chronic users of recreational drugs should be one of the target populations. However, many studies have demonstrated that marijuana depresses immune responses (7). Therefore, our goal is to determine whether recreational drug users would be able to respond successfully to a vaccine for syphilis or if drugs they are using would interfere extensively with their ability to develop protective immunity. Two animal models have been used to investigate this question: initially, the Syrian hamster and, currently, the rabbit.

HAMSTER MODEL FOR EXPERIMENTAL SYPHILIS

In the 1940s, Turner and Hollander showed that hamsters are variably susceptible to infection with *Treponema pallidum* subsp. *pallidum* (the Nichols strain isolated

Drugs of Abuse, Immunity, and AIDS, Edited by
H. Friedman *et al.*, Plenum Press, New York, 1993

originally from human venereal syphilis, 8) (9). They found that some wild-type individual hamsters developed skin lesions after intradermal inoculation of suspensions of treponemes, but that lesions did not form routinely in this species as they did in rabbits. In later studies, Schell and his colleagues observed that other subspecies of *T. pallidum*, namely, *pertenue* the agent of yaws and *endemicum* the agent of endemic non-venereal syphilis, provoked skin lesion formation fairly uniformly in two different inbred strains of hamsters (10,11), but that the Nichols strain did not produce skin lesions, although subclinical infection occurred (12). We confirmed these findings with Nichols treponemes in the LSH inbred strain of hamsters and have been studying immunomodulation of syphilitic infection in hamsters. Infection was persistent though subclinical and the spirochetes could be recovered from hamster lymph nodes for a year or more after inoculation of rabbit-cultivated treponemes. However, no skin or obvious deep tissue lesions formed. Previously, we showed that treatment of infected hamsters with cyclophosphamide before and during infection reduced host defenses sufficiently that ulcerative skin lesions, typical of syphilitic infection in humans and rabbits, formed at sites of intradermal inoculation of the microorganisms.

EFFECT OF THC ON HAMSTER TREPONEMAL INFECTION

Since immunosuppressive treatment resulted in activation of disease in *T. pallidum*-infected hamsters, we investigated the effect of treatment with the active component of marijuana, delta-9-tetrahydrocannabinol (THC). All animals were maintained in an American Association for Accreditation of Laboratory Animal Care-approved facility at the University of South Florida under the care of a veterinarian.

Male hamsters received treatment by gavage with THC in dimethyl sulfoxide (DMSO) emulsified in sesame seed oil 1 day prior to inoculation of 1.25 x 10^6 *T. pallidum* intradermally into shaved skin on the right side of the abdomen. THC-treatment continued on alternate days for 1 to 5 weeks. At no time, with no dosage (levels ranged from 0.5 to 10 mg THC/kg body weight) were skin lesions of any form observed. Groups of hamsters were anesthetized with carbon dioxide after 1 to 3 weeks of treatment. After euthanasia, lymph nodes were removed. Both draining (right) and contralateral (left) lymph nodes were ground separately in RPMI 1640 medium (Sigma, St. Louis MO) in sterile mortars. The suspensions were centrifuged at 500 x *g* for 3 minutes and the number of treponemes was counted by darkfield microscopy (12). In Figure 1 the results observed for animals treated with 10 mg THC/kg body weight for 3 weeks are presented. Maximal effects were observed with this dosage. Vehicle controls (DMSO controls) and sham-treated controls, which were intubated but received nothing via the tubing, are included.

At 2 weeks post-infection (wpi), there were almost ten times more treponemes in lymph nodes of THC-treated hamsters than in controls. This effect had waned considerably by 3 wpi. Counts of treponemes in the opposite lymph nodes were made to see if dissemination of the treponemes from the initial area of inoculation had been enhanced by THC-treatment. There was no evidence that this had occurred; it did not differ significantly.

RABBIT MODEL FOR EXPERIMENTAL SYPHILIS

When results for hamsters showed limited enhancement of infection, experiments were continued in rabbits, since (a) they are more susceptible to infection with *T. pallidum* subsp. *pallidum* and skin lesions can be induced with a very few treponemes, (b) analysis of dose-response assays would be facilitated, and (c) number of animals required for the experiments would be greatly reduced.

Since the early years of this century rabbits have been the animal model for human syphilis (8). Rabbits can be infected with *T. pallidum* subsp. *pallidum* the etiologic agent of human venereal syphilis by intratesticular, intravenous or intradermal inoculation. These organisms are routinely cultivated in rabbits by intratesticular inoculation for investigational and diagnostic purposes, since they have not been grown successfully in bacteriologic or tissue culture. Ten to 14 days after intratesticular inoculation of 1.5 x 10^7 treponemes orchitis develops. Extracts from the tissues at this stage provide treponemes for experiments (13).

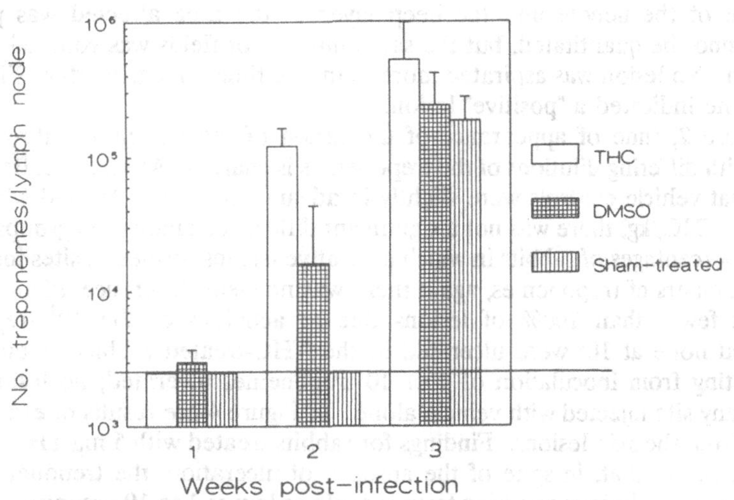

Fig. 1. Effect of THC-treatment on numbers of *T. pallidum* observed in draining lymph nodes. Male Syrian hamsters reeived THC in DMSO emulsified in sesame seed oil by gavage every other day for 3 wks starting 1 day prior to inoculation of 1.25 x 10^6 *T. pallidum* intradermally. Lymph nodes were triturated in RPMI 1640 medium and centrifuged at 500 x g; treponemes present in supernatant fluid were counted by darkfield microscopy. The horizontal line indicates the minimum number of treponemes detectable by the protocol used; bars show SE of the means.

EFFECT OF THC ON RABBIT TREPONEMAL INFECTION

THC is being administered intravenously in DMSO in 1% Tween 80 in physiologic saline 3 times a week for about 5 weeks. After pre-treatment, serial tenfold dilutions of *T. pallidum* are inoculated intradermally into the dorsal skin. There are 8 sites/rabbit from 0 to 10^6 treponemes/inoculum. Results for 0 (vehicle controls), 1 and 5 mg THC/kg body weight are being reported here.

Several observations are being made to define the development of skin lesions at the sites of inoculation of the treponemes. Rabbits are much more highly sensitive to infection with treponemes intradermally than are hamsters; 1 treponeme is considered to be sufficient to evoke ulcer development in the rabbit. Skin lesions present initially as small zones of erythema. Soon induration develops and at some time thereafter ulceration begins and progresses until an ulcerative lesion about 1 inch in diameter with underlying induration is present. This stage persists for several weeks. Development through these stages was recorded. Since we were interested in any change in pathogenesis which could be observed in THC-treated animals in comparison with controls, as soon as swelling appeared, two perpendicular diameters of the lesion were measured with vernier calipers. Height of the lesions is not readily measurable, but flatness of lesions was noted since this tended to correspond to difficulty in recovering treponemes by aspiration. The spirochetes are present in the base of the lesion. Usually, in untreated rabbits, treponemes are not present in sufficient numbers in the local lesion for detection in aspirates prior to development of ulceration. In these experiments, aspirates were made as soon as the lesion had enough depth that emplacement of the needle into the deep layer of the area affected was possible. Aspirates cannot be quantitated, but the same number of fields was counted for each sample taken. No lesion was aspirated more than one time on a given day. Finding of one treponeme indicated a "positive" lesion.

In Figure 2, time of appearance of ulceration of the lesions resulting at sites inoculated with differing dilutions of the treponemes is charted. Although at first glance it appears that vehicle controls were slightly in advance of rabbits treated with either 5 mg or 1 mg THC/kg, there was not a significant difference among the groups. If one looks at the percentages of rabbits in which ulcerative lesions formed at sites inoculated with given numbers of treponemes, again there was no clear difference, Figure 3. It is notable that fewer than 100% of lesions due to activities of the 10^3 treponemal inoculum and none at 10^2 were ulcerated in the THC-treated rabbits. None of the lesions resulting from inoculation of 1 or 10 treponemes ulcerated; no lesions were observed at any site injected with vehicle alone. In Figure 4 are results of examination of aspirates from the skin lesions. Findings for rabbits treated with 5 mg THC/kg body weight demonstrate that, in spite of the absence of ulceration, the treponemes were proliferating in some lesions resulting from inocula as low as 1 to 10 organisms. On the other hand, in DMSO controls, treponemes were not detected after inoculation of fewer than 10^3 organisms. By this measure, there was a thousandfold difference in THC-treated and control groups of rabbits, therefore.

These dose-response experiments pointed out that there seem to be optimal combinations of initial inoculum of spirochetes and dosage of THC for the effect on infectivity to occur. This can be observed in Figure 5, which shows results of treatment with 5 mg THC/kg body weight and inoculation of 10^5 treponemes. The time of maximum difference between treated and control rabbits is during the period 2 to 3 weeks after infection.

The significance of the 2-to-3 week post-infection period for observation of effectiveness of treatment is not clear. It seems to be fairly characteristic for both hamster and rabbit infections and for administration of cyclophosphamide as well as THC. In the untreated hamster, we observed that this was the period when proliferation of the treponemes is progressing rapidly - perhaps this is their maximal growth phase in the local lesion. It also may be that development of tolerance to THC after the 3 week period is responsible for the discontinuation of inhibition of host defenses.

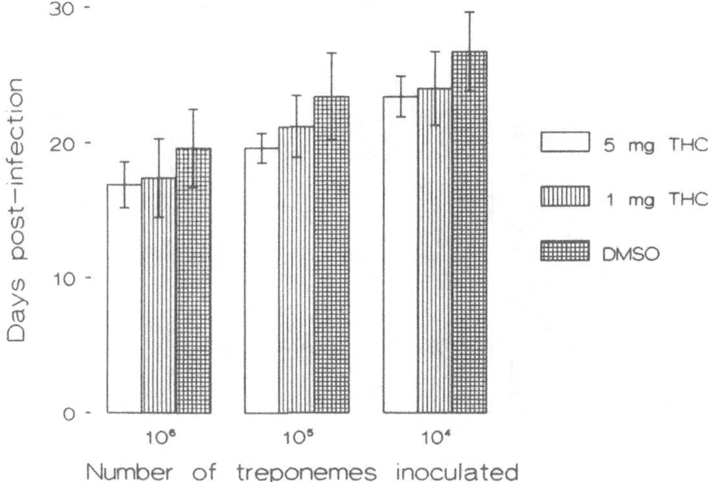

Fig. 2. Time (days post-infection) of ulcer-formation in rabbits treated with THC. Administration of 5-mg (7 rabbits), 1-mg (5) or 0-mg (vehicle controls, 8) doses of THC in 4% DMSO in 1% Tween 80 in 0.85% NaCl solution intravenously started one day before intradermal inoculation of New Zealand male rabbits with tenfold serial dilutions of *T. pallidum* in medium RPMI 1640 containing 10% normal rabbit serum. Treatment was continued 3 times per week for 35-36 days. DMSO indicates vehicle controls.

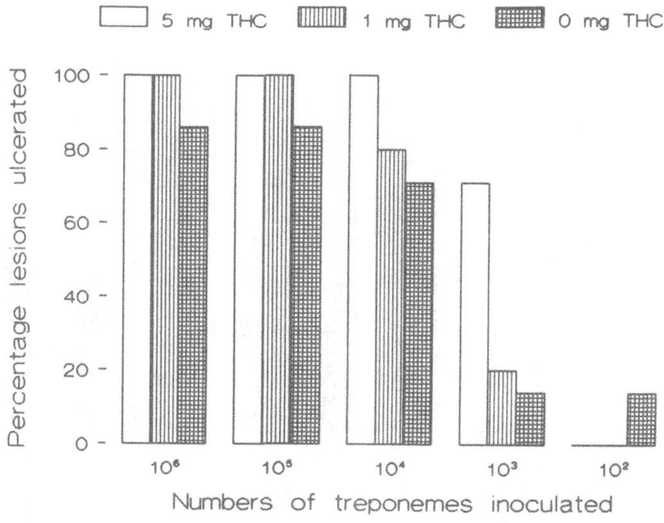

Fig. 3. Incidence of ulcerative lesions in rabbits treated with THC. These are the same rabbits described in Fig. 2.

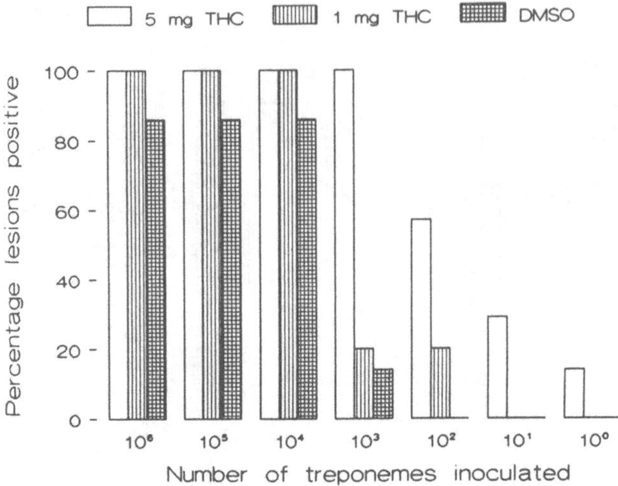

Fig. 4. Recovery of treponemes from intradermal lesions of rabbits treated with THC. These are the same rabbits described in Fig. 2. These dose-response experiments pointed out that there seem to be optimal combinations of initial inoculum of spirochetes and dosage of THC for observation of the effect on infectivity. This can be observed in Fig. 5 which shows results of treatment with 5 mg THC/kg body weight and inoculation of 10^5 treponemes. The time of maximum difference between treated and control rabbits is during the period 2 to 3 wks after infection.

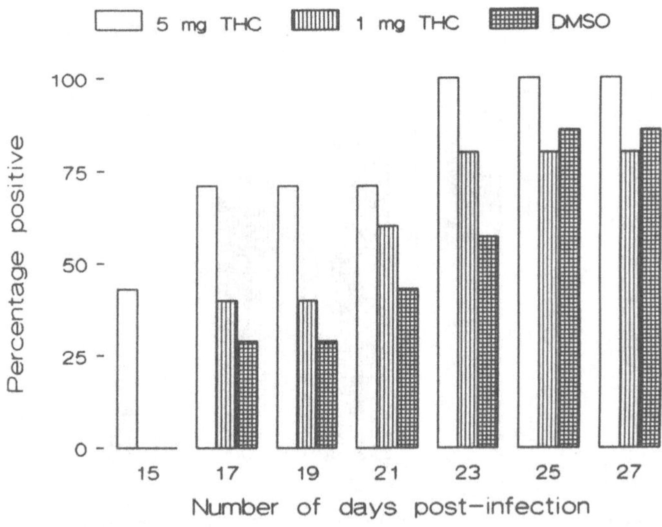

Fig. 5. Effect of THC-treatment on time of appearance of treponemes in aspirates from intradermal lesions. This is one of the groups of rabbits described in Fig. 2.

SUMMARY AND CONCLUSIONS

In summary, treponemal infections in hamsters treated with THC were slightly enhanced in comparison with vehicle controls. A greater degree of enhancement was exhibited in rabbits; treponemes proliferated more readily during treatment with THC than in control animals. Contrary to expectations, this occurred even in lesions which were not developed fully, i.e., were not ulcerated. Thus, treponemes were present in aspirates earlier during infection and from sites which had received smaller inocula of treponemes in these rabbits than in controls. Lesions in control groups developed ulcerations earlier than did the THC-groups, but treponemes were too scarce to be seen in pre-ulcerative lesions in these animals.

It appears that THC-treatment enhanced infection with *T. pallidum*. It may be that in the local skin lesion, macrophages which are vitally important in early host responses to treponemal infection may not have been functioning optimally and mediators of tissue damage may not have been produced and, therefore, ulceration was delayed in spite of enhanced infectivity of the treponemes.

Acknowledgememts

This work was supported in part by NIDA grant DA07303.

REFERENCES

1. Centers for Disease Control, USPHS, "Summary of Notifiable Diseases, United States, 1990" USDHHS, Atlanta (1990).
2. Centers for Disease Control, USPHS, Relationship of syphilis to drug use and prostitution - Connecticut and Philadelphia, Pennsylvania. MMWR 37:755 (1989).
3. R. Marx, S.O. Aral, R.T. Rolfs, C.E. Sterk and J.G. Kahn, Crack, sex, and STD, *Sex. Transm. Dis.* 18:92 (1991).
4. L. A. Borenstein, J.D. Radolf, T.E. Fehniger, D.R. Blanco, J.N. Miller and M.A. Lovett, Immunization of rabbits with recombinant *Treponema pallidum* surface antigen 4D alters the course of experimental syphilis, *J. Immunol.* 140:2415 (1988).
5. C. I. Champion, J.N. Miller, M.A. Lovett and D.R. Blanco, Cloning, sequencing, and expression of two class B endoflagellar genes of *Treponema pallidum* subsp. *pallidum* encoding the 34.5- and 31.0-kilodalton proteins, *Infect. Immun.* 58:1697 (1990).
6. R. Strugnell, A. Cockayne and C.W. Penn, Molecular and antigenic analysis of treponemes, *Crit. Rev. Microbiol.* 17:231 (1990).
7. H. Friedman, T.Klein and S. Specter, "Immunosuppression by marijuana and its components. Psychoneuroimmunology", 2d ed. Academic Press, Inc., pp. 931 (1991).
8. H. J. Nichols, Observations on a strain of *Spirochaeta pallida* isolated from the nervous system. *J. Exper. Med.* 19:362 (1914).
9. T. B. Turner and D.H. Hollander, "Biology of the Treponematoses", WHO Monogr. Ser. no. 35, World Health Organization, Geneva (1957).
10. R. F. Schell, J.L. LeFrock, J.P. Babu and J.K. Chan, Use of CB hamsters in the study of *Treponema pertenue*, *Br. J. Vener. Dis.* 55:316 (1979).
11. R. F. Schell, J.L. LeFrock, J.K. Chan, and O. Bagasra, LSH hamster model of syphilitic infection, *Infect. Immun.* 28:909 (1980).
12. R. F. Schell, A.A. Azadegan, S.G. Nitskansky, and J.L. LeFrock, Acquired resistance of hamsters to challenge with homologous and heterologous virulent treponemes, *Infect. Immun.* 37:617 (1982).
13. J. N. Miller, "Spirochetes in Body Fluids and Tissues," Charles C Thomas, Springfield, Illinois (1971).

SERUM PROTEINS AFFECT THE INHIBITION BY DELTA-TETRAHYDROCANNABINOL OF TUMOR NECROSIS FACTOR ALPHA PRODUCTION BY MOUSE MACROPHAGES

Zhi-Ming Zheng, Steven Specter and Herman Friedman

Department of Medical Microbiology and Immunology
University of South Florida College of Medicine
Tampa, FL 33612

INTRODUCTION

In vitro studies of the effects of marijuana's major psychoactive component, delta-9-tetrahydrocannabinol (THC), on immune functions show that THC is able to inhibit a variety of immune functions (1,2). However, the effect of THC on tumor necrosis factor (TNF) production by macrophages has not been reported until recent work in our laboratory (3). TNF-α, which is secreted principally by activated macrophages (4), has recently been shown to be produced in greater amounts if stimulation of murine peritoneal macrophages is performed in medium containing *Salmonella enteritidis* lipopolysaccharide (LPS) and 0.5% bovine serum albumin (BSA) in place of 10% fetal bovine serum (FBS) (Z. M. Zheng & S. Specter, unpublished observations). The use of BSA resulted in a reduction in the serum protein in the medium used to examine the effect of THC on TNF-α production (3). This reduction of serum is important since increasing the serum concentration in culture medium has been shown to inhibit *in vitro* activity of THC (5). In the current report, we present the effect of FBS and BSA on the inhibition by THC of TNF-α production by mouse resident peritoneal macrophages.

MATERIALS AND METHODS

Mouse Macrophage Culture and TNF-α Induction

Macrophages were obtained by washing the peritoneal cavity of female BALB/c mice with 5 ml of cold Hanks' balanced salt solution (HBSS) containing 50 mM HEPES. The cells were washed twice by centrifugation at 300 g for 10 min at room temperature and resuspended in standard RPMI 1640 medium. The cells were counted, adjusted to 1 x 10^6 cells/ml, and then plated in flat-bottom 96-well plates (Costar, Cambridge, MA) at 100 µl/well. After incubation for 2 h at 37°C in 5% CO_2, 95% air, nonadherent cells were removed by washing with standard RPMI 1640 medium. Adherent cells were treated with a final volume of 100 µl induction medium (standard RPMI 1640 medium with BSA [Sigma] or FBS [Hyclone] plus LPS [10 ng/ml, Sigma]

Drugs of Abuse, Immunity, and AIDS, Edited by
H. Friedman *et al.*, Plenum Press, New York, 1993

and murine IFN-γ [100 u/ml, Genzyme]) per well. Treatments included induction medium only or medium containing 0.05% DMSO (the diluent for THC), or 1, 5, or 10 μg (3.2×10^{-5} M) THC/ml at 37°C in 5% CO_2. Supernatant fluids from adherent cell cultures were collected after the designated incubation period for each experiment and stored at -20°C for use in the TNF-α assay.

Titration of TNF-α by Bioassay

Lysis of a TNF-sensitive murine cell line, WEHI-164, using a ^{51}Cr release cytotoxicity assay (6) was used to measure TNF-α activity. WEHI-164 cells (1×10^6) were labeled with 100 μCi of $Na[^{51}Cr]O_4$ (Amersham) for 1 hr at 37°C. One hundred μl TNF (macrophage supernatant fluids) was added to 100 μl of labeled WEHI-164 cells (5×10^4 cells/ml) in 96-well flat-bottom microtiter plates. After 6 h at 37°C, the ^{51}Cr released into 100 μl of the supernatant fluid from lysed target cells was collected and counted in a gamma counter as a measure of cell death. Results in triplicate wells of each macrophage supernatant are averaged and expressed as percent specific cytotoxicity as previously reported (3).

Confirmation that the cytotoxic activity of macrophage supernatant fluids for WEHI-164 cells was due to TNF-α was by neutralization using anti-mouse TNF-α polyclonal antibody (Genzyme).

Statistical Analysis

Statistical analysis was done using the one-tailed analysis of a pooled two sample *t*-test (7). Experimental values were compared with the vehicle control value only. P values <0.05 were considered significant.

RESULTS

Effect of FBS on the Inhibition by THC of TNF-α Production

In these experiments, 10% FBS was included in TNF-α induction medium with or without THC. Ten experiments were carried out, using 7-10 wk old BALB/c mice (8 experiments) and 14-19 wk old BALB/c mice (2 experiments). In 3 out of 8 experiments using young mice, THC did not show any effect on TNF-α production by macrophages at the concentrations of 1-10 μg/ml (data not shown). Although, in the remaining 5 experiments, THC caused a decrease in TNF-α production, there was no significant difference between drug-treated and -nontreated groups (Table 1). However, macrophages from 14-19 wk old mice were sensitive to THC inhibition at 10 μg/ml ($P<0.05$); therefore, TNF-α production by these macrophages could be inhibited by THC (Table 1).

Effect of BSA on the Inhibition by THC of TNF-α Production

In these experiments, BSA at 0.5% and 5% was included in TNF-α induction medium with or without THC. Addition of THC to macrophage cultures during TNF-α induction in 5 experiments using 8-10 week old BALB/c mice consistently showed that THC significantly decreased TNF-α production by macrophages after a 6 hr induction period ($P<0.025$ at 5 μg THC/ml and $P<0.005$ at 10 μg THC/ml, respectively) (Fig. 1). However, when the induction medium containing 5% BSA and THC at 5-10 μg/ml was used, there was no inhibition of TNF-α production and in some cases there was increased TNF-α production by macrophages (Fig. 2).

Table 1. Effect of THC on TNF-α production by resident peritoneal macrophages from BALB/c mice

	Age of mice (weeks)			
	7-10		14 - 19	
THC (μg/ml)	TNF units/ml	% of controls	TNF units/ml	% of controls
0[a]	104.6 ± 52.7[b]	100.0	80.0 ± 22.6[c]	100.0
1	104.6 ± 59.1	100.0	53.0 ± 15.6	66.3
5	78.2 ± 42.7	74.8	32.2 ±42.1	40.3
10	54.3 ± 29.9	51.9	9.3 ±12.3	11.6

[a]0.05% DMSO vehicle only.
[b]Data shown represent the mean ± SD from 5 experiments each performed in triplicate when supernatant fluids were collected from cultures of adherent cells in induction medium with 10% FBS for 6 hr. Each experiment contained the pooled macrophages from at least 5 animals.
[c]Data shown represent the mean ± SD from 2 experiments each performed in triplicates. Other experimental conditions were as above.

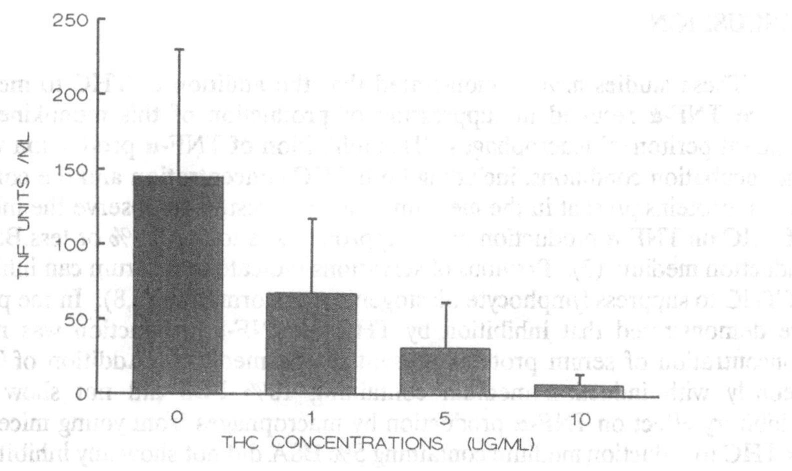

Fig. 1. Inhibition by THC of TNF-α production by murine macrophages. Macrophage supernatants were collected after 6 hr incubation in 0.5% BSA-containing-induction medium with or without THC and then assayed for TNF-α production using WEHI-164 cells labeled with ^{51}Cr. Data were calculated from triplicate cultures from 5 experiments. Each experiment contained the pooled macrophages from at least 5 animals. $P<0.025$ at 5 μg THC/ml and $P<0.005$ at 10 μg THC/ml compared with 0.05% DMSO vehicle after 6 h induction.

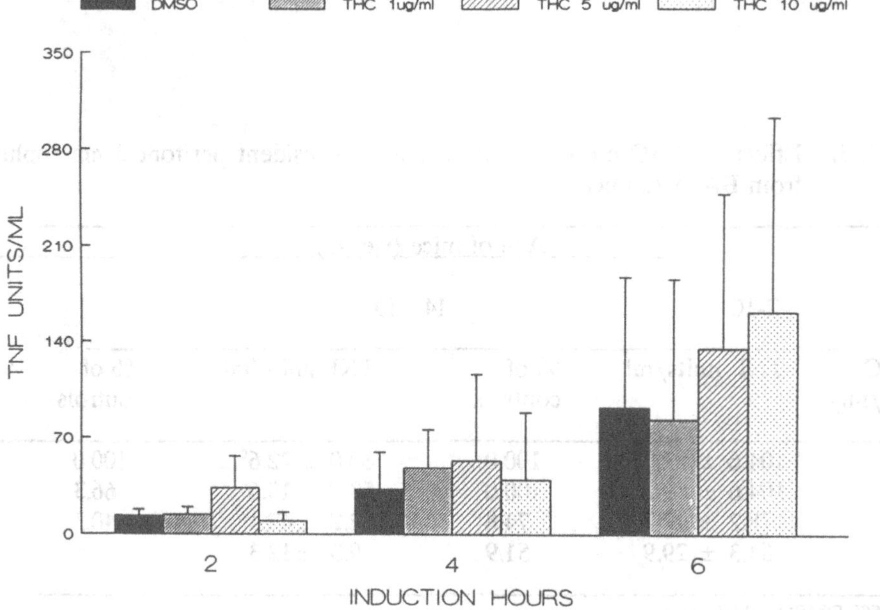

Fig. 2. Effect of 5% BSA concentration on THC inhibitory activity to TNF-α production by murine macrophages. Macrophage supernatants were serially collected after 2, 4, or 6 h incubation in induction medium with or without THC and then assayed for TNF-α production. Data in this figure were calculated from three experiments. Each experiment contained the pooled macrophages from at least 10 animals.

DISCUSSION

These studies have demonstrated that the addition of THC to medium used to induce TNF-α resulted in suppression of production of this monokine from mouse resident peritoneal macrophages. This inhibition of TNF-α production was related to the incubation conditions, including both THC concentration and the concentration of serum proteins present in the medium. The best results to observe the inhibitory effect of THC on TNF-α production in our approach was to use 0.5% or less BSA-containing induction medium (3). Previous observations indicate that serum can inhibit the ability of THC to suppress lymphocyte blastogenic transformation (5,8). In the present report, we demonstrated that inhibition by THC of TNF-α production was related to the concentration of serum proteins present in the medium. Addition of THC simultaneously with induction medium containing 10% FBS did not show a significant inhibitory effect on TNF-α production by macrophages from young mice and addition of THC to induction medium containing 5% BSA did not show any inhibitory effect and sometimes increased this TNF production. In addition, the data suggest that macrophages from older mice (14-19 week) appear more sensitive to THC treatment than younger ones, although they produce less TNF-α. A similar age related observation was reported by Pross et al., regarding the inhibitory effect of THC on mouse lymphocyte proliferation (9). Thus, the report by others that THC did not inhibit TNF-α production (10) may be due to the induction conditions (using 10% FBS-containing medium) and collection time (24 hr post-stimulation by LPS) when TNF-α levels are likely to have diminished (11, 12). We have observed that the optimal TNF-α production by macrophages was after 4-8 h stimulation by LPS. Thereafter, the activity of TNF-α in macrophage cultures was decreased dramatically and little TNF-α activity could be detected using a bioassay (Z. M. Zheng & S. Specter, unpublished observations).

The mechanism by which THC inhibits TNF production is not yet clear. Because THC is lipophilic and can be incorporated into cell membranes (2) it is possible that cell membrane alterations may contribute to the inhibitory effects of the drug for macrophages. In addition, inhibition of TNF production might be due to the alterations by THC of LPS-induced signal transduction and gene regulation. The mechanism(s) by which THC affects TNF-α production is currently the focus of research efforts.

Acknowledgements

This study was supported by grants DA 04141, DA 05363, and DA 07245 from the National Institute on Drug Abuse, Public Health Service.

REFERENCES

1. T. W. Klein and H. Friedman, Modulation of murine immune cell function by marijuana components. *in*: "Drugs of abuse and immune function", R. R. Watson, ed., pp. 87-111. CRC Press, Boca Raton, FL (1990).
2. S. Specter, G. Lancz, and H. Friedman, Marijuana and immunosuppression in man, *in*: "Drugs of abuse and immune function, R. R. Watson, ed., pp.73-85. CRC Press, Boca Raton, FL (1990).
3. Z. M. Zheng, S. Specter, and H. Friedman, Inhibition by delta-9-tetrahydrocannabinol of tumor necrosis factor alpha production by mouse and human macrophages, *Int. J. Immunopharmacol.* 14:1445 (1992).
4. L. J. Old, Tumor necrosis factor, *Scientific Amer.* 258:59 (1988).
5. G. G. Nahas, A. Morishima, and B. Desoize, Effects of cannabinoids on macromolecular synthesis and replication of cultured lymphocytes, *Fed. Proc.* 36:1748 (1977).
6. M. K. Eskandari, D. T. Nguyen, S. L. Kunkel, and D. G. Remick, WEHI 164 subclone 13 assay for TNF: sensitivity, specificity, and reliability, *Immunol. Invest.* 19:69 (1990).
7. R. C. Duncan, R. G. Knapp, and M. C. Miller. (eds). "Introductory Biostatistics for the Health Sciences", John Wiley & Sons, New York (1983).
8. T. W. Klein, C. A. Newton, R. Widen, and H. Friedman, The effects of delta-9-tetrahydrocannabinol and 11-hydroxy-delta-9-tetrahydrocannabinol on T-lymphocyte and B-lymphocyte mitogen responses, *J. Immunopharmacol.* 7:451 (1985).
9. S. Pross, C. Newton, T. W. Klein, and H. Friedman, Age-associated differences in cannabinoid-induced suppression of murine spleen, lymph node and thymus cell blastogenic responses, *Immunopharmacol.* 14:159 (1987).
10. B. Watzl, P. Scuderi, and R. R. Watson, Influence of marijuana components (THC and CBD) on human mononuclear cell cytokine secretion *in vitro*, *Adv. Exp. Med. Biol.* 288:63 (1991).
11. M. Barak and N. Gruener, Neopterin augmentation of tumor necrosis factor production, *Immunol. Lett.* 30:101 (1991).
12. D. T. Nguyen, M. K. Eskandari, L. E. DeForge, C. L. Raiford, R. M. Strieter, S. L. Kunkel, and D. G. Remick, Cyclosporin A modulation of tumor necrosis factor gene expression and effects *in vitro* and *in vivo*, *J. Immunol.* 144:3822 (1990).

MARIJUANA AND HOST RESISTANCE TO HERPESVIRUS INFECTION

G. A. Cabral, D. A. Dove Pettit, and K. Fischer-Stenger

Department of Microbiology and Immunology
Medical College of Virginia/Virginia Commonwealth University
Richmond, Virginia 23298-0678

INTRODUCTION

The marijuana plant contains in excess of 400 chemical entities, of which 60 or more are cannabinoids (1). Delta-9-tetrahydrocannabinol (THC) is the major psychoactive cannabinoid in marijuana and has been shown to induce immunosuppressive effects both *in vivo* and *in vitro*. The drug inhibits lymphocyte responsiveness to mitogens and particulate antigens (2), decreases T-cell rosette formation (3,4), suppresses leukocyte migration (5), and alters macrophage morphology, function, motility, and protein expression (6-8).

It has been reported that THC exposure suppresses host resistance to viral infection (9-11) and that marijuana use is associated with an increased incidence of recurrent viral infection (10,12). Mice and guinea pigs treated with various doses of THC, which are achievable in humans, experienced more severe primary herpes simplex virus type 2 (HSV2) vaginal infection (13). The exacerbated disease was characterized by rapid onset, greater number of genital lesions, higher quantities of viral yields, and higher mortalities.

Although many studies have been undertaken to define the alterations in immune function which result from THC exposure, little has been reported on the molecular mechanism responsible for such changes. Since THC is a highly lipophilic molecule, one can speculate that THC elicits membrane perturbation thereby altering cell surface membrane selective permeability. The attendant increase in intracellular sodium could result in disruption of the assembly and orientation of cytoskeletal elements and alter a variety of cell functions. Alternatively, structural requirements for immunosuppression suggest the involvement of a cannabinoid receptor. THC inhibition of mitogen-mediated proliferation of lymphocytes has led to the hypothesis that cannabinoids interfere with an early signal transduction event (14-17). Transduction of such a signal may be mediated by a receptor homologous to that found in neural tissue. Indeed, neurotransmitter receptors have been identified on cells of the immune system which, upon

Drugs of Abuse, Immunity, and AIDS, Edited by
H. Friedman *et al.*, Plenum Press, New York, 1993

binding to the neurotransmitter, have been shown to elicit both immunosuppression and immunomodulatory effects (18,19).

In the present study, the effect of THC on cytolytic T-lymphocyte (CTL) functional competence against herpes simplex virus infection was assessed. In addition, Northern Analysis was performed using total RNA from rat spleen, thymus and lung to determine if cells of the immune system possess a cannabinoid receptor homologous to that found in neural tissue. The lung tissue was used as a crude sample to address receptor expression in alveolar macrophages.

METHODS

Mouse Virus Infection and Drug-Dosing Regimen

Eight-week old virus-free female C3H/HeJ mice (H-2^k) (Charles River Breeding Laboratories, Wilmington, MA) were quarantined for one week. Mice (N=4 per group) were administered THC (15 mg/kg to 100 mg/kg), or vehicle (ethanol:emulphor:saline; 1:1:18), in a volume of 0.01 ml/g body weight intraperitoneally (ip) on days 1-4, 8-11, and 15-18. On day 21, mice receiving virus were injected with 10^7 plaque-forming units (PFU) of herpes simplex virus type 1 (HSV1). Seven days later, mice were killed by cervical dislocation and their spleens were aseptically removed. THC administration had little effect on spleen mass. Spleen mass averaged 142 mg for mice not exposed to virus and treated with drug, vehicle, or placebo (0.85% saline). An approximate 25% increase in spleen mass was noted for mice receiving HSV1 even when treated with THC. Single-cell suspensions were prepared by teasing cells through 80-mesh sieves into Hanks' balanced salt solution (HBSS) (GIBCO, Grand Island, NY) and were depleted of erythrocytes with distilled H_20 (20). Total viable cell counts were performed with a hemacytometer using the trypan blue exclusion method (21). Cells were resuspended in RPMI 1640 (GIBCO) containing 5% heat-inactivated fetal calf serum (FCS) (Flow Laboratories, McLean, VA) to serve as effector cells in the cytotoxicity assays.

Target Cells and Virus

L929 mouse fibroblasts (H-2^k) (American Type Culture Collection, Rockville, MD; ATCC: CCL-1) were grown in RPMI 1640 supplemented with 10% FCS, 1.5% sodium bicarbonate, 25 mM Hepes buffer, 1% glutamine, 1% MEM vitamins, 1% non-essential amino acids, penicillin (100 U/ml), and streptomycin (100 μg/ml). The cells were maintained at 37°C in 5% CO_2 in 75-cm^2 tissue culture flasks and were subcultured twice weekly.

HSV1, strain KOS (22), was propagated in green monkey kidney (Vero) cells and was shown by plaque assay (23) to contain 4 x 10^8 PFU/ml. HSV1 stocks were stored at -80°C until used in experiments. Virus suspensions to be used for *in vivo* infection were sonicated (70 kcycles/sec, 1 min), diluted in HBSS (5 x 10^7 PFU/ml) and 0.2 ml was injected ip into mice. A replicate inoculum was assessed for infectivity by plaque assay in order to confirm the number of PFU introduced into mice.

Cytotoxicity Assay

L929 target cells were suspended in 1 ml of RPMI 1640 containing 5% FCS and were infected with HSV1 at a multiplicity of infection (moi) of 10 and simultaneously labeled with 100 μCi of $Na_2{}^{51}CrO_4$/(1 x 10^6) cells for a total of 4 hr at 37°C. Cells, then, were washed three times with warm medium and suspended at a concentration of 1 x 10^5 cells/ml in RPMI 1640 with 5% FCS. Uninfected, radiolabeled L929 cells were used as control target cells in the cytotoxicity assays. Target cells were added to effector cells in 96-well round-bottom microtiter plates at a concentration of 1 x 10^4 cells/well for an effector cell:target cell (E:T) ratio of 100:1 or 50:1. Cytotoxicity assays began 6 hr post-infection and were carried out for 4 hr at 37°C in a 5% CO_2 humidified incubator. All assays were performed in quadruplicate. Results were reported as % Specific Release according to the following formula:

$$\% \text{ Specific Release} = \frac{\text{experimental release - spontaneous release}}{\text{total release - spontaneous release}} \times 100\%$$

Total releasable ^{51}Cr was obtained by exposing radiolabeled target cells to 1N NaOH.

FACScan Analysis

Spleen cells from each treatment group were collected, depleted of erythrocytes, washed and suspended (1 x 10^7 cells/ml) in cold phosphate buffered saline (PBS) containing 1% bovine serum albumin (BSA) and 0.1% sodium azide. Cells (100 µl) were incubated with 2 µl each of phycoerythrin-labeled anti-L3T4 (clone GK1.5) and fluorescein-labeled anti-Lyt-2 (clone 53-6.7) antibodies (Becton Dickinson, Mountain View, CA) for 30 min at 4°C in the dark. Cells were washed twice with cold PBS and data on 10^5 viable cells were obtained using a FACScan flow cytometer (Becton Dickinson) equipped with an Argon laser emitting 15 mW at 488 nm. Data were analyzed by a Hewlett-Packard 9000 computer (Portland, OR) using Consort 30 and LYSIS Programs (Becton Dickinson).

Microscopy

For Nomarski optics microscopy, L929 target cells at 70% confluency on coverslips, were infected with HSV1 at a moi of 10 for 4 hr. Spleen cells from each of the treatment groups, were depleted of erythrocytes (20) and macrophages (24) and were added to target cells to yield an E:T ratio of 5:1. Co-cultures were incubated for 1 hr, 4 hr, or 6 hr, and fixed with 2% glutaraldehyde in 0.2 M sodium cacodylate buffer (pH 7.0) for 30 min at room temperature. Coverslips were mounted onto glass slides in the fixative solution and monolayers were examined and photographed on an Olympus BH-2 light microscope equipped with Nomarski optics (Opelco, Washington, D.C.). For each treatment group four random microscopic fields (20X magnification) were examined. A total of at least 100 conjugates for each treatment group was examined.

Northern Analysis

Total RNA was isolated from brain, spleen, thymus, and lung of Sprague Dawley rats and from a rat neuroblastoma cell line, B103, using the guanidinium isothiocyanate-/cesium chloride method (25). The RNA obtained was separated by electrophoresis in a 1% agarose-formaldehyde gel and was blot-transferred onto a nitrocellulose membrane. The blots were baked for 2 hr at 80°C in a vacuum oven and then were incubated for 4 hr at 37°C in prehybridization buffer containing 50% formamide, 5X SSC (20X SSC = 3.0M NaCl, 0.3M $Na_3C_6H_5O_4$, pH 7.0), 0.1% BSA, 0.1% polyvinylpyrrolidone, 0.1% Ficoll, 0.1 M NaH_2PO_4 and 20 µg/ml sheared and denatured salmon sperm DNA. Following this treatment, blots were hybridized for 18 hr at 37°C in hybridization buffer (prehybridization buffer containing 5% dextran sulfate and nick-translated cannabinoid receptor cDNA) and were washed using the following regimen: four 5 min washes in 2X SSC and 0.2% sodium dodecyl sulfate (SDS) at 37°C; one 20 min wash in 2X SSC and 0.2% SDS at 37°C; a final 20 min wash in 0.5X SSC and 1% SDS at 37°C. Autoradiography was carried out at -70°C using XRP-5 X-ray film and intensifying screens. Equivalent loading and the quality of the RNA were determined by ethidium bromide staining of the gel before Northern transfer.

The Probe

The plasmid containing the cannabinoid receptor cDNA, SKR6 (26), was kindly provided by Dr. Lisa Matsuda (Department of Psychiatry and Behavioral Sciences, Medical University of South Carolina). The SKR6 clone was digested with BamHI and EcoRI. The resulting fragments were separated using gel electrophoresis and a 2.4 kb fragment containing receptor cDNA was excised, eluted (Centrilutor, Amicon, Beverly, MA), and purified using organic solvent extractions. The receptor cDNA, then, was ^{32}P-labeled by means of nick translation (Bethesda Research Laboratories Life Technologies, Inc. Bethesda, MD) and was used as a probe in hybridization experiments.

RESULTS

Effect of THC on CTL Activity

The effect of THC on anti-HSV1 CTL function following *in vivo* priming with 10^7 PFU HSV1 was assessed using a chromium release assay (Table 1). C3H/HeJ mice (H-2^k) upon infection with HSV1 generated CTL activity (29%) towards H-2 restricted, virus-infected L929 (H-2^k) target cells but not towards uninfected target cells. The anti-herpes CTL activity was decreased in a dose-related manner when mice were exposed to 15 mg/kg or 100 mg/kg THC. The CTL response generated from mice exposed to 100 mg/kg THC was decreased more than two-fold when compared with that generated from virus-infected mice receiving vehicle.

Table 1. Effect of delta-9-tetrahydrocannabinol (THC) on anti-Herpes CTL activity.

Treatment[a]	Virus	% Cytolysis ± S.E.	
L929-HSV1	Inoculum	L929-HSV1	L929
vehicle	-	4.6 ± 2.6	2.1 ± 0.5
vehicle	+	28.9 ± 2.4	6.7 ± 1.6
15 mg/kg THC	+	19.2 ± 5.6	0.9 ± 0.9
100 mg/kg THC	+	12.7 ± 2.0	2.4 ± 1.3

[a] C3H/HeJ mice (H-2^k) were subjected to 3 rounds of 4 days each of i.p. injections of vehicle (ethanol:emulphor:saline; 1:1:18) or THC interspersed with 3 day rest periods (i.e., days 1-4, 8-11, and 15-18). Mice receiving HSV1 were inoculated i.p. on day 21 with 10^7 PFU. Splenocytes were harvested 7 days later and were assessed for cytolytic activity against ^{51}Cr-labeled HSV1-infected or uninfected murine L929 cells (H-2^k).

Effect of THC on Murine Splenocytes

Spleen cells from each treatment group were analyzed by two-color FACScan analysis using phycoerythrin-labeled anti-L3T4 and fluorescein-labeled anti-Lyt-2 antibodies to discriminate between T-helper and T-cytotoxic cells, respectively (Fig. 1). Vehicle controls were composed of approximately 16% $L3T4^+$ lymphocytes and 6% Lyt-2^+ lymphocytes yielding a $L3T4^+$/Lyt-2^+ ratio of approximately 2.5:1. Consistent with the induction of anti-HSV1 CTL activity, the percent of Lyt-2^+ lymphocytes increased in the splenocyte populations obtained from mice infected with HSV1. For these splenocytes an $L3T4^+$/Lyt-2^+ ratio of approximately 1.3:1 was obtained. Although THC

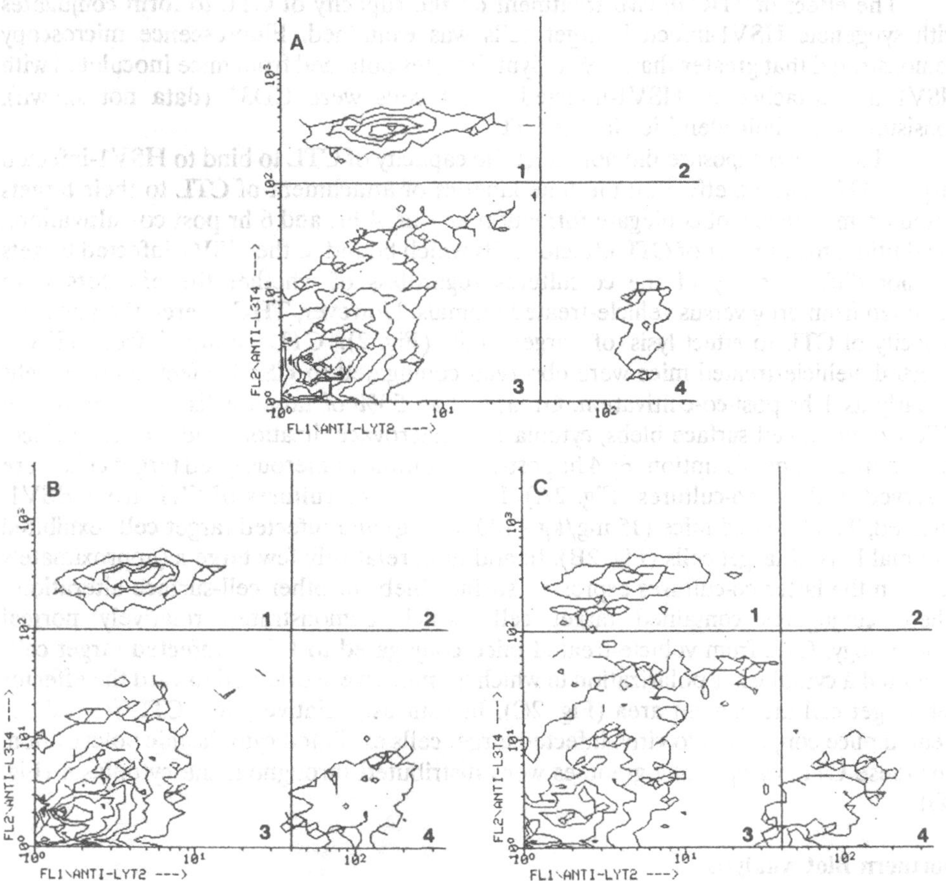

Fig.1. FACScan Contour Plot Analysis of Splenocytes Simultaneously Stained for Murine T-Helper ($L3T4^+$) and T-Cytotoxic (Lyt-2^+) cells. Phycoerythrin-labeled anti-L3T4 was employed to identify T-helper cells on the ordinate (quadrant 1) while fluoresceinated anti-Lyt-2 was used to identify T-cytotoxic cells on the abscissa (quadrant 4). The contour plot at the origin of each graph (quadrant 3) designates cells which are L3T4, Lyt-2^-. (A). Profile of splenocytes of vehicle-treated mice; quadrant 1: 16.3%, quadrant 2: 0.6%, quadrant 3: 76.3%, and quadrant 4: 6.8%. (B). Profile of splenocytes of vehicle-treated mice inoculated with virus; quadrant 1: 15.8%, quadrant 2: 0.4%, quadrant 3: 71.9%, and quadrant 4: 11.9%. Note the increase in Lyt-2^+ cells in quadrant 4. (C). Profile of splenocytes of mice receiving 100 mg/kg THC and inoculated with virus; quadrant 1: 14.6%, quadrant 2: 0.6%, quadrant 3: 73.0%, and quadrant 4: 11.8%. THC had no effect on the number of T-helper cells or on the intensity of L3T4 cell-surface expression from either HSV1-infected or uninfected mice and did not affect the approximate two-fold increase in Lyt-2^+ cells for HSV1-infected mice. However, the drug diminished the intensity in staining of Lyt-2^+ cells.

administration did not affect the approximate two-fold increase in the number of Lyt-2^+ cells from vehicle-treated HSV1 inoculated mice, differences in the intensity of Lyt-2^+ staining were noted when compared with splenocytes from HSV1-infected vehicle-treated mice. Vehicle-treated mice exhibited a contour plot for which Lyt-2^+ staining exceeded $\log_{10}$ 2 intensity. Splenocytes of HSV1-infected mice not receiving drug, exhibited Lyt-2^+ staining for which the intensity ranged from $\log_{10}$ 1.4 to $\log_{10}$ 2.1. In contrast, a decrease in the intensity of Lyt-2^+ staining was noted for splenocytes obtained from mice treated with 100 mg/kg THC.

Effect of THC on Effector: Target Cell Attachment

The effect of THC *in vivo* treatment on the capacity of CTL to form conjugates with syngeneic HSV1-infected target cells was examined. Fluorescence microscopy demonstrated that greater than 90% of lymphocytes obtained from mice inoculated with HSV1 and attached to HSV1-infected target cells were $CD3^+$ (data not shown), consistent with their identification as CTL.

THC *in vivo* exposure did not affect the capacity of CTL to bind to HSV1-infected targets. THC had no effect on the time kinetics of attachment of CTL to their targets based on monitoring of conjugate formation at 1 hr, 4 hr, and 6 hr post co-cultivation. In addition, the number of CTL effector cells which bound to the HSV1-infected targets did not differ for any of the co-cultures regardless of whether the effectors were obtained from drug versus vehicle-treated animals. However, THC altered the apparent capacity of CTL to effect lysis of target cells (Fig. 2). CTL obtained from HSV1-infected, vehicle-treated mice were observed conjugated to HSV1-infected target cells as early as 1 hr post-co-cultivation. Greater than 50% of target cells conjugated with CTL exhibited cell surface blebs, cytoplasmic macrovacuolization, and/or cell surface plasma membrane disruption. By 4 hr post-conjugation, numerous lysed target cells were observed in these co-cultures (Fig. 2A). In contrast, co-cultures of CTL from HSV1-infected, THC-treated mice (15 mg/kg - 100 mg/kg) and infected target cells exhibited minimal lysis of target cells (Fig. 2B). In addition, relatively few targets (approximately 10%) in the latter co-cultures expressed surface blebs or other cell-surface alterations. These conjugates contained target cells which demonstrated relatively normal morphology. CTL from vehicle-treated mice conjugated to HSV1-infected target cells exhibited a cytoplasmic polarization in which granules were oriented toward the effector cell-target cell attachment area (Fig. 2C). In contrast, relatively few CTL from drug-treated mice conjugated to virus-infected target cells exhibited cytoplasmic polarization. For these CTL, cytoplasmic granules were distributed throughout the cytoplasm (Fig. 2D).

Northern Blot Analysis

To determine whether cells of the immune system express a cannabinoid receptor homologous to that previously identified in a rat cerebral cortex cDNA library, total RNA was isolated from rat tissue and cell lines. A single 5.8 kb transcript was detected in rat brain and lung and in a rat neuroblastoma cell line, B103 (Fig. 3). No message was detected in rat spleen or thymus.

DISCUSSION

Delta-9-tetrahydrocannabinol (THC), the major psychoactive component of marijuana, has been shown to be immunosuppressive *in vitro* (2,27) and to suppress the immune system in a number of animal models. The cannabinoid decreases host

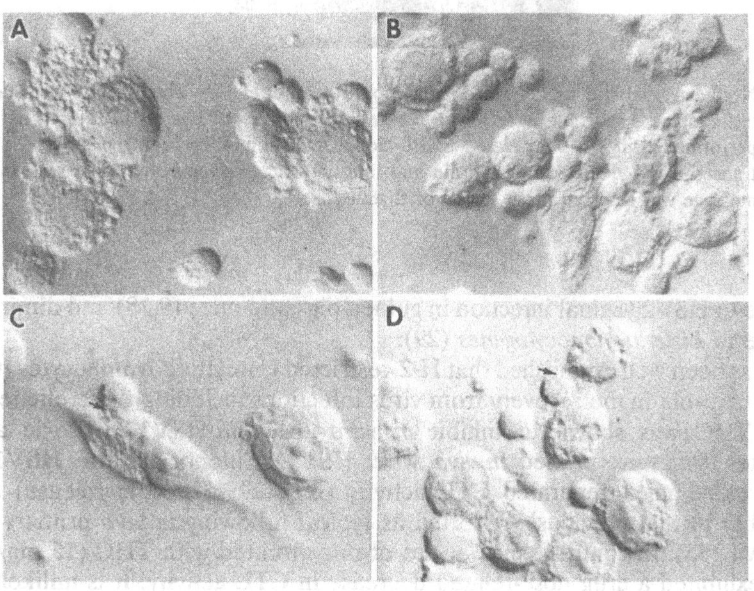

Fig. 2. Nomarski Optics Microscopy of CTL:HSV1-infected L929 Conjugates. Mice (H-2^k) were subjected to the drug dosing regimen described in Materials and Methods. Splenocytes were depleted of erythrocytes and macrophages, and co-cultured with HSV1-infected or uninfected L929 target cells (H-2^k) for 1 hr, 4 hr, or 6 hr. (A) CTL and HSV1-infected L929 cell co-cultures at 4 hr postcultivation. CTL from vehicle-treated, HSV1-infected mice conjugate to, and readily lyse, HSV1-infected L929 cells. (B) CTL from THC-treated mice (100 mg/kg) and HSV1-infected L929 cell co-cultures at 6 hr post-incubation. Note that CTL bind to target cell but do not effect lysis. (C) CTL from vehicle-treated, HSV1-infected mice conjugated to a target HSV1-infected L929 cell showing cytoplasmic polarization as evidenced by granule reorientation toward the effector cell-target cell attachment junction. (D) CTL from drug-treated (100 mg/kg) mice showing that the cytoplasmic granules are not oriented toward the effector cell:target cell junction. Arrows identify CTL granules.

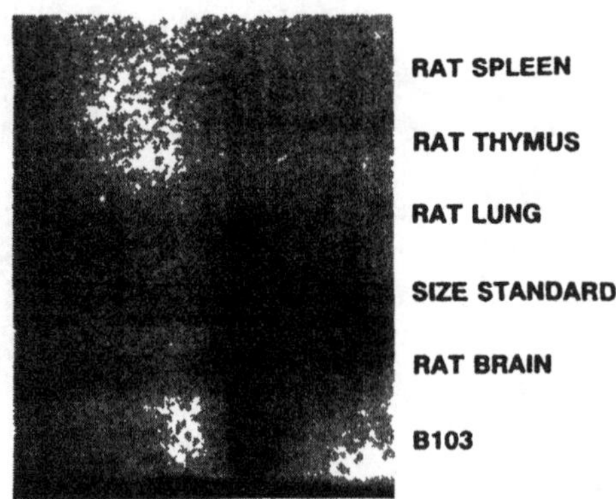

Fig. 3. Northern Analysis Probing with Cannabinoid Receptor cDNA. Total RNA was isolated from rat brain, spleen, and lung and from a rat neuroblastoma cell line, B103. Northern analysis was performed using nick-translated SKR6-cloned cannabinoid receptor cDNA. A single 5.8 kb transcript was detected in rat brain and lung and in a rat neuroblastoma cell line, B103. No message was detected in rat spleen or thymus.

resistance to HSV2 vaginal infection in guinea pigs and mice (9,28) and diminishes host resistance to *Listeria monocytogenes* (29).

It has been well established that H-2-restricted cytolytic T-lymphocytes (CTL) play an important role in the recovery from virus infections including those elicited by HSV (30-35). THC was shown to inhibit *in vitro* the anti-HSV1 cytotoxic activity of splenocytes from mice primed *in vivo* with HSV1. Splenocytes of HSV1-infected, vehicle-treated mice generated CTL activity (e.g., 29% specific release) at a level comparable to that previously reported as typical following *in vivo* primary induction with HSV1 (35). In contrast, splenocytes of mice treated with THC (15 mg/kg or 100 mg/kg) exhibited a drug dose-related decrease in CTL activity. It is unlikely that NK cells were responsible for the cytolytic activity in our system since the effector cells which were bound to virally-infected targets were small, $CD3^+$ lymphocytes. NK cells, on the other hand, are typically large granular lymphocytes which do not express CD3 on their surface.

The most obvious alterations in T-cell function from drug exposure could be due to a decrease in the total number of reactive T-cells. In order to determine whether THC affected total T-lymphocyte cell numbers of mice in the different experimental groups, spleen masses and total T-cell numbers of virus-infected drug-treated or untreated mice were calculated. THC did not exert a major effect on spleen mass. In addition, no major differences in total splenocyte numbers among the experimental groups in relation to spleen mass were noted. These observations indicate that the drug at the doses employed did not exert a toxicological effect on virus-exposed animals which could have accounted for a decrease in total cell number.

Since THC had little affect on either spleen mass or total splenocyte numbers, experiments were conducted using FACScan analysis in order to determine whether the drug affected individual populations of T-lymphocytes. Results of double staining with fluorescein-labeled anti-Lyt-2 and phycoerythrin-labeled anti-L3T4 antibodies to identify T-cytotoxic and T-helper cells, respectively, indicated that THC had no major effect on the number of T-helper cells from either uninfected or HSV1-infected mice. Splenocytes of drug-treated mice exhibited an approximate two-fold increase in Lyt-2^+ cells following exposure to virus. THC treatment did not affect the expected increase in Lyt-2^+ cell number in mice exposed to HSV1. This increase was comparable to that recorded for HSV1-infected vehicle-treated mice.

Effector cell-target cell contact-dependent antiviral activities are multistep processes in which conjugation of the effector cell to its target is followed by post-conjugation events which either effect cytolysis of the target cell or inhibit virus replication within that cell (36,28). CTL versus NK cell or macrophage cell contact-dependent events are distinctive, however, in that CTL activities are MHC-restricted. In order to determine the step in CTL contact-dependent effector function affected by THC, experiments were conducted to determine whether the drug altered the capacity of anti-HSV1 CTL to attach to their syngeneic HSV1-infected targets. THC did not alter the capacity of CTL to attach to virus-infected murine L929 cells. CTL from virus-infected vehicle-treated mice induced cell surface blebs on, and macrovacuolization within, HSV1-infected target cells by as early as 1 hr post-conjugation. By 6 hr post-conjugation, numerous lysed target cells with CTL attached to them were observed. In contrast, conjugates containing CTL from drug-treated mice rarely exhibited blebs or lysed target cells even by 6 hr post-co-cultivation. These results are in agreement with our cytotoxicity data indicating a decrease in cytolytic activity of CTL from HSV1-infected mice treated with THC. The ability of CTL to attach to target cells in spite of drug exposure is in agreement with previous studies which indicated that peritoneal macrophages of mice treated with THC and receiving *Propionibacterium acnes* (*P. acnes*) exhibited decreased antiviral activity but, nevertheless, were capable of attaching to tumor cells or to virus-infected cells (37). These observations suggest that THC may exert a common mode of action on effector cell mediators of both MHC-restricted and non-MHC-restricted cell contact-dependent cytolytic activities.

In the present study, Nomarski optics microscopy revealed that cytoplasmic granules of CTL conjugated to target HSV1-infected cells were found directed toward the proximal edge of the effector cell:target cell attachment junction. In contrast, conjugates containing CTL from drug-treated mice exhibited granules which were randomly distributed in the cytoplasm and not necessarily oriented towards the effector cell:target cell junction. These observations suggest that THC may alter the capacity of CTL to undergo cytoplasmic polarization and cytoskeletal reorientation following conjugation with the virus-infected target cell.

The mechanism responsible for such THC-induced alterations has not been determined. However, THC has been shown to bring about a morphological disruption of cellular membranes (38,39) and of cytoskeletal elements (40). Perturbations of cellular membranes could cause a disruption of cytoskeletal elements within the effector cell resulting in the failure to transport CTL granules containing effector molecules to the virus-infected cell. Indeed, we have shown that THC administered *in vitro* elicits membrane perturbation of cell surface and cytoplasmic membranes and disrupts the assembly and orientation of cytoskeletal elements in rat neuroblastoma cells (40). Perturbations in cellular membranes may be attributed to the interaction of the highly lipophilic THC molecule. Such binding has been shown to affect membrane fluidity and subsequently alter selective permeability (41). Alterations in cell surface membrane selective permeability with the attendant increase in intracellular sodium have been proposed as a mode which results in disruption of cytoskeletal elements (42).

Although the above mechanism is plausible, the involvement of a cannabinoid receptor is appealing since immune dysfunction is not observed in experiments utilizing cannabidiol, a non-psychoactive cannabinoid with structural similarities to THC (43). Thus, to address the issue of receptor involvement in immunosuppression, standard Northern blot analysis was employed. The failure to detect message for the cannabinoid receptor in rat spleen and thymus demonstrates that it is either absent in these tissues or is present in low quantities which are not detected when total RNA is used for blotting. The presence of a hybridization signal in rat brain and a rat neuroblastoma cell line, B103, is not surprising since similar results have been previously reported (26); however, the presence of a signal in rat lung is an interesting finding since Northern blot analysis of dog lung tissue using a human cannabinoid receptor cDNA revealed no hybridization (44). This discrepancy may reflect differences in experimental methodologies or species divergence. The presence of receptor mRNA in rat lung could be the result of receptor expression in alveolar macrophages in the lung tissue used. Studies are in progress to define the cellular specificity of cannabinoid receptor expression in lung tissue.

Acknowledgements

The authors thank Drs. B R. tin and L. S. Harris of the Department of Pharmacology and Toxicology, Virginia Commonwealth University for providing Delta-9-tetrahydrocannabinol and Mr. Alan Updegrove for excellent technical assistance. This research was supported by National Institute on Drug Abuse (NIDA) grant R01-DA05832 and by NIDA individual national service award DA05448 to K. Fischer-Stenger.

REFERENCES

1. C. E. Turner, Marijuana and cannabis: research. Why the conflict, *in*: "Marihuana '84," D. J. Harvey ed., IRL Press, Oxford (1985).
2. G. E. Nahas, N. Sucia-Foca, J. P. Armand, and A. Morishima, Inhibition of cellular mediated immunity in marihuana smokers, *Science* 183:419 (1974).
3. G. Gupta, M. Grieco, and P. Cushman, Impairment of rosette forming T-lymphocytes in chronic marijuana users, *New Engl. J. Med.* 291:874 (1974).
4. P. Cushman and R. Khurana, Marijuana and T-lymphocyte rosettes, *Clin. Pharmacol. Ther.* 19:310 (1976).
5. L. Schwartzfarb, N. Needle and M. Chavez-Chase, Dose related inhibition of leukocyte migration by marijuana and Delta-9-tetrahydrocannabinol, *J. Clin. Pharmacol.* 14:35 (1974).
6. M. Lopez-Cepero, M. Friedman, T. Klein, and H. Friedman, Tetrahydrocannabinol-induced suppression of macrophage spreading and phagocytic activity in vitro, *J. Leuk. Biol.* 39:679 (1986).
7. G. A. Cabral and E. M. Mishkin, Delta-9-tetrahydrocannabinol inhibits macrophage protein expression in response to bacterial immunomodulators, *J. Tox. Environ. Health*, 26:175 (1989).
8. G. A. Cabral, A. L. Stinnett, J. Bailey, S. F. Ali, M. G. Paule, A. C. Scallet, and W. Slikker Jr, Chronic Marijuana Smoke Alters Alveolar Macrophage Morphology and Protein Expression, *Pharm. Biochem. Behav.* 40:643 (1991).
9. E. M. Mishkin and G. A. Cabral, Delta-9-tetrahydrocannabinol decreases host resistance to herpes simplex virus type 2 vaginal infection in the $B_6C_3F_1$ mouse, *J. Gen. Virol.* 66:2639 (1985).
10. G. A. Cabral, E. M. Mishkin, F. Marciano-Cabral, P. Coleman, L. Harris, and A. E. Munson, Effect of delta-9-tetrahydrocannabinol on herpes simplex virus type 2 vaginal infection in the guinea pig, *Proc. Soc. Exp. Biol. Med.* 182:181 (1986).
11. G. A. Cabral, J. C. Lockmuller, and E. M. Mishkin, Delta-9-tetrahydrocannabinol decreases alpha/beta interferon response to herpes simplex virus type 2 in the $B_6C_3F_1$ mouse, *Proc. Soc. Exp. Biol. Med.* 181:305 (1987).
12. B. E. Juel-Jensen, Cannabis and recurrent herpes simplex, *Br. Med. J.* IV:296 (1972).
13. M. P. Holsapple, E. M. Mishkin, A. E. Munson, and G. A. Cabral, *In vivo* and *in vitro* effects of Delta-9-tetrahydrocannabinol on immune responsiveness and vaginal resistance to herpes simplex virus type II (HSV2) infection by $B_6C_3F_1$ mice, *in*: "Marihuana '84," D. J. Harvey ed., IRL Press, Oxford (1985).
14. S. Pross, T. Klein, C. Newton, and H. Friedman, Differential effects of marijuana components on proliferation of spleen, lymph node and thymus cells *in vitro*, *Intl. J. Immunopharmac.* 9(3):363 (1987).
15. Y. Kawakami, T. W. Klein, C. Newton, J. Y. Djeu, G. Dennert, S. Specter, and H. Friedman, Suppression by cannabinoids of a cloned cell line with natural killer cell activity, *Proc. Soc. Exp. Biol. Med.* 187(3):355 (1988).
16. S. Specter, G. Lancz, and J. Hazelden, Marijuana and Immunity: Tetrahydrocannabinol mediated inhibition of lymphocyte blastogenesis, *Int. J. Immunopharmac.* 12(3):261 (1990).

17. T. W. Klein and H. Friedman, Modulation of murine immune cell function by marijuana components, *in*: "CRC Drugs of Abuse and Immune Function," R.R. Watson ed., CRC Press, Boca Raton (1990).
18. C. R. Plata-Salaman, Immunoregulators in the nervous system, *Neurosci. Biobehav. Rev.* 15:182 (1991).
19. B. McEwen, Influences of hormones and neuroactive substances on immune function, *in*: "The Neuro-Immune-Endocrine-Connection," C.W. Cotman ed., Raven Press, New York (1987).
20. B. B. Mishell, S. M. Shiigi, C. Henry, E. L. Chan, J. North, R. Gallily, M. Slomich, K. Miller, J. Marbrook, D. Parks, and A. H. Good, Preparation of mouse cell suspensions, *in*: "Selected Methods in Cellular Immunology," B. B. Mishell and S. M. Shiigi eds., WH Freeman and Company, San Francisco (1980).
21. B. B. Mishell, S. M. Shiigi, C. Henry, E. L. Chan, J. North, R. Gallily, M. Slomich, K. Miller, J. Marbrook, D. Parks, and A. H. Good, Determination of viability by trypan blue exclusion, *in*: "Selected Methods in Cellular Immunology," B. B. Mishell and S. M. Shiigi eds., WH Freeman and Company, San Francisco (1980).
22. K. O. Smith, Relationship between the envelope and the infectivity of herpes simplex virus, *Proc. Soc. Exp. Biol. Med.* 115:814 (1964).
23. F. Rapp, Variants of herpes simplex virus: isolation, characterization and factors influencing plaque formation, *J. Bacteriol.* 86:985 (1963).
24. D. L. Beller, Collection of Macrophages from the spleen, thymus, and bone marrow, *in*: "Manual of Macrophage Methodology," H. B. Herscowitz, T. H. Holden, J. A. Bellanti, and A. Ghaffar, eds., Marcel Dekker, Inc., New York (1981).
25. J. M. Chirgwin, A. E. Przybyla, R. Y. MacDonald, and W. J. Rutter, Isolation of biologically active ribonucleic acid from sources enriched in ribonuclease, *Biochem.* 18:5284 (1977).
26. L. A. Matsuda, S. J. Lolait, M. J. Brownstein, A. C. Young, and T. I. Bonner, Structure of a cannabinoid receptor and functional expression of the cloned cDNA, *Nature* 346:561 (1990).
27. T. W. Klein, C. A. Newton, R. Weden, and H. Friedman, The effect of delta-9-tetrahydrocannabinol and 11-hydroxy-delta-9-tetrahydrocannabinol on T-lymphocyte and B-lymphocyte mitogen responses, *J. Immunopharm.* 7(4):451 (1985).
28. P. S. Morahan, S. S. Morse, and M. B. McGeorge, Macrophage extrinsic antiviral activity during herpes simplex virus infection, *J. Gen. Virol.* 46:291 (1980).
29. P. S. Morahan, P. C. Klykken, S. H. Smith, L. S. Harris, and A. E. Munson, Effects of cannabinoids on host resistance to Listeria monocytogenes and herpes simplex virus, *Infect. Immun.* 23:670 (1979).
30. R. V. Blanden, T cell response to viral and bacterial infection, *Transplant. Rev.* 19:56 (1974).
31. K. L. Yap and G. L. Ada, The recovery of mice from influenza A virus infection: adoptive transfer of immunity with immune T lymphocytes, *Scand. J. Immunol.* 7:389 (1978).
32. H. W. Kreth, V. ter Meulen, and G. Eckert, Demonstration of HLA restricted killer cells in patients with acute measles, *Med. Micobiol. Immunol.* (Berl) 165:203 (1979).
33. L. Y. Lin and B. A. Askonas, Cross-reactivity for different type A influenza viruses of a cloned T killer cell line, *Nature* 288:164 (1980).
34. B. T. Rouse and M. Lawman, Induction of cytotoxic T Iymphocytes against herpes simplex virus type 1: role of accessory cells and amplifying factor, *J. Immunol.* 124:2341 (1980).
35. M. J. Lawman, B. T. Rouse, R. J. Courtney, and R. D. Walker, Cell-mediated immunity against herpes simplex induction of cytotoxic T lymphocytes, *Infect. Immun.* 27:133 (1980).
36. E. Martz, Mechanism of specific tumor cell lysis by alloimmune T lymphocytes: resolution and characterization of discrete steps in the cellular interaction, *Contemp. Topics Immunobiol.* 7:301 (1977).
37. G. A. Cabral and R. Vasquez, Effects of marihuana on macrophage function, *in*: "Drugs of Abuse, Immunity, and Immunodeficiency," H. Friedman, S. Specter, T. Klein, eds., Plenum Press, New York (1991).
38. M. K. Poddar, G. Mittra, and J. J. Ghosh, Delta-9-tetrahydrocannabinol-induced changes in brain ribosomes, *Toxicol. Appl. Pharmacol.* 46:737 (1978).
39. W. A. Meyers and R. G. Heath, Cannabis sativa: ultrastructural changes in organelles and neurons in brain septal region of monkeys, *J. Neurosci. Res.* 4:9 (1979).
40. G. A. Cabral, P. J. McNerney, and E. M. Mishkin, Interaction of delta-9-tetrahydrocannabinol with rat B103 neuroblastoma cells, *Archiv. Toxicol.* 60:438 (1987).
41. D. R. Wing, J. T. Leuschner, G. A. Brent, D. J. Harvey, and W. D. Paton, Quantification of in vivo membrane associated delta-1-tetrahydrocannabinol and its effect on membrane fluidity, *in*: "Proc. of 9th Internatl. Cong. of Pharmacol. 3rd Satellite Symp. on Cannabis" D. J. Harvey ed., IRL Press, Oxford (1985).
42. E. Leopardi, D. S. Friend, and W. Rosenau, Target cell lysis: ultrastructural and cytoskeletal alterations, *J. Immunol.* 133:3429 (1984).

43. G. A. Cabral and R. Vasquez, Marijuana decreases macrophage antiviral and antitumor activities, *Adv. Biosc.* 80:93 (1991).

44. C. M. Gerard, C. Mollereau, G. Vassart, and M. Parmentier, Molecular cloning of a human cannabinoid receptor which is also expressed in testis, *Biochem. J.* 279(1):129 (1991).

MARIJUANA AND HEAD AND NECK CANCER

James N. Endicott, Paulette Skipper and Lizette Hernandez

University of South Florida, Division of Otolaryngology
P.O. Box 280179, Tampa, FL 33618

Although head and neck cancer comprises only 5 to 7% (1) of human cancer, the devastating functional, psychosocial, and cosmetic affects as a result of standard therapy has delegated special importance to these tumors. Eighty-five percent of head and neck tumors have a squamous cell carcinoma histology and characteristically grow slowly with eventual regional lymphatic spread to cervical lymph nodes. Distant metastasis (below the clavicles) occurs in a late or more advanced stage and is generally considered incurable. Squamous cell carcinoma occurs in the mucosal lining of the upper aerodigestive tract including larynx, hypopharynx, oropharynx, oral cavity, nasopharynx and nose. Early cancers may be cured with radiation therapy or conservative surgical procedures. Advanced cancers without distant metastasis may require wide-field resection with post-operative radiation for cure.

Heavy cigarette smoking and alcohol consumption are major independent etiologic factors (2) for squamous cell carcinoma of the head and neck. Pathophysiologic mechanisms may occur by a direct chemical carcinogenic affect or indirectly by local immunosuppression or by genetic influences. The average age of the head and neck cancer patient was 58 in several large prospective studies (3,4). A trend has been recently noted in our literature for an increased incidence of squamous cell carcinoma in adults younger than 40, suggesting a new pattern of possible etiologic association (5, 6, 7, 8). Marijuana has been suggested as one of the common risk factors in several reports (9, 10, 11).

Recent nationwide surveys demonstrate a decline in marijuana use (12, 13), although marijuana is still the most widely abused drug in our society. In a 1987 survey (12) among high school seniors, about 50% had smoked marijuana at one time, slightly less than 40% used it within the past year, 23% used it within the past month, and 4% (6% of male students) reported using it daily.

Cannabis products may be taken orally but are usually smoked exposing the upper aerodigestive tract and the lungs to respiratory irritants and carcinogens. A synergistic action has been observed for tobacco and marijuana smoke for histologic changes in the mucosa of the respiratory tract (14). Donald first reported 6 cases of head and neck cancer in young marijuana smokers in 1986 (9) and 5 more cases in 1991 (1). Six head and neck and two lung cancers in young marijuana smoking patients were reported by Taylor in 1988 (10). Other isolated cases have been reported, (8), however, cancer in

Drugs of Abuse, Immunity, and AIDS, Edited by
H. Friedman *et al.*, Plenum Press, New York, 1993

children with *in utero* exposure to marijuana has been reported in acute monoblastic leukemia (15) and in childhood astrocytoma in a case controlled study (16).

METHODS AND MATERIALS

We report 23 cases (age range 17-41; median age is 36) of head and neck cancer squamous cell carcinoma in the young patients arbitrarily defined as age 41 or younger during the author's 16 year practice (Table 1). Twenty-one of the 23 or 92% of young patients used marijuana; only one patient stated he did not use marijuana, two of the patients were not questioned with regard to marijuana use. Two case reports are illustrative of the history and clinical course of these patients.

Case Reports

Case 1. A 30 year old legal assistant (patient #2 in table) was first diagnosed with severe dysplasia of the right true vocal cord and severe dysplasia of the left true vocal cord on September 3, 1975, when she was 17 years old. On January 10, 1987, a biopsy revealed severe dysplasia with focal cancer in situ of the left true vocal cord and severe dysplasia with squamous cell carcinoma in situ including foci of microscopic invasion of the right true vocal cord.

The patient underwent 33 treatments of radiation therapy between January 29, 1987 and March 17, 1987. The patient began smoking one and one-half packs of cigarettes per day at the age of 13. She quit smoking in November 1986, but began again with 1 cigarette a day in June 1987. The patient began drinking at the age of 15 and is presently drinking approximately a six pack a month. She began at the age of 15 with at least one joint per day, but between 1972 and 1979, she smoked at least one joint per day or did 2 bowls per day. Between 1981 and 1987, the patient smoked one joint every three months. Between 1974 and 1979 the patient was extensively using cocaine, speed, valium, heroin and many other drugs.

In April 1988 a microsuspension laryngoscopy biopsy and laser excision was performed; the right anterior cord revealed squamous cell carcinoma in situ.

In May 1989 she was diagnosed with Bowenoid dysplasia, severe in some areas, bordering on cis Vin II and Vin III of cervix and treated with cryosurgery. In addition, she developed a left upper labium minora vulvar lesion, squamous cell carcinoma in situ on biopsy, which was excised in the office.

In August 1990 a direct laryngoscopy with removal of leukoplakia on left cord was performed. The biopsy revealed squamous cell carcinoma in situ.

Human papilloma virus (HPV) like changes were noted focally; stromal invasion cannot be ruled out. HPV stains were negative. Laser excision was then performed in October 1990 for this primary.

The patient has been in follow up since October 1990 with no evidence of disease.

Case 2. A 37 year old white male (patient # 16 in table) presented to his primary care physician with a one-year history of hoarseness. The patient stated that the hoarseness had waxed and waned over the last year, and over the past month had gotten significantly worse. Past medical history was unremarkable, and the patient had enjoyed good overall health. Family history was negative for carcinoma. Significant in his social history was the fact that the patient was a daily user of marijuana. He stated he smoked an average of 6-10 joints a day for the past ten years. He had a history of moderate alcohol use. He had never smoked cigarettes, and had no history of exposure to chemical or fumes. He was employed as a camera salesman, and he used to travel with a country rock band. Review of systems was otherwise negative. He denied

Table 1

Patient	Stage	Age Dx	MJ HX	Alive w/o Disease
1	I	38	Y	Y
2	I	17	Y	Y
3	III	40	?	N
4	IV	40	Y	Y
5	III	40	N	N
6	IV	27	Y	Y
7	II	30	?	?
8	II	33	Y	?
9	III	32	Y	N
10	IV	41	Y	Y
11	II	37	Y	?
12	IV	35	Y	Y
13	III	20	Y	N
14	IV	39	Y	N
15	IV	38	Y	N
16	III	37	Y	Y
17	II	29	Y	?
18	III	22	Y	Y
19	IV	34	Y	N
20	III	28	Y	Y
21	IV	37	Y	Y
22	IV	40	Y	N
23	II	35	Y	N

weight loss, fever, or dysphagia. Physical exam revealed a well-developed, well-nourished white male who was noticeably hoarse. On indirect exam a fungating mass arising from the left true vocal cord was seen. The mass extended from the area of the false cord to the subglottis. The left arytenoid moved on phonation, but the left cord was fixed by the mass. The anterior commissure was not involved. Examination of the neck was negative. The remainder of the physical exam was unremarkable. Direct laryngoscopy revealed a transglottic squamous cell carcinoma staged T_3N_0. A wide-field laryngectomy was performed. The patient had an uncomplicated postoperative course and received XRT ten days after discharge. He is free of disease at 10 years.

DISCUSSION

Smoking popularity is generally attributed to the pleasure derived from the psychoactive components within smoke, such as nicotine in tobacco and delta-9-tetrahydrocannabinol (THC) in cannabis which also serve to reinforce smoking through addiction, psychogenic dependence or both (17). Although marijuana has similar respiratory irritants found in tobacco smoke (ammonia, hydrocyanic acid, acetone, acetaldehyde and toluene), the carcinogenic factors including napthalenes, benzopyrene, benzanthracene, and nitrosamine are 50% to 70% greater in marijuana (18). Techniques for smoking marijuana and tobacco differ substantially, with marijuana inhalation or "puff" volume about 2/3 larger, the depth of smoke inhalation about 40% greater, and breath holding about four times longer than those characteristic of tobacco smoking (19). Marijuana cigarettes do not contain filters and generate about twice as much tar as tobacco per unit of weight, assuming a similar smoking profile (20). These differences in filtration and smoking technique can result in a 4 fold greater amount of tar delivered to the respiratory tract from smoking marijuana than from a comparable amount of tobacco (17). Carcinogens may be concentrated by the paraphernalia used to enhance the euphoric affect of marijuana by increasing the actual amount of drug in the smoke (1).

Numerous human and animal experiments have been performed to study the relationship of marijuana smoking and its effects on humoral and T-cell mediated immune function and though results have been conflicting, there has been an observed trend toward immunosuppression by THC. A lower T-cell count, a reduced lymphocyte response to phytohemagglutinin (PHA), a reduced phagocytic activity of the polymorphonuclear leukocytes, (21) and a marked reduction in T-cell rosette in formation has been observed (22). A dose related suppression of natural killer cells has been observed when human peripheral blood mononuclear cells are exposed to delta-9-THC (23). The blood of healthy, non-drug taking volunteers had suppression of interleukin-1, interleukin-2 and cytokine production when it was exposed to delta-9-THC and cannabidiol (24). However, Dax et al., were unable to demonstrate alterations in tests of lymphocyte subset formation on exposing human subjects to controlled administration of THC. They concluded that THC may act through specific receptors or via non-specific membrane perturbation and by prostonoid mechanisms singly or in concert to account for the highly varied results of previous studies of THC induced modulation of the immune and endocrine systems (25).

Leuchtenberger et al., demonstrated a variability of nuclear sizes and shapes, ploidy and DNA content, and an increased number of mitosis and mitotic abnormalities (26). Other studies have shown chromosome ruptures, a hypoploid cell synthesis and a cell with micronuclei in cultured human epithelial cells exposed to marijuana smoke (27).

One theory on delta-9-THC mechanism of action is the effect of marijuana influenced depletion of arginine, an important component of DNA and RNA enzyme metabolism. Secondary results of the arginine deficiency include chromosome abnormalities, growth retardation, altered gametogenesis, and immunosuppression.[18]

Malignant transformation occurred earlier in marijuana and tobacco smoke exposed hamster lung cell cultures than in controls, suggesting that smoking may have accelerated rather than initiated the malignant change (28).

Several questions need to be answered regarding marijuana as a risk factor in young patients. Why would patients develop an early malignancy from marijuana instead of tobacco smoking alone? The long term respiratory consequences of tobacco smoking generally do not become clinically apparent until two or more decades after the smoking habit is initiated (29). The age of our patients and the short period of at-risk cigarette smoking argue against this etiology.

Why would some marijuana smoking young adults acquire head and neck cancer, but peers with the same risk factor remain disease free? A mutational event must take place in paired genes on homologous chromosomes for carcinogenesis to occur in post-zygotic life. A higher mutation rate is thought to be a determining factor for neoplastic transformation. Persons with defects in any step of DNA or chromosome repair should be classified in the at-risk category. Chromosome fragility is an indicator of high mutation rates. DNA repair competence can be indirectly measured by the bleomycin chromosome fragility assay where bleomycin is used as a mutagen in cultured lymphocytes (30). Hsu studied a large series of patients over a 6 year period and found that mutagen sensitivity may play an important role in determining carcinogenesis of organs and tissues that have direct contact with the external environment (lung, colon, & head and neck cancer) (31).

Schantz notes that young adults may become environmentally genetically predisposed by environmental carcinogens stating that genetically susceptible individuals who have chronic mucosal carcinogenic exposure may acquire head and neck cancer. He compared 20 head and neck patients to controls and found that young adults with squamous cell carcinoma of the upper aerodigestive tract express chromosome hypersensitivity to the clastogen bleomycin. No marijuana smoking patients were studied (32). This hypothesis provides an explanation for the site specificity of tumor development.

A better explanation in young marijuana smokers may be that the potential morphotic and cytologic disturbances caused by chronic marijuana smoking may predispose patients to the later development of head and neck cancer with or without a genetic cellular predisposition. Minimal smoking of marijuana may result in mutagenic change in the genetically predisposed patient or chronic marijuana smoking may result in a future risk for early mutagenic change in non-genetically predisposed individuals. Two of our marijuana smoking young patients were found to have higher breakage rates than older head and neck squamous cell carcinoma patients as compared to controls with *Ataxia Telangiectasia*. Our preliminary work is underway to further define marijuana as a risk factor for development of head and neck cancer in young patients.

REFERENCES

1. P. J. Donald, Advanced malignancy in the young marijuana smoker, *in*: "Drugs of Abuse, Immunity, and Immunodeficiency", H. Friedman et al., eds, Plenum Press, New York (1991).
2. M. R.Spitz, J. J.Fueger, H. Goepfert, W. K. Hong, G. R. Newell, Aquamous cell carcinoma of the upper aerodigestive tract. a case comparison analysis, *Cancer* 61:203 (1988).
3. J. N. Endicott, R. Jensen, G. Lyman, P. Skipper, et al., Adjuvant chemotherapy for advanced head and neck squamous carcinoma-final report of the head and neck contracts program, *Cancer* 60:301 (1987).

4. G. Wolf, W. K. Hong, S. Fisher, S. Urba, J. Endicott, L. Close, et al., Induction chemotherapy plus radiation compared with surgery plus radiation in patients with advanced laryngeal cancer, *N. Engl. J. Med.* 324:1685 (1991).
5. L. J. Shemen, J. Klotz, D. Schottenfeld, E. W. Strong, Increase of tongue cancer in young men, *JAMA* 252:1857 (1984).
6. R. H. Depue, Rising mortality from cancer of the tongue in young white males, *N. Engl. J. Med.* 315:647 (1986).
7. R. J. Cusmano, M. S. Persky, Squamous cell carcinoma of the oral cavity and oropharynx in young adults, *Head and Neck Surgery* 10:229 (1988).
8. J. B. Jones, M. B. Lampe, H. W. Cheung, Carcinoma of the tongue in young patients, *J. of Otolaryngol.* 18:105 (1989).
9. P. J. Donald, Marijuana smoking-possible cause of head and neck carcinoma in young patients, *Otol, Head and Neck Surg.* 94:517 (1986).
10. F. M. Taylor, Marijuana as a potential respiratory tract carcinogen: a retrospective analysis of a community hospital population, *South. Med J.* 81:1213 (1988).
11. R. P. Fergusson, J. Hasson, S. Walker, Metastatic lung cancer in a young marijuana smoker, *JAMA* 261:41 (1989).
12. National Trends in Drug Use and Related Factors Among American High School Students and Young Adults, 1975-1986, US DHHS Publication No. (ADM) 87-1535, *Public Hlth Serv.* (1987).
13. National Household Survey on Drug Abuse: Population Estimates 1988, US DHHS Publication No. (ADM) 89-1636, Rockville, MD, *Natl. Inst. on Drug Abuse* (1989).
14. D. P. Tashkin, A. H. Coulson, V. A. Clark, M. Simmons, L. B. Bourque, S. Duann, G. H. Spivey, H. Gong, Respiratory symptoms, and lung function in habitual heavy smokers of marijuana alone, smokers of marijuana and tobacco, smokers of tobacco alone, and non-smokers, *Am. Review of Resp. Dis.* 135: 209 (1987).
15. L. F. Odom, B. C. Lampkin, R. Tannous, J. D. Buckley, G. D. Hammond, Acute monoblastic leukemia: a unique subtype-A review from the childrens cancer study group, *Leukemia Res.* 14:1 (1990).
16. R. R. Kuijten, G. R. Bunin, C. C. Nass, A. T. Meadows, Gestational and familial risk factors for childhood astrocytoma: results of a case-control study, *Cancer Res.* 50:2608 (1990).
17. D. P. Tashkin, Pulmonary complications of smoked substance abuse, *in:* "Addiction Medicine" [Special Issue], *West J. Med.* 152:525 (1990).
18. K. O. Fehr and H. Kalant, Cannabis health hazards: proceedings of an ARF/WHL scientific meeting on adverse health and behavioral consequences of cannabis use, Toronto, *Addiction Res. Found.* 501 (1983).
19. T. C. Wu, D. P. Tashkin, B. Djahed, et al., Pulmonary hazards of smoking marijuana as compared with tobacco, *N. Engl. J. Med.* 318:347 (1988).
20. W. S. Rickert, J. C. Robinson, B. Rogers, A comparison of tar, carbon monoxide and pH levels in smoke from marijuana and tobacco cigarettes, *Can. J. Public Hlth.* 73:386 (1982).
21. B. H. Petersen, L. Lemberger, J. Graham, B. Dalton, Alterations in the cellular-mediated immune responsiveness of chronic marijuana smokers, *Psychopharmacol. Commun.* 1:67 (1975).
22. P. Cushman, M. Grieco, S. Gupta, Reduction in T-lymphocytes forming active rosettes in chronic marijuana smokers, *Int. J. Clin. Pharmacol. Biopharm.* 12:217 (1975).
23. S. Specter, Effects of marijuana on natural killer cell activity in man, Presented at: "Drugs of Abuse, Immunity, and Immunodeficiency", Clearwater, FL, Dec. 13-15 (1989).
24. B. Waltz, P. Scuderi, R. R. Watson, Influence of marijuana components (THC and CBD) on human mononuclear cells cytokine secretion *in vitro*, Presented at "Drugs of Abuse, Immunity, and Immunodeficiency", Clearwater, FL, Dec. 13-15 (1989).
25. E. N. Dax, N. S. Pilotte, W. H. Adler, J. E. Nagel, W. R. Lange, The effects of 9-ene-tetrahydrocannabinol on hormone release and immune function, *J. Steroid Biochem.* 34(1-6):263 (1989).
26. C. Leuchtenberger, R. Leuchtenberger, Morphological and cytochemical effects of marijuana cigarette smoke on epithelioid cells of lung explain from mice, *Nature* 234:227 (1971).
27. S. S. Mitsuyama, L. F. Jarvek, T. K. Fu, F. S. Yen, Chromosome studies before and after supervised marijuana smoking, *in*: "Pharmacology of Marijuana," M. C. .Braude and S.Szara, eds., Raven Press, New York (1976).
28. C. Leuchtenberger, R. Leuchtenberger, Cytological and cytochemical studies of the effects of fresh marihuana cigarette smoke on growth and DNA metabolism of animal and human lung cultures, *in*: "Pharmacology of Marijuana," M. C. Braude and S. Szara, eds., Raven Press, New York (1976),
29. "Smoking and Health": A Report of the Surgeon General, US DHEW publication No. 79-50066. US Dept. of Hlth, Education, and Welfare, Public Health Service, Office on Smoking and Health, (1979).
30. T. C. Hsu, L. M. Cherry, N. A. Samaan, Differential mutagen susceptibility in cultured lymphocytes of normal individuals and cancer patients, *Cancer Genet. Cytogenet.* 17:307 (1985).

31. T. C. Hsu, D. A. Johnston, L. M. Cherry, et al., Sensitivity to genotoxic effects of bleomycin in humans: possible relationship to environmental carcinogenesis, *Int J Cancer.* 43:403 (1989).
32. S. P.Schantz, T. C. Hsu, N. Ainslie, R. Moser, Young adults with head and neck cancer express increased susceptibility to mutagen-induced chromosome damage, *JAMA* 262:23 3313 (1989).

EVIDENCE FOR A CANNABINOID RECEPTOR IN IMMUNOMODULATION BY CANNABINOID COMPOUNDS

Norbert E. Kaminski

Department of Pharmacology and Toxicology
Box 613/MCV Station, Medical College of Virginia, Virginia Commonwealth University, Richmond, Virginia 23298

INTRODUCTION

A number of structurally related cannabinoid compounds, including the major psychoactive component of marihuana, delta-9-tetrahydrocannabinol (Δ^9-THC), have been widely established as being immunosuppressive. Although much has been learned with respect to which immune responses demonstrate sensitivity to modulation by cannabinoids, the mechanism(s) responsible for these effects has remained elusive. Over the past decade, significant insight has been forthcoming regarding the cellular and biochemical mechanisms which mediate the effects of cannabinoids on the central nervous system (CNS). From these investigations at least three lines of evidence have emerged which strongly implicated a role by a cannabinoid receptor in CNS association cannabinoid activity and include: (i) stereoselective effects; (ii) a high degree of specific binding by the synthetic bicyclic cannabinoid, CP-55,940, to various brain tissue preparation as analyzed by radioligand binding; and (iii) cannabinoid modulation of adenylate cyclase-cAMP second messenger system. The existence of a cannabinoid receptor in association with neuronal tissue has been recently confirmed by Matsuda and coworkers (1) through the isolation and cloning of a G-protein coupled receptor from a rat brain cDNA library. When cloned, this receptor demonstrate all of the characteristics predicted for a putative cannabinoid receptor. More recently, an almost identical receptor has been cloned from human brain which possessed more than 97% homogeneity (2) to that isolated by Matsuda and coworkers. In light of these findings, the objective of the presently reported studies was to explore the possibility that immune inhibition by cannabimimetic agents is mediated through a cannabinoid receptor present on immunocytes. Our approach was to determine whether mouse spleen cells exhibit the same characteristics as those previously demonstrated for the cannabinoid receptor in neuronal tissue, stereoselectivity, high degree of cannabinoid binding, and modulation of adenylate cyclase-cAMP second messenger system.

MATERIALS AND METHODS

Chemicals

Δ9-THC was provided by the National Institute on Drug Abuse. CP-55,940 and CP-56,667(±cis-3-[2-hydroxy-4-(1,1-dimethylheptyl)phenyl]-trans-4-(3-hydroxypropyl)cyclohexanol]) were gifts of Dr. Lawrence Melvin (Pfizer, Inc., Groton, CT). Dr. Raphael Mechoulam, (Hebrew University, Israel) supplied HU-210 and HU-211 (± 11OH-Δ8-tetrahydrocannabinol-dimethylheptyl).

Mice

Virus-free female B6C3F1 mice, 5-6 wks of age (Frederick Cancer Research Center) were housed in plastic cages containing a saw dust bedding (4 mice per cage) at 21-24°C and 40-60% relative humidity with a 12 hr light/dark cycle. Mice received food (Purina Certified Laboratory Chow) and water *ad libitum* and were not used for experimentation until their body wt. was 17-20 g.

In vitro Antibody Assays

Spleens from untreated mice were isolated aseptically, made into a single spleen cell suspension, adjusted to 1.0 x 10^7 cells/ml in complete RPMI 1640 and transferred in 500 µl aliquots to the wells of the 48 well culture plate. Cannabinoid compounds were added directly in 5 µl of vehicle (0.01% DMSO or 0.1% ethanol, final culture concentration) to the respective wells and sensitized with SRBC. The *in vitro* antibody forming cell (AFC) response was performed as previously described (3).

In vitro Binding of [^{3}H]-CP-55,940 to Mouse Spleen Cells

The filtration procedure used for [^{3}H]-CP 55,940 binding was a modification of the centrifugation method described by Devane and coworkers (4) and has been previously described (5). A scatchard analysis was performed to determine the affinity (K_D) and the number of binding sites per spleen cell (Bmax). Scatchard and Hill analysis were run on the EBDA/LIGAND computer program.

cAMP Determination

Single spleen cell suspensions were prepared as described above. The cells were washed once with RPMI 1640 and centrifuged at 800 x g for 10 min to form a pellet. EBSS without HEPES buffer containing 5% FBS at 1 ml/spleen in addition to Gey's solution was added to the cell pellet to lyse the red blood cells. The remaining intact spleen cells were pelleted by centrifugation at 1600 x g for 15 min and the supernatant containing the lysates discarded. The cells were washed twice in EBSS without HEPES buffer and adjusted to 5 x 10^6 cells/ml in RPMI containing 1% FBS. Forskolin-stimulated accumulation of intracellular cAMP was measure in the presence of 100 µM 3-isobutyl-1-methyl xanthine (IBMX) (Sigma, St. Louis, MO) and Δ9-THC using a cAMP assay kit (Diagnostic Products Inc., Los Angles, CA) as previously described (3).

Statistical Analysis of Data

The mean ± SE was determined for each treatment group of a given experiment. The homogeneity of the results was determined using Bartlett's test for homogeneity (6). Homogeneous data were evaluated by a parametric analysis of variance When significant differences occurred, treatment groups were compared to the vehicle controls using a Dunnett's two-tailed t-test (7). Nonhomogeneous data was evaluated for significance using Wilcoxon's rank test (8).

RESULTS AND DISCUSSION

To assess whether mouse spleen cells functionally demonstrate enantiomer selective sensitivity to cannabinoids, the immunomodulatory potencies of two enantiomeric cannabinoid pairs, CP-55,940 vs. CP-56,667 and HU-210 vs. HU-211, were compared to each other and to Δ^9-THC, as measured by the *in vitro* SRBC AFC response. Historically, (-) cannabinoid enantiomers characteristically demonstrate significantly greater CNS potency than the (+) enantiomers. Table 1 shows a comparison between Δ^9-THC, CP-55,940 and CP-56,667 and their inhibitory effect on the IgM antibody forming cells response. Interestingly, the (-) enantiomers consistently possessed significantly greater immunosuppressive potency than the respective (+) enantiomer (data not shown for HU-210 and HU-211). No effect on spleen cell number or viability was observed with any of the cannabinoid congeners at any of the test concentrations. Most striking, was the complete lack of activity found with CP-56,667 even at relatively high concentrations (18.6 μM). It is also important to emphasize that both of the (-) synthetic enantiomers tested (i.e., CP-55,940 and HU-210) demonstrated significantly greater immunosuppressive potency than Δ^9-THC which is in agreement with their reported CNS activity.

Radioligand-binding experiments revealed a high degree of specific binding of [^{3}H-CP55,940 to mouse spleen cells. The saturation isotherm indicated approximately 45-65% specific binding of the tritiated ligand to spleen cells. The scatchard analysis demonstrated single site binding on spleen cells possessing a KD of 910 pM and a BmaX of approximately 900 - 1500 receptors per spleen cell (data not shown). Because a heterogeneous spleen cell preparation was utilized for these studies, it is presently unclear whether this receptor is present on all spleen cells in relatively low abundance or whether the receptor is present in higher abundance than predicted by these studies but expressed only on select spleen cell subpopulations. Nonetheless, the K_D values were quite similarly to those reported by Herkenham (K_D ˜ 1 nM for [^{3}H]-CP-55,940) in rat brain slices (9).

Lastly, the effect of Δ9-THC on forskolin-stimulated adenylate cyclase activity in cultured mouse spleen cells was determined. Enzyme activity was measured by quantitating intracellular cAMP accumulation in the presence of the phosphodiesterase inhibitor, IBMX. IBMX was used to ensure that changes in intracellular cAMP were not merely attributable to changes in phoshodiesterase-catalyzed cAMP breakdown. Intracellular cAMP was measured over a broad Δ^9-THC concentration range (100 nM - 20 μM) after 5 and 15 min stimulation of spleen cells with forskolin. In the presence of forskolin, Δ^9-THC markedly inhibited direct stimulation of adenylate cyclase in a dose related manner (Table 2). Following 5 min forskolin stimulation, 10-20 μM Δ^9-THC treated cells demonstrated approximately a 33% decrease in cAMP, as compared to controls (forskolin + IBMX). This inhibition of adenylate cyclase by Δ9-THC was even more pronounced following 15 min forskolin stimulation resulting in approximately a 66% decrease in intracellular cAMP at 20 μM ΔTHC, as compared to the forskolin + IBMX control. These results are strikingly reminiscent of those originally reported by Howlett (4) in which the author described a rapid inhibition of secretin stimulated adenylate cyclase by Δ^9-THC in N18TG2 neuroblastoma cell membranes (approximately 21% decrease at 2 μM Δ^9-THC).

In summary, the results described in this report, although providing indirect evidence, are consistent with a model of cannabinoid immunomodulation mediated

Table 1. A Comparison of Immunosuppressive Potency of Δ9-THC, CP-55940 and CP-56667 (Day 5 IgM Antibody Forming Cell Response)

Treatment	AFC/10^6 SPLC	Treatment	AFC/10^6 SPLC	Treatment	AFC/10^6 SPLC
NA	673 ± 30[c]				
VH (DMSO)[a]	725 ± 46	VH (EtOH)[b]	711 ± 77		
Δ^9-THC (μM)		CP-55940 (μM)		CP-56667 (μM)	
0.32	661 ± 48	0.27	556 ± 37	0.27	618 ± 92
1.60	536 ± 41	1.3	526 ± 29	1.3	530 ± 39
3.3	638 ± 66	2.7	327 ± 66*	2.7	608 ± 36
6.3	547 ± 48	5.3	226 ± 53*	5.3	697 ± 130
12.6	356 ± 32*	10.6	126 ± 45*	10.6	715 ± 57
22.0	228 ± 69*	18.6	103 ± 13*	18.6	548 ± 73

[a]0.01% DMSO, final concentration in culture; vehicle for Δ9-THC.
[b]0.01% ethanol, final concentration in culture; vehicle for CP-55940 and CP-56667.
[c]mean ± standard error for quadruplicate samples.
***$p<0.05$ as determined by Dunnett's T-test as compared to vehicle control.**
Results are from one of three representative experiments.

Table 2. **Inhibition of Forskolin-Stimulated Intracellular cAMP Accumulation in Spleen Cells**

Treatment	5 min stimulation[a] cAMP (pMoles)			15 min stimulation[b] cAMP (pMoles)		
NA	1.206	±	0 038[c]	1.918	+	0.091
VH	1.251	±	0.235	2.030	+	0.211
VH + IBMX	1.981	±	0.119	3.308	+	0.127
Forsk	6.385	±	0.346	15.142	+	0.466
Forsk + IBMX	8.521	±	0.163	18.864	+	1.288
Forsk + IBMX + Δ^9-THC (μM)						
0.1	11.437	±	0.435	19.496	±	0.938
0.5	9.464	±	0.101	18.175	±	0.403
1.0	9.121	±	0.356	17.264	±	0.374
10.0	4.878	±	0. 144**	7.603	±	0.656*-
15.0	5.405	±	0.369-*	5.367	±	0.473-
20.0	5.492	±	0.207**	5.343	±	0.292**

[a] 5 min stimulation with 50 μM forskolin.
[b] 15 min stimulation with 50 μM forskolin.
[c] mean ± standard error for quadruplicate samples
** $p < 0.01$ as determined by Dunnett's T-test as compared to forskolin + IBMX control.
Results are from one of three representative experiments.

through a G protein-coupled cannabinoid receptor. This interpretation is supported by striking parallels between previously reported results describing cannabinoid-neuronal tissue interactions and our present findings with mouse lymphoid tissue. Studies are presently underway in our laboratory to further characterize the role of the cannabinoid receptor in immune modulation by cannabinoids.

ACKNOWLEDGEMENT

This work was supported by the National Institute on Drug Abuse Grant RO1 DA07908.

REFERENCES

1. L. A. Matsuda, S. J. Lolait, M. J. Brownstein, A. C. Young, and T. I. Bonner, Structure of a cannabinoid receptor and functional expression of the cloned cDNA, Nature, 346:561 (1990).
2. C. M. Gerard, C. Mollereau, G. Vassart and M. Parmentier, Nucleotide sequence of a human cannabinoid receptor cDNA, *Nucleic Acids Res.*, 18:7142 (1990).
3. A. R. Schatz, F. K. Kessler, and N. E. Kaminski, Inhibition of adenylate cyclase by Δ-9 tetrahydrocannabinol in mouse spleen cells: A potential mechanism for cannabinoid mediated immunosuppression, *Life Sci.*, 51:25 (1992).

4. W. A. Devane, F. A. Dysarz, M. R. Johnson, L. S. Melvin, and A. C. Howlett, Determination and characterization of a cannabinoid receptor in rat brain, *Mol. Pharmacol.*, 34:605 (1988).
5. N. E. Kaminski, M. E. Abood, F. K. Kessler, B. R. Martin, and A. R. Schatz, Identification of a functionally relevant cannabinoid receptor on mouse spleen cells involved in cannabinoid-mediated immune modulation, *Mol. Pharmacol.*, (submitted).
6. M. S. Bartlett, Sub-sampling for attributes, *J. Roy. Stat. Soc, Suppl.*, 4:131 (1937).
7. C. W. DuMett, A multiple comparison procedure for comparing several treatments with a control, *J. Amer. Stat. Assoc.*, 50:1096 (1955).
8. Gehan-Wilcoxon, *in*: "Survival Distributions: Reliability Applications in the Biomedical Sciences," A. J. Gross and V. A. Clark, eds. John Wiley and Sons, New York (1975).
9. M. Herkenham, A. B. Lynn, M. D. Little, M. R. Johnson, L. S. Melvin, B. R. de Costa, and K. C. Rice, Cannabinoid receptor localization in brain, *Proc. Natl. Acad. Sci.*, 87:1932 (1990).

COCAINE AND IMMUNOCOMPETENCE: POSSIBLE ROLE OF REACTIVE METABOLITES

Michael P. Holsapple, Ray A. Matulka, Eric D. Stanulis and Stephen D. Jordan

Department of Pharmacology and Toxicology, Medical College of Virginia/Virginia Commonwealth University, Richmond, VA 23298

INTRODUCTION

Although drug abuse has been widely discussed as a possible co-factor in the onset and/or progression of AIDS, available literature is not consistent with cocaine use being associated with marked effects on immunocompetence. The initial objective of the present investigation was to determine the effects of cocaine on immunocompetence following direct addition to cultured splenocytes from female B6C3F1 mice. Because cocaine is a potent local anesthetic, we used procaine as a comparative control in these studies. As discussed below, the results from these studies were not consistent with a role by direct immunomodulatory actions of cocaine. We speculated that the *in vivo* effects of cocaine on the immune system may be an indirect consequence of exposure. The overall purpose of this study was to begin to examine possible indirect mechanism(s) for the effects of cocaine on the immune system, with an emphasis on a role by reactive metabolites. Cocaine is metabolized to norcocaine and, ultimately to more reactive intermediates, via a minor metabolic pathway mediated by the cytochrome P-450 system. The generation of these metabolites is associated with hepatotoxicity, which is both sex- and strain-dependent (i.e., dependent on the relative activity of the P-450 system). To provide evidence for a role by P-450-dependent metabolites in cocaine's actions on the immune system, we have compared the effects of subchronic (14 day) exposure to cocaine on the T-dependent antibody response in female B6C3F1 mice, female DBA/2 mice and male B6C3F1 mice.

MATERIALS AND METHODS

Chemicals

Cocaine hydrochloride was provided by the National Institute on Drug Abuse. Procaine hydrochloride was purchased from Sigma Chemical Co. (St. Louis, MO).

Drugs of Abuse, Immunity, and AIDS, Edited by
H. Friedman *et al.*, Plenum Press, New York, 1993

Mice

All mice were purchased virus-free from the Frederick Cancer Research Center at 5-6 wks of age. For the *in vivo* studies, we compared the effects of cocaine in female B6C3F1 mice, male B6C3F1 mice and female DBA/2 mice. All mice were quarantined for one wk and were used at between 6 and 8 wks of age. Mice were housed in plastic cages containing a saw dust bedding (4 mice per cage) at 21-24°C and 40-60% relative humidity with a 12 hr light/dark cycle. Mice received food (Purine Certified Laboratory Chow) and water *ad libitum* and were not used for experimentation until their body wt. was 17-20 g.

***In vitro* Antibody Assays**

Spleens from untreated female B6C3F1 mice were isolated aseptically, made into a single spleen cell suspension, adjusted to 1.0 x 10^7 cells/ml in complete RPMI 1640 and transferred in 500 μl aliquots to the wells of the 48-well culture plate. Cocaine and procaine were prepared in sterile saline and serial dilutions were made. Both drugs were added directly in 5 μl aliquots to the respective wells so that the final concentrations ranged from 10^{-8} M to 10^{-4} M. All wells were immediately sensitized with sheep erythrocytes (sRBC). The sRBC were added at a 1:1 ratio with the splenocytes. The *in vitro* antibody forming cells (AFC) response was quantitated on Day 5, which is the optimal response, as previously described (1). Viability was determined on the day of assay by the pronase method, as previously described (2).

***In vivo* Antibody Assays**

For the *in vivo* studies, cocaine stock solutions of 1 mg/ml to 8 mg/ml were prepared fresh daily in saline. Female and male B6C3F1 mice were administered either saline or 10, 20, 40, 60 or 80 mg/kg cocaine/day via intraperitoneal (i.p.) injection for 14 consecutive days. Female DBA/2 mice were administered either saline or 40, 60 or 80 mg/kg cocaine/day via i.p. injection for 14 consecutive days. Preliminary results in female B6C3F1 mice demonstrated that a 14 day exposure was necessary to observe any effects on the antibody response, in that we saw no effects on the antibody response following either a single injection or a 7-day dosing regimen. On day 11 of the 14 day exposure, all mice were sensitized to 5 x 10^8 sRBC in 1 ml via i.p. injection. On day 15, animals were terminated and anti-sRBC antibody responses were determined, as previously described (3). We have historically observed that the *in vivo* antibody response to sRBC peaks 4 days after sensitization.

Statistical Analysis of Data

The mean ± S.E. was determined for each treatment group of a given experiment. The AFC results were analyzed for homogeneity using Bartlett's test for homogeneity (4). All data was determined to be homogeneous and was evaluated by a parametric analysis of variance. When significant differences occurred, treatment groups were compared to the vehicle controls using a Dunnett's two tailed *t*-test (5).

RESULTS AND DISCUSSION

In one of the earliest studies to address the possible effects of cocaine on immunocompetence, previous results from our laboratory indicated that in spite of the fact that behaviorally active doses of cocaine were tested, the effects on immune function were quite modest (6). In these studies, male CD-1 mice, a randomly-bred strain, were injected (i.p.) with cocaine at either 25 or 50 mg/kg/day for 14 consecutive days. All mice became hyperactive at these doses, and a number of mice convulsed and died at the high dose. The delayed hypersensitivity response to sRBC was unaffected, while the antibody response to the same antigen was significantly suppressed (35%) only at the lowest dose. The overall goal of the current studies was to characterize the effects of cocaine on the immunocompetence of female B6C3F1 mice, an inbred strain which is the animal model recommended for immunological studies by the National Toxicology Program (7).

The initial objective of these studies was to assess the direct effects of cocaine on the *in vivo* antibody response. Because cocaine is a potent local anesthetic, we used procaine, a local anesthetic, which shares with cocaine the presence of an ester linkage; but which lacks the abuse potential of cocaine, as a comparative control. The results are presented in Table 1 and indicate that the potency of the two drugs was very comparable, if anything, procaine was more active than cocaine at most of the concentrations tested. Neither drug produced any significant reductions in viability over the concentration range tested. Cocaine produced a modest, but not significant suppression of 41% at the highest concentration tested, 10^{-4} M. In subsequent studies, we have determined that higher concentrations of cocaine ($>10^{-3}$ M) did produce significant reductions; but these high doses were also associated with marked decreases in viability. In order to put this concentration range of cocaine into some sort of perspective, it is important to emphasize that one laboratory (8) has estimated that the peak plasma levels of cocaine in man are between 2×10^{-7} M and 1.7×10^{-6} M; and that another laboratory (9) has estimated that the lethal blood level of cocaine in man is 6×10^{-6} M. As indicated in Table 1, cocaine produced no better than a nonsignificant 20% suppression at these concentrations. Taken together, this profile of activity raises serious questions about the biological significance of the results presented in Table 1 and suggest that any effects on immunocompetence associated with *in vivo* exposure to cocaine are not mediated by the direct effects of this drug on lymphocyte function.

Table 1. Comparison of the direct effects of cocaine and procaine on the *in vitro* antibody response.

Treatment		Antibody response[1]	% control
Vehicle		1057 ± 147	-
Cocaine	10^{-8} M	957 ± 133	91%
	10^{-7} M	1010 ± 215	96%
	10^{-6} M	821 ± 189	78%
	10^{-5} M	831 ± 148	79%
	10^{-4} M	621 ± 103	59%
Procaine	10^{-8} M	1043 ± 208	99%
	10^{-7} M	730 ± 231	69%
	10^{-6} M	790 ± 76	75%
	10^{-5} M	643 ± 150	61%
	10^{-4} M	537 ± 142	51%

[1]Results are presented as the number of antibody forming cells (AFC) per 10^6 recovered cells, and are based on four replicate wells.

Our initial results from studies measuring the effects of cocaine on the *in vivo* antibody response in female B6C3F1 mice were equally unspectacular. The results from a number of *in vivo* studies are summarized in Table 2. In first trial, we tested cocaine from 10 mg/kg/day to 40 mg/kg/day for 14 consecutive days. Although it appeared that the lowest dose tested was the threshold for behavioral activity, no parameters were included in these studies to specifically quantitate this action. Mice did display obvious hyperexcitability when exposed to 10 mg/kg cocaine. The antibody response in the control mice was 1159 ± 161 AFC/10^6 spleen cells. The only effect observed in this first trial was a significant enhancement of 77% at the middle dose. In our second trial, we tested cocaine at either 60 mg/kg/day or 80 mg/kg/day for 14 consecutive days. The antibody response in the control mice was 1547 ± 140 AFC/10^6 spleen cells. In spite of the fact that one mouse convulsed and died at the low dose, there was only a slight suppression of 20%. In the high-dose group, 3 out of 5 mice convulsed and died; but there was a significant suppression of 80% observed in the remaining mice. These results indicated that cocaine was immunosuppressive in female B6C3F1 mice; but only at very high concentrations.

Coincidentally with these initial studies in female B6C3F1 mice, we scanned the literature concerning cocaine's profile of activity for clues regarding a basis for a possible indirect mechanism of action. A number of laboratories have demonstrated that cocaine's effects on the liver are mediated by the generation of reactive metabolites by the cytochrome P-450 pathway, specifically the oxidative N-demethylation of cocaine to norcocaine. As reviewed by Boesterli and Goldin (10), mice are the species most susceptible to cocaine-induced hepatotoxicity. However, in mice there are both sex- and strain-dependent differences in cocaine-induced hepatotoxicity which are correlated with differences in P-450 metabolic capability: males are more sensitive than females; and DBA/2 mice are more sensitive than C57BL/6 mice (<u>NOTE</u>: B6C3F1 mice are the F1 generation of a cross between C57BL/6 mice and C3H mice). We were struck by the fact that female B6 mice were most resistant to the hepatotoxic effects of cocaine, and by our observation that these mice were also very resistant to cocaine-induced immunotoxicity. We therefore formulated a working model centered around a parallel profile of activity between cocaine-induced hepatotoxicity and cocaine-induced immunotoxicity. As a critical part of this working model, we formulated the following hypothesis: Cocaine's effects on immunocompetence are an indirect consequence of exposure mediated by the generation of reactive intermediates by the cytochrome P-450 system.

In order to test this hypothesis, we decided to take advantage of the sex- and strain-dependent differences described above for hepatotoxicity. These results are also summarized in Table 2. Male B6C3F1 mice were exposed to cocaine from 10 mg/kg/day to 80 mg/kg/day for 14 consecutive days. The behavioral effects of cocaine at the low end of the dose-response curve in male B6C3F1 mice appeared to be identical to the profile described above for female B6C3F1 mice. The antibody response in the control mice was 1634 ± 163. The results indicated that male B6 mice were more sensitive than female B6 mice for all parameters. There was greater lethality at the higher doses (i.e., 9/10 mice died at the two highest concentrations). Significant changes in the antibody response, both enhancement (i.e., 41% at 10 mg/kg/day, which was essentially devoid of activity in females) and suppression (i.e., <50% at 40 mg/kg/day, a dose which was a no effect dose in females), occurred at lower doses. Female DBA/2 mice were exposed to cocaine from 40 mg/kg/day to 80 mg/kg/day for 14 consecutive days. The pattern of lethality by cocaine was different in the two strains of female mice. DBA/2 mice appeared to be more resistant to the lethal effects of cocaine in that fewer animals died over this dose range and the time to death was markedly delayed. Nonetheless, the results of the antibody response

Table 2. Summary of results from subchronic (14 day) studies with cocaine

Mouse strain and sex	Parameter	Cocaine dose (mg/kg/day) 10	20	40	60	80
Female B6C3F1	Lethality[1]	0/5	0/5	0/5	1/5	3/5
	Antibody response[2]	12% **I**	77% **I***	2% **D**	20% **D**	80% **D****
Male B6C3F1	Lethality	0/5	0/5	0/5	4/5	5/5
	Antibody response	41% **I***	17% **I**	55% **D****	84% **D**	-
Female DBA/2	Lethality	NT[3]	NT	0/5	0/5	1/5
	Antibody response	NT	NT	20% **D**	48% **D***	55% **D***

[1]Lethality - number of mice from N=5/group, which died during the 14 day treatment. All B6C3F1 mice which died, did so during days 3-6 of exposure. All DBA/2 mice which died, did so during days 8-10 of exposure.

[2]Antibody response - presented as percent of control (i.e., the control values are indicated in the text) with "I" reflecting an increase and "D" reflecting a decrease. * and ** are results which were significantly different from control at $p<0.05$ and $p<0.01$, respectively.

[3]NT - not tested

were consistent with the hypothesis. The antibody response in the control mice was 564 ± 73. As shown in Table 2, we observed a significant suppression of about 50% at 60 mg/kg/day in female DBA/2, a dose which was essentially devoid of activity in female B6C3F1 mice. Taken together, these results offer at least preliminary support for a role by the generation of reactive intermediates in cocaine-induced immunosuppression. We believe that it is premature to speculate on a similar role for metabolism in the enhanced antibody response that we observed in both male and female B6C3F1 mice; and to conclude that an enhancement cannot be observed in DBA/2 mice. Additional work is necessary to expand the dose-response curve in the various mouse models, and to begin to characterize the effects of cocaine in male DBA/2 mice, which should be exquisitely sensitive to the immunological effects of cocaine.

REFERENCES

1. M. P. Holsapple, P. J. McNerney, D. W. Barnes and K. L. White, Jr., Suppression of humoral antibody production by exposure to 1,2,3,6,7,8-hexachlorodibenzo-p-dioxin, *J. Pharmac. Exp. Ther.*, 231:518 (1984).
2. K. W. Johnson, A. E. Munson, D. H. Kim and M. P. Holsapple, Role of reactive metabolites in suppression of humoral immunity by N-nitrosodimethylamine, *J. Pharmac. Exp. Ther.*, 240:847 (1987).
3. M. P. Holsapple, J. A. McCay and D. W. Barnes, Immunosuppression without liver induction by subchronic exposure to 2,7-dichlorodibenzo-p-dioxin in adult female B6C3F1 mice, *Toxicol. Appl. Pharmac.* 83:445 (1986).
4. M. S. Bartlett, Sub-sampling for attributes, *J. Roy. Stat. Soc. Suppl.*, 4-131 (1937).
5. C. W. Dunnett, A multiple comparison procedure for comparing several treatments with a control, *J. Amer. Stat. Assoc.*., 50:1096 (1955).
6. M. P. Holsapple and A. E. Munson, Immunotoxicology of abused drugs, *in*: "Immunotoxicology and Immunopharmacology," J. H. Dean, M. I. Luster, A. E. Munson and H. Amos, eds., Raven Press, New York (1985).
7. M. I. Luster, A. E. Munson, P. T. Thomas, M. P. Holsapple, J. D. Fenters, K. L. White, Jr., L. D. Lauer, D. R. Germolec, G. J. Rosenthal and J. H. Dean, Development of a testing battery to assess chemical-induced immunotoxicity: National Toxicology Program's guidelines for immunotoxicity evaluation in mice, *Fundam. Appl. Toxicol.* 10:2 (1988).
8. E. J. Cone, K. Kumor, L. K. Thompson and M. Sherer, Correlation of saliva cocaine levels with plasma levels and with pharmacologic effects after intravenous cocaine administration in human subjects, *J. Anal. Toxicol.*, 12:200 (1988).
9. R. G. Smart and L. Anglin, Do we know the lethal dose of cocaine? *J. Forensic Sci.*, 32:303 (1987).
10. U. A. Boelsterli and C. Goldin, Biomechanisms of cocaine-induced hepatocyte injury mediated by the formation of reactive metabolites, *Arch. Toxicol.*, 65:351 (1991).

MOLECULAR MECHANISMS ASSOCIATED WITH COCAINE-INDUCED MODULATION OF HUMAN T LYMPHOCYTES PROLIFERATION

Katsuhiko Matsui, Herman Friedman and Thomas W. Klein

Department of Medical Microbiology and Immunology
University of South Florida College of Medicine
Tampa, Florida 33612

INTRODUCTION

The increasing abuse of cocaine by young adults and the many deaths attributed to cocaine overdose have prompted questions concerning the public health risk of abusing the drug. These deaths result from a combination of drug effects on both the central and sympathetic nervous systems (1). In addition to the lethal toxic effects of cocaine, previous reports demonstrated that cocaine has various influences, both suppression and enhancement, on the immune function of humans and experimental animals (2, 3, 4, 5). However, the mechanisms of immunomodulation *in vivo* are unclear, because cocaine can act either as a local anesthetic or systemically through the central nervous system.

Previously, we reported that high concentrations of cocaine (300 μM to 600 μM) suppressed the proliferation of human peripheral blood mononuclear cells to optimal concentrations of the polyclonal mitogenic lectin phytohemagglutinin (PHA) (6). The present study was undertaken to extend our initial findings by employing pharmacologically achievable cocaine concentrations and by using purified T cell populations. Also, cocaine effects were compared between anti-CD3 and PHA-stimulated cells, because the constellation of receptor activation mechanisms is incompletely understood for PHA (7). The CD3 molecule of human peripheral blood T lymphocytes is associated with the T cell antigen receptor (TCR), and is an important signal transducer during the process of T cell activation to a specific antigen (8).

Activation of T cells by either PHA or anti-CD3 antibody involves interleukin-2 (IL-2) secretion and IL-2 receptor expression, and these two events are essential for the subsequent lymphoproliferation (9). Furthermore, increases in cytosolic free calcium (Ca^{2+}) are required for the production of IL-2, but not for the expression of the IL-2 receptor (10). In this study, we demonstrate that the cocaine effects on anti-CD3 and PHA-induced proliferations of human T lymphocytes are accompanied by modulation of Ca^{2+} mobilization and subsequent IL-2 production, but the expression of IL-2 receptor may not be influenced by cocaine treatment. It is also suggested that the molecular mechanism of divergent drug effects on anti-CD3 and PHA-induced proliferations may involve the activation of Na^+/H^+ antiport.

Drugs of Abuse, Immunity, and AIDS, Edited by
H. Friedman *et al.*, Plenum Press, New York, 1993

EFFECTS OF COCAINE ON PROLIFERATION AND IL-2 PRODUCTION

Human peripheral blood T lymphocytes were purified from the blood of random donors. The leukocyte buffy coat cells were layered onto Ficoll-Hypaque gradients and centrifuged. The peripheral blood leukocytes at the interface were collected and were allowed to adhere to plastic petri dishes to remove adherent cells. The nonadherent cells were recovered and further purified on discontinuous percoll density gradients (11). The resulting purified T lymphocytes (2 x 10^6 cells/ml) were prepared in RPMI 1640 medium containing 10% fetal calf serum and antibiotics (6). The cells were cultured with either mouse anti-human CD3 antibody (IgG1 subclass; 50 ng/ml) or PHA (0.2 µg/ml) at 37oC for 48 hr in 96-well plates and tested for drug susceptibility. Some of the wells were pre-coated with anti-mouse IgG1 which provides a framework for binding and immobilizing the Fc part of anti-CD3 antibody (12). The cultures were subsequently pulsed for 18 hr with ^{3}H-thymidine (0.5 µCi per well) and the incorporated radioactivity was determined by liquid scintillation counting. Figure 1 shows the effects of cocaine on anti-CD3 and PHA-induced proliferation of human peripheral blood T lymphocytes. The suppression of the PHA-induced proliferation of T cells by cocaine showed a bell-shaped dose response to cocaine treatment with maximum suppression (27.9%) of proliferation occurring at 3 µM cocaine ($P < 0.05$). However, cocaine treatment augmented lymphocyte proliferation induced by anti-CD3 as much as 150% of control at a drug concentration of 3 µM ($P < 0.01$).

The proliferation of T cells in response to anti-CD3 and PHA involves the production of and response to IL-2 (9, 13). Therefore, the amounts of IL-2 in the culture supernatant of T cells, which were cultured at 37°C for 48 hr in the presence

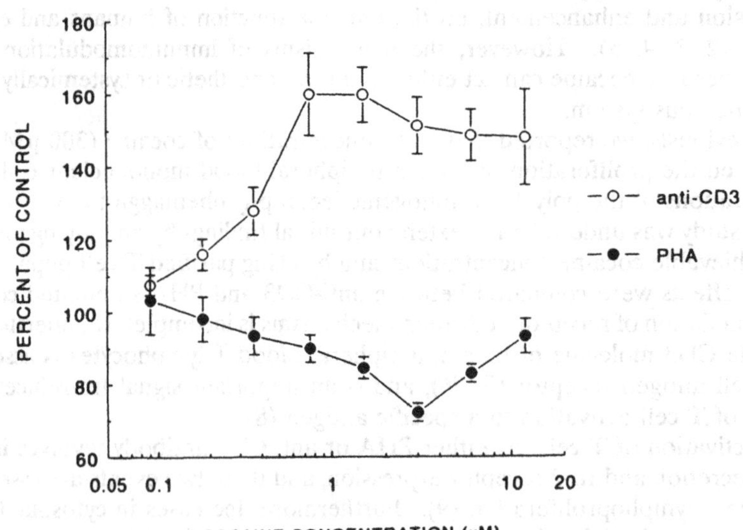

Fig. 1. Cocaine modulates the proliferative response of human peripheral blood T lymphocytes stimulated with anti-CD3 antibody or PHA. Results are presented as mean percent of control ± S.E.M. (n=5) obtained by dividing delta cpm values from drug treated cultures by those from non-drug treated cultures x 100. The cpm range for the non-drug cultures stimulated with anti-CD3 and PHA was 20,080-37,074 and 11,000-25,000 cpm, respectively.

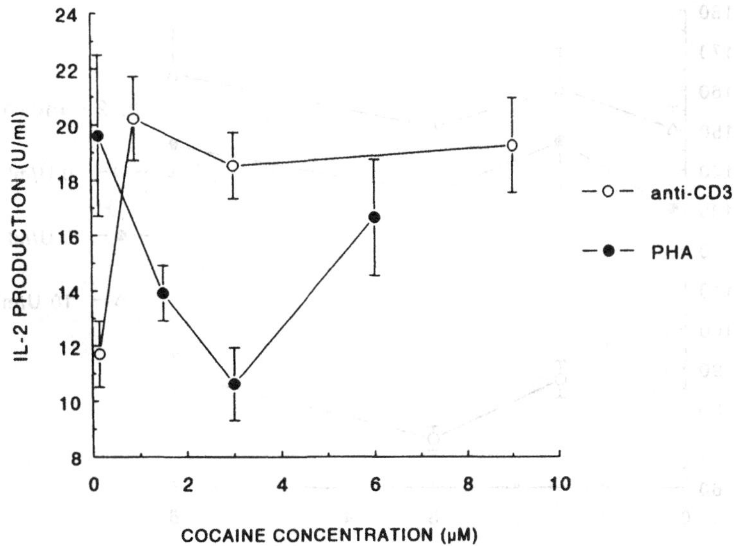

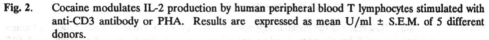

Fig. 2. Cocaine modulates IL-2 production by human peripheral blood T lymphocytes stimulated with anti-CD3 antibody or PHA. Results are expressed as mean U/ml ± S.E.M. of 5 different donors.

of cocaine and mitogens according to the method of Baroja & Ceuppens (14), were measured by ELISA (Intertest-2X; Genzyme, Cambridge, MA). As shown in Fig. 2, the level of IL-2 production by T cell cultures following ligand stimulation and drug treatment paralleled the proliferative response. The maximum augmentation of IL-2 production was observed at 0.9 μM of cocaine ($P< 0.01$) when T cells were stimulated with anti-CD3, and then reached a plateau at higher drug concentrations. On the other hand, IL-2 production observed in the PHA-activated cultures was maximally inhibited ($P< 0.01$) at 3.0 μM cocaine with higher drug concentrations having less of an effect. These results suggested that cocaine modulation of proliferation was linked to effects on the cellular synthesis and release of IL-2. The results in Fig. 3 support this conclusion and demonstrate that the addition of recombinant IL-2 to suppressed cultures restores the proliferative response. Drug effects on IL-2 receptor expression, however, are apparently not involved because no differences were observed by flow cytometry in the expression of the 55 KDa, low-affinity, IL-2 receptor (data not shown).

INVOLVEMENT OF CYTOSOLIC CALCIUM MOBILIZATION IN COCAINE EFFECTS

Lymphocyte proliferation in response to anti-CD3 or PHA is accompanied by an increase in the concentration of intracellular free Ca^{2+} (15, 16), and the Ca^{2+} mobilization is strongly related with IL-2 production. Therefore, the effect of cocaine on Ca^{2+} mobilization in anti-CD3 and PHA-activated T cells was studied. Human T lymphocytes (1×10^8 cells/ml) were loaded with 10 μM Fura 2/AM in tissue culture medium as previously described (15). A portion of the loaded cells was incubated for 40 min at 4°C with anti-CD3 (1 μg/ml), and then these cells were resuspended at 2×10^7 cells/ml in Dulbecco's phosphate buffered saline (PBS) containing 1.0 mM $CaCl_2$

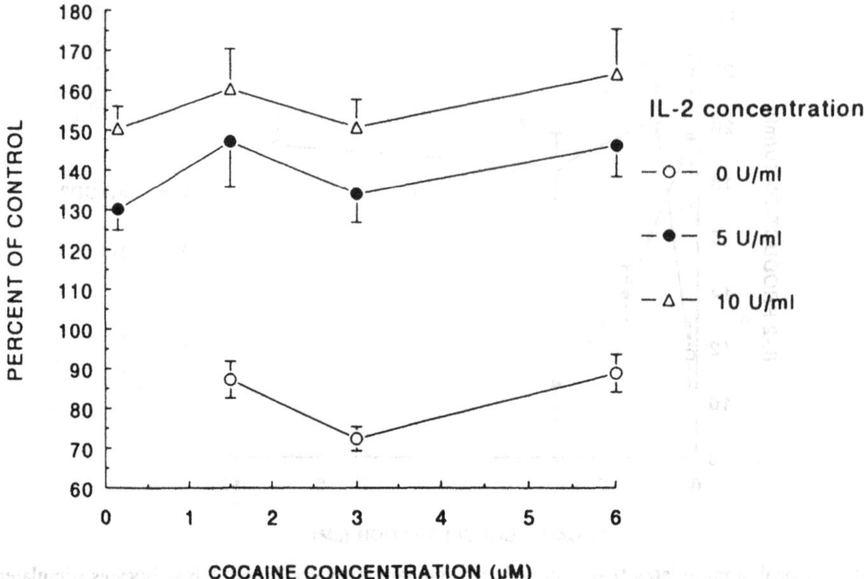

Fig. 3. Exogenous IL-2 restores the cocaine suppressive effect on PHA-induced proliferation of human peripheral blood T lymphocytes. T cells were cultured at 37°C for 48 hr with cocaine, PHA (0.2 μg/ml) and IL-2, and then pulsed with 0.5 μCi of ^{3}H-thymidine for 18 hr. Data are presented as mean percent of control ± S.E.M. of 5 different donors (see Figure 1 for details). The cpm range for the non-drug and non-IL-2 culture was 19,000-28,000 cpm.

and 0.5 mM $MgCl_2$. The cells were then incubated with 3 μM cocaine at 37°C for 15 min, and subsequently treated with PHA (10 μg/ml) or anti-mouse IgG1 (5 μg/ml) to crosslink the cell-surface anti-CD3. The fluorescence was measured at 37°C by using a Perkin Elmer LS-3B spectrofluorometer. The excitation and emission wavelengths were 350 and 500 nm, respectively. As shown in Fig. 4, in the absence of drug, the free Ca^{2+} mobilization following stimulation by anti-CD3 and PHA increased from 96.5 nM to 210.6 nM and 199.3 nM, respectively. However, as seen in the proliferation and IL-2 production studies, pre-treating the cells with 3 μM cocaine augmented Ca^{2+} mobilization following anti-CD3 treatment ($P < 0.01$) and depressed Ca^{2+} mobilization following PHA treatment ($P < 0.01$). The drug alone did not have any effects on cytosolic Ca^{2+} levels. Furthermore, the suppression of Ca^{2+} mobilization in PHA-stimulated cells was restored to 280.0 nM by addition of 0.25 μM ionomycin which is an ionophore for Ca^{2+}. The addition of 0.25 and 0.5 μM ionomycin also attenuated the cocaine-induced suppression of proliferation (Fig. 5), suggesting the drug effect is strongly associated with a lowering of Ca^{2+} mobilization.

Mills et al., (10) reported that chelation of Ca^{2+} with EGTA suppressed the PHA-induced proliferation and IL-2 production of purified T cells but had no effect on the expression of the low affinity, IL-2 receptor (Tac antigen). This finding suggests that Ca^{2+} mobilization is required for lymphoproliferation and IL-2 secretion but not required for IL-2 receptor expression. The treatment of T lymphocytes with suboptimal concentrations of PHA also demonstrated the association between Ca^{2+} mobilization and both proliferation and IL-2 secretion (17). In that study, the suboptimal concentration of PHA caused a lowering of proliferation, which coincided with a

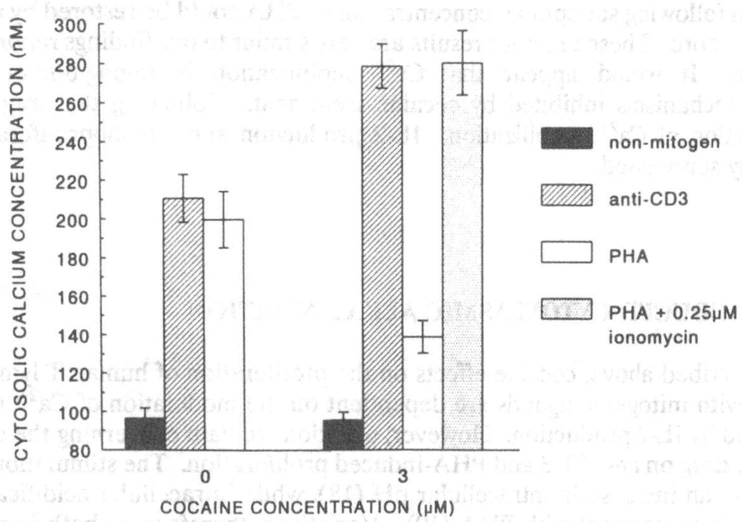

Fig. 4. Cocaine modulates intracellular Ca^{2+} mobilization of T lymphocytes in response to anti-CD3 antibody or PHA. Data are expressed as mean value ± S.E.M of 5 experiments.

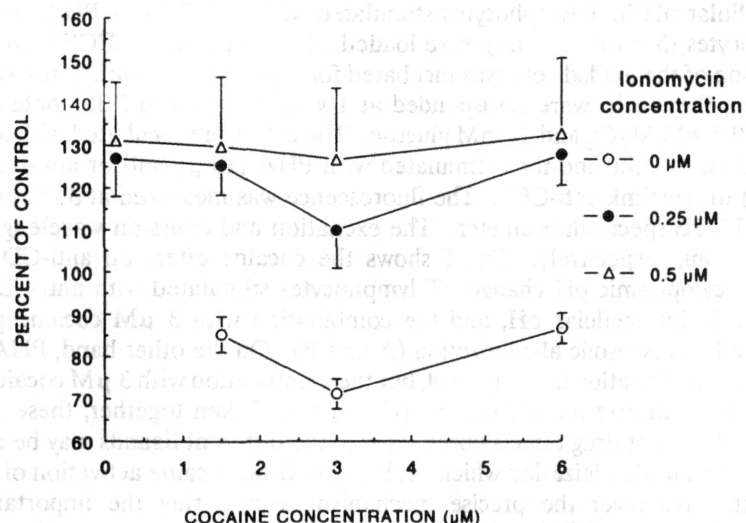

Fig. 5. Ionomycin restores the cocaine suppressive effect on PHA-induced proliferation of human peripheral blood T lymphocytes. T cells were cultured at 37°C for 48 hr with cocaine, PHA (0.2 μg/ml) and ionomycin, and then pulsed with 0.5 μCi of ^{3}H-thymidine for 18 hr. Data are expressed as mean value ± S.E.M. of 5 experiments (see Fig. 1 for details). The cpm range for the non-drug, non-ionomycin group was 12,000-25,000 cpm.

lowering of Ca^{2+} mobilization and IL-2 production. However, the lowering of proliferation following suboptimal concentration of PHA could be restored by addition of Ca^{2+} ionophore. These previous results are very similar to our findings reported here with cocaine. It would appear that Ca^{2+} mobilization is among one of the first molecular mechanisms inhibited by cocaine treatment. Following the drug-induced down-regulation of Ca^{2+} mobilization, IL-2 production and lymphoproliferation are subsequently suppressed.

COCAINE-INDUCED CYTOPLASMIC ALKALINIZATION

As described above, cocaine effects on the proliferation of human T lymphocytes stimulated with mitogenic ligands are dependent on the modulation of Ca^{2+} mobilization followed by IL-2 production. However, questions remain concerning the divergent effect of the drug on anti-CD3 and PHA-induced proliferation. The stimulation by anti-CD3 leads to an increase in intracellular pH (18), while intracellular acidification was noted following treatment with PHA (19). Variations, therefore, in both intracellular Ca^{2+} and intracellular pH (through activation of the amiloride sensitive Na^+/H^+ antiport) are believed to be important in T cell activation. In our studies, cocaine treatment alone had no effect on the concentration of Ca^{2+} suggesting that the drug probably acts only in conjunction with the signals generated by mitogenic ligands. Involvement of Ca^{2+} in the activation of the Na^+/H^+ antiport has been observed in T lymphocytes stimulated with anti-CD3 or PHA (18, 19). Therefore, the drug effect on intracellular pH in T lymphocytes stimulated with anti-CD3 or PHA was studied. T lymphocytes (3 x 10^7 cells/ml) were loaded with 2.5 μg/ml BCECF/AM in PBS (19). A portion of the loaded cells was incubated for 40 min at 4°C with anti-CD3 (1 μg/ml), and then these cells were resuspended at 1 x 10^7 cells/ml in PBS containing 1.0 mM $CaCl_2$, 0.5 mM $MgCl_2$ and 10 mM glucose. The cells were incubated with 3 μM cocaine at 37°C for 15 min, and then stimulated with PHA (10 μg/ml) or anti-mouse IgG1 (5 μg/ml) to crosslink anti-CD3. The fluorescence was measured at 37°C using a Perkin Elmer LS-3B spectrofluorometer. The excitation and emission wavelengths were 495 and 526 nm, respectively. Fig. 6 shows the cocaine effect on anti-CD3 and PHA-induced cytoplasmic pH change. T lymphocytes stimulated with anti-CD3 caused an increase in intracellular pH, and the combination with 3 μM cocaine pretreatment enhanced this cytosolic alkalinization (A and B). On the other hand, PHA stimulation caused an acidification in the cytosol, but the combination with 3 μM cocaine treatment tended to neutralize the pH decline (C and D). Taken together, these data indicate that the divergent drug effects observed with the different ligands may be accompanied by cytoplasmic alkalinization which could result from cocaine activation of the Na^+/H^+ antiport. Whatever the precise mechanism, considering the importance of Ca^{2+} mobilization and Na^+/H^+ antiport in T lymphocytes, it seems reasonable to suspect that the cocaine effects on these ions is at least partially responsible for the modulation of lymphocyte activation.

In conclusion, our results demonstrate that cocaine modulates the proliferation of human T lymphocytes by affecting Ca^{2+} mobilization and cytoplasmic alkalinization with subsequent effects on production of the T cell growth factor, IL-2. These *in vitro* results may explain several *in vivo* studies demonstrating that cocaine treatment leads to both augmentation and diminution of immune function.

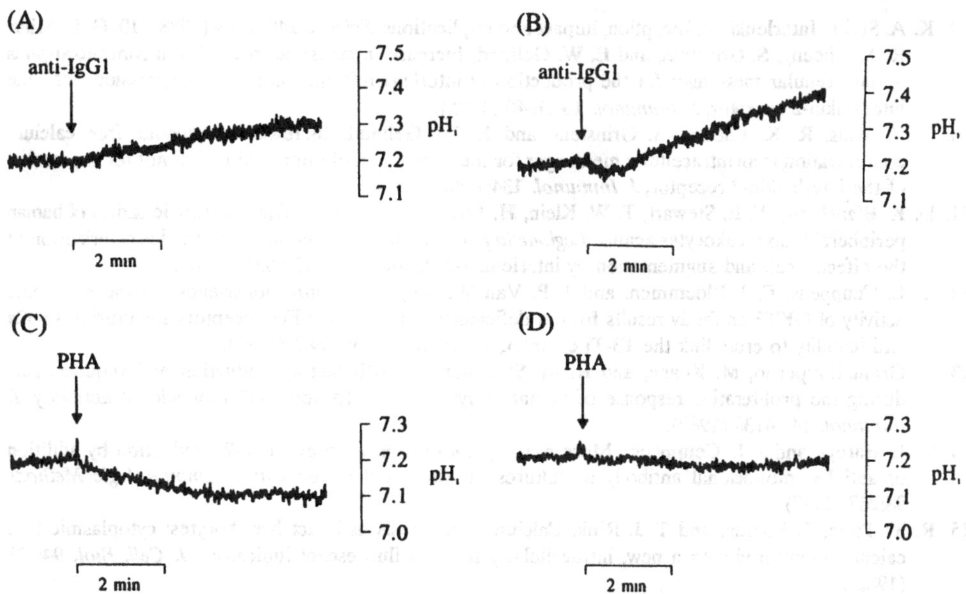

Fig. 6. Cocaine alkalinizes intracellular pH of T lymphocytes in response to anti-CD3 antibody or PHA. The concentrations of cocaine are (A and C) 0 μM and (B and D) 3 μM. (A) and (B) were stimulated with 5 μg/ml anti-IgG1 to crosslink the cell-surface anti-CD3, and (C) and (D) were stimulated with 10 μg/ml PHA. The results are from a single, representative donor.

ACKNOWLEDGEMENTS

This work was supported by Public Health Service Grant DA05568 from the National Institute on Drug Abuse.

REFERENCES

1. K. Pearman, Cocaine: A review, *J. Laryngol. Ontol.* 93:1191 (1979).
2. P. DiFrancesco, F. Pica, C. Croce, C. Favalli, E. Tubaro, and E. Garaci, Effect of acute or daily cocaine administration on cellular immune response and virus infection in mice, *Natn.Immun. Cell Growth Regul.* 9:397 (1990).
3. D. W. Ou, M. L. Shen, and Y. D. Luo, Effects of cocaine on the immune system of BALB/c mice, *Clin. Immunol. Immunopathol.* 52:305 (1989).
4. O. Bagasra, and L. Forman, Functional analysis of lymphocytes subpopulations in experimental cocaine abuse. I. Dose-dependent activation of lymphocyte subsets, *Clin. Exp. Immunol.* 77:289 (1989).
5. H. F. Havas, M. Dellaria, G. Schiffman, E. B. Geller, and M. W. Adler, Effect of cocaine on the immune response and host resistance in BALB/c mice, *Int. Arch. Allergy Appl.Immunol.* 83:377 (1987).
6. T. W. Klein, C. A. Newton, and H. Friedman, Suppression of human and mouse lymphocyte proliferation by cocaine, *in*: "Psychological, Neuropsychiatric and Substance Abuse Aspects of AIDS", T. P. Bride, ed., pp. 319, Raven Press, New York (1988).
7. J. M. Kanellopoulas, S. Depetris, G. Lecca, and M. J. Crumpton, The mitogenic lectin from *Phaseolus vulgaris* does not recognize the T3 antigen of human T lymphocytes, *Eur. J. Immunol.*15:479 (1985).
8. S. C. Meuer, K. A. Fitzgerald, R. E. Hussey, J. C. Hodgdon, S. F. Schlossman, and E. L. Reinherz, Clonotypic structures involved in antigen-specific human T cell function, J. Exp. Med. 157:705 (1983).

9. K. A. Smith, Interleukin-2: Inception, impact and implications, *Science* 240: 1169 (1988). 10. G. B. Mills, R. K. Cheung, S. Grinstein, and E. W. Gelfand, Increase in cytosolic free calcium concentration is an intracellular messenger for the production of interleukin-2 but not for expression of the interleukin-2 receptor, *J. Immunol.* 134:1640 (1985).
10. G. B. Mills, R. K. Cheung, S. Grinstein, and E. W. Gelfand, Increase in cytosolic free calcium concentration is an intracellular messenger for the production of interleukin-2 but not for expression of the interleukin-2 receptor, *J. Immunol.* 134:1640 (1985).
11. D. K. Blanchard, W. E. Stewart, T. W. Klein, H. Friedman, and J. Y. Djeu, Cytolytic activity of human peripheral blood leukocytes against *Legionella pneumophila*-infected monocytes: characterization of the effector cell and augmentation by interleukin-2, *J. Immunol.* 139:551 (1987).
12. J. L. Ceuppens, F. J. Bloemmen, and J. P. Van Wauwe, T cell unresponsiveness to the mitogenic activity of OKT3 antibody results from a deficiency of monocytes Fcr receptors for murine IgG2a and inability to cross-link the T3-Ti complex, *J. Immunol.* 135:3882 (1985).
13. A. Granelli-Piperno, M. Keane, and R. M. Steinman, Growth factor production and requirements during the proliferative response of human T lymphocytes to anti-CD3 monoclonal antibody, *J. Immunol.* 142:4138 (1989).
14. M. L. Baroja, and J. L. Ceuppens, More exact quantification of interleukin-2 production by addition of anti-Tac monoclonal antibody to cultures of stimulated lymphocytes, *J.Immunologic Methods* 98:267 (1987).
15. R. Y. Tsien, T. Pozzan, and T. J. Rink, Calcium homeotasis in intact lymphocytes: cytoplasmic free calcium monitored with a new, intracellularly trapped fluorescent indicator, *J. Cell. Biol.* 94:325 (1982).
16. A. Weiss, J. Imboden, D. Shoback, and J. Stobo, Role of T3 surface molecules in human T-cell activation: T3 dependent activation results in an increase in cytoplasmic free calcium, *Proc. Natl. Acad. Sci.* USA, 81:4169 (1984).
17. G. B. Mills, J. W. W. Lee, R. K. Cheung, and E. W. Gelfand, Characterization of the requirements for human T cell mitogenesis by using suboptimal concentrations of phytohemagglutinin, *J. Immunol.* 135: 3087 (1985).
18. P. M. Rosoff, and L. C. Cantley, Stimulation of the T3-T cell receptor-associated Ca^{2+} influx enhances the activity of the Na^+/H^+ exchanger in a leukemic human T cell line, *J. Biol. Chem.* 260:14053 (1985).
19. E. W. Gelfand, R. K. Cheung, and S. Grinstein, Calcium-dependent intracellular acidification dominates the pH response to mitogen in human T cells, *J. Immunol.* 140:246 (1988).

EFFECTS OF COCAINE ON THE RESPIRATORY BURST OF MURINE MACROPHAGES

Austin Vaz,[1] Stanley S. Lefkowitz,[1,2] and Doris L. Lefkowitz[2,3]

Dept. of Med. Microbiol.,[1] and Dept. of Psychiatry,[2] Texas Tech Univ. Hlth. Sciences Ctr., Lubbock, TX 79430; Dept. of Biol. Sciences,[3] Texas Tech Univ., Lubbock TX 79409

SUMMARY

Cocaine is a central nervous stimulant with a major potential for abuse. It is used clinically as a local anesthetic and vasoconstrictor. The effects of cocaine on the immune system have not been studied in depth. In this study, we have investigated the effects of cocaine on the respiratory burst (RB) of murine macrophages (Mø). The RB was measured by determining the increase in chemiluminescence. Both peritoneal and alveolar Mø were isolated from cocaine-exposed mice and saline-exposed controls. Cocaine was administered by the intraperitoneal, intravenous, and intramuscular route. Both peritoneal and alveolar Mø from cocaine-exposed mice showed an increase in chemiluminescence when compared with Mø from matched controls. This effect was seen as early as one hour after cocaine exposure and lasted for up to 48 hours. Intraperitoneal injection of cocaine metabolites did not affect the RB. Macrophages exposed to cocaine *in vitro* failed to respond by an increase in RB. These findings indicate that cocaine induces the production of reactive oxygen intermediates (ROI) and suggests possible changes in Mø functions.

INTRODUCTION

Cocaine is an alkaloid derived from the leaves of *Erythroxylon coca*. It is readily absorbed through the mucus membranes of the respiratory and the gastrointestinal tracts. Cocaine abuse causes various negative effects on body function. These include cardiovascular toxicity, cerebrovascular accidents, pulmonary problems and obstetrical complications. Cocaine toxicity to the fetus has also been well documented (1).

The effects of cocaine on the immune system have not been fully studied. A recent review (2) showed that cocaine has suppressive as well as enhancing effects on the immune system. The present study evaluates the effects of cocaine on the respiratory burst (RB) of both peritoneal and alveolar macrophages. Macrophages are widely distributed throughout most tissues. They play a major role in both cellular and humoral immunity and are involved in phagocytosis, antigen presentation, and production of

Drugs of Abuse, Immunity, and AIDS, Edited by
H. Friedman *et al.*, Plenum Press, New York, 1993

various cytokines. They also play a key role in inflammation and healing of tissues following injury.

One of the most important functions of the macrophage is to ingest and kill microorganisms. Allen and coworkers have shown that these cells emit light while ingesting particles (3,4). The production of high-energy compounds during bactericidal activity can result in the production of light. This spontaneous luminescence can be used as an assay of phagocytic function or as a sensitive means to quantitate microbicidal metabolic activity. These measurements, however, require large numbers of cells as well as a very sensitive light detector, such as present in a scintillation counter or luminometer.

Phagocytosis by macrophages also is accompanied by an increase in the production of superoxide anion. Superoxide which is released into the medium, spontaneously dismutates into 0_2 and H_20_2 as follows:

$$20_{2^-} + 2H^+ \rightarrow H_20_2 + 0_2$$

Chemiluminescence can be enhanced using luminol (5-amino-2,3-dihydro-1,4-phthalazinedione) which is oxidized by H_20_2. The addition of a stimulant such as opsonized zymosan to macrophages, *in vitro*, results in an increase in the RB. The latter can be readily measured, by determining the increase in chemiluminescence. The increase in chemiluminescence is rapid and occurs within minutes of the addition of the stimulating agent.

MATERIALS AND METHODS

Animals

Male or female 8-16 wk old C57BL/6 mice, were obtained from Charles River Laboratories.

Drug

Cocaine HCl was obtained from the National Institute of Drug Abuse (NIDA). Metabolites of cocaine (ecgonine methylester HCl and ecgonine HCl) were also obtained from NIDA. Both were dissolved in phosphate buffered saline (PBS) and injected intraperitoneally, intravenously or intramuscularly using various schedules. Control mice were injected with PBS.

Collection of Peritoneal Macrophages

The method described by Lefkowitz *et al.*, was used (5). Briefly, mice were sacrificed by cervical dislocation. With the ventral side up, the skin was swabbed with 70% alcohol, cut along the midline and removed. Each animal was injected with 8 ml of cold PBS at pH 7.2. The abdomen was gently massaged, with the needle still left i.p. for one minute and the fluid slowly withdrawn. Cells were centrifuged at 150 x g for 10 minutes at 5°C and resuspended in the appropriate medium.

Collection of Alveolar Macrophages

The method described by Holt (6) was used and is briefly described as follows. Mice were sacrificed using an i.p. injection of 0.5 ml sodium pentobarbital (65 mg/ml;

Anthony Products Co., CA) The trachea of the mice were exposed and a lavage tube (O.D. < 1 mm was inserted through a small incision made in the trachea. A 10 ml vertical syringe filled with 9.1 ml PBS and 0.9 ml Xylocaine solution (40 mg/ml; Astra, Westborough, MA), an empty 10 ml horizontal syringe and the lavage tube were inter-connected via a three-way stopcock. The lungs were filled with 0.5 ml fluid from the vertical syringe at a time. The chest was massaged gently and fluid withdrawn into the horizontal syringe by changing the direction of the stopcock. This process was repeated until the lungs were lavaged with 10 ml of fluid. The cells were centrifuged at 150 x g and resuspended in the appropriate medium.

Measurement of Respiratory Burst by Chemiluminescence

The method as described by Lefkowitz *et al.*, (7) was used and is described briefly as follows: Peritoneal or alveolar Mø, suspended in 10 ml cold PBS at pH 7.2 were centrifuged and washed 2 x with cold PBS. They were then resuspended in medium and the cell concentration adjusted to 1 x 10^6 cells /ml for the peritoneal cells and 2.5 x 10^5 cells /ml for the alveolar Mø. Chemiluminescence medium contains Auto-Pow EMEM (Flow Lab Inc., McLean, VA); Bovine Serum Albumin (essentially globulin-free) 1.0 g/dl (Sigma, Kansas City, MO); HEPES 0.6 g/dl (Sigma); and Sodium Bicarbonate 0.2 g/dl (Sigma). Exactly 100 µl cell suspension were added to each 8 x 50 mm tube (Evergreen Scientific, Los Angeles, CA). Cell monolayers were incubated at 37°C under 5% CO_2 for one hour. Supernatants were discarded and the monolayer in each tube was washed and 100 µl media, 100 µl of zymosan (Sigma) opsonized with guinea pig complement (GIBCO, Long Island, NY), and 30 µl of luminol (Eastman Kodak, Rochester, NY) were added to each tube. The tubes were read in a luminometer (Turner designs, Mountain View, CA, Model 20e) which was programmed for 5 consecutive two-minute readings.

RESULTS

The RB was measured as chemiluminescence or emission of light per unit time. All figures show the Y-axis measuring the relative emission of light as counts obtained directly from the luminometer. The X-axis represents the time intervals of 2, 4, 6, 8, and 10 minutes. At each interval Mø cultures were assayed in triplicate and results expressed as the mean ± S.E.M.

In Figure 1, two mice injected i.p. with 2.5 mg/kg cocaine were compared with two control mice injected with saline. The peritoneal Mø from the cocaine-treated mice showed an increase in the RB when cells were harvested 60 minutes after exposure. This increase was in the range of 3000-5000 count range which was at least 10 fold greater than the controls.

Figure 2 illustrates that this enhancement of the respiratory burst could still be measured 24 hrs after exposure to cocaine. A "dose-dependent" increase was noted using 2.5 mg/kg and 5 mg/kg.

Figure 3 shows that an enhancement of the RB was also obtained using the i.v. route of administration. Mice injected with 2.5 or 5 mg/kg i.v. also showed an increase in the respiratory burst of peritoneal Mø measured 24 hrs after injection. The intramuscular route of administration of cocaine also gave similar results with effects persisting for at least 24 hrs after exposure (data not shown).

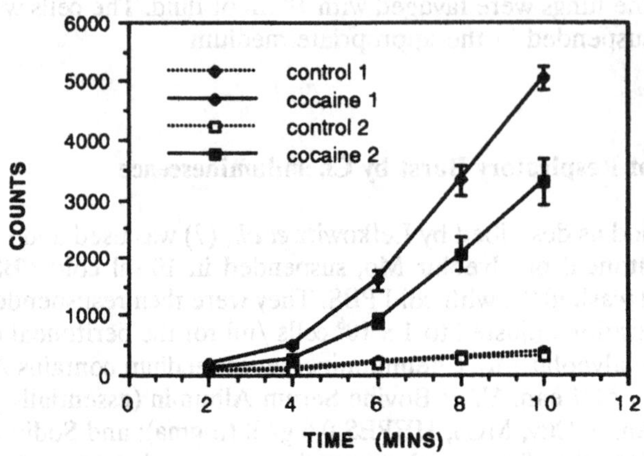

Fig. 1. **Enhancement of the respiratory burst of peritoneal macrophages 60 min. after a single i.p. injection of 2.5 mg/kg of cocaine.**

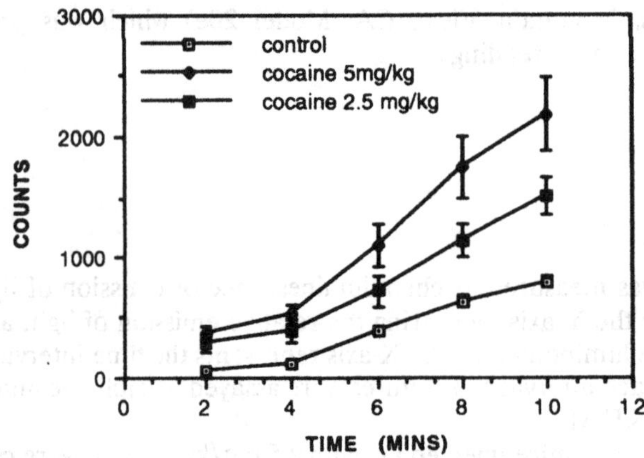

Fig. 2. **Enhancement of the respiratory burst of peritoneal macrophages 24 hr after a single i.p. injection of cocaine.**

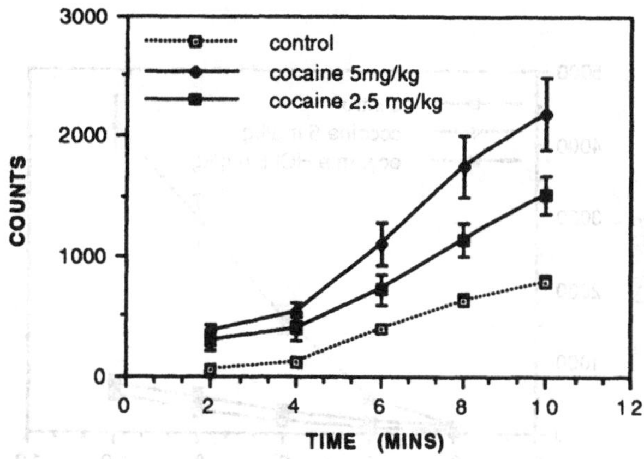

Fig. 3. Enhancement of the respiratory burst of peritoneal macrophages 24 hr after a single i.v. injection of cocaine.

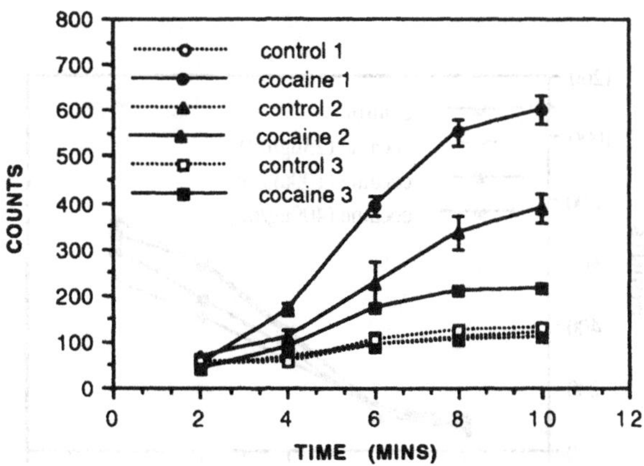

Fig. 4. Enhancement of the respiratory burst of alveolar macrophages 60 min. after a single i.p. in section of 10 mg/kg cocaine.

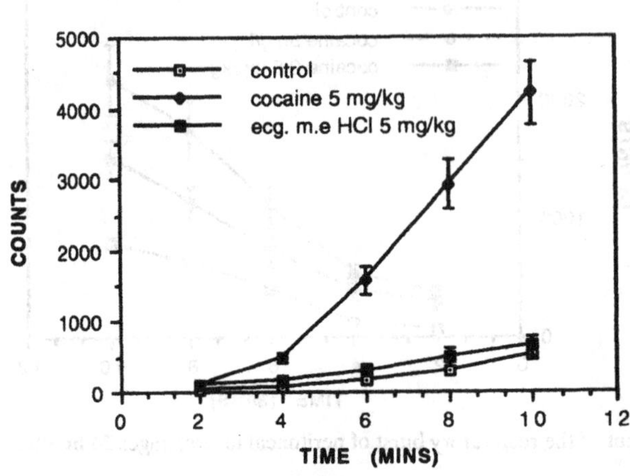

Fig. 5. Enhancement of the respiratory burst 1 hr after a 5 mg/kg injection of cocaine or ecgonine methyl ester HCl.

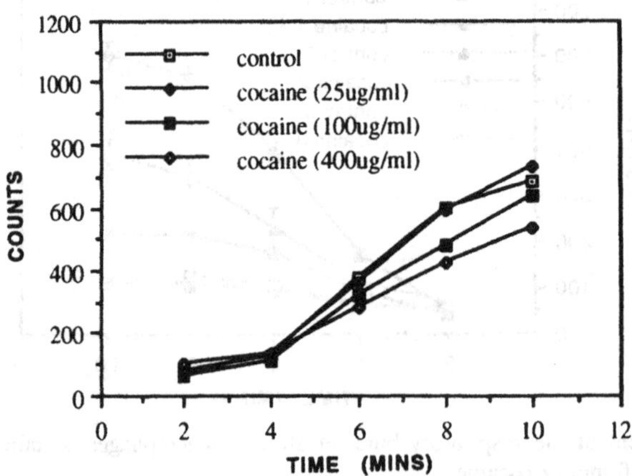

Fig. 6. Effect of cocaine on the respiratory burst of peritoneal macrophages 60 min. after exposure *in vitro*.

Alveolar Mø were also tested for their responses to injections of cocaine *in vivo*. A similar increase in the RB of alveolar Mø was obtained when measured at 60 min (Fig. 4) and 24 hrs (data not shown) after a single i.p. injection of 10 mg/kg cocaine. Luminescence was generally lower than that obtained with peritoneal Mø.

The next question addressed was whether the metabolites of cocaine induced a similar increase in the RB When 5 mg/kg of ecgonine methyl ester HCl (Fig. 5) or ecgonine HCl (data not shown), were injected i.p., neither affected the RB after 1 hr (Fig. 5). Twenty-four hours after exposure to cocaine *in vivo*, neither metabolite affected the RB of peritoneal Mø (data not shown).

Since a major increase in the RB of isolated Mø was observed when mice were exposed to cocaine *in vivo*, it was necessary to determine if cocaine affects Mø directly. *In vitro* exposure of peritoneal Mø to cocaine (25-400 μg/ml) for 60 min. had no apparent effect on the RB (Fig. 6). Experiments were also done exposing Mø to cocaine *in vitro* for 15 and 120 mins, however, no detectable effect was observed (data not shown).

DISCUSSION

The RB or "oxidative burst" measures the increase in superoxide and other reactive oxygen intermediates (ROI). The capacity to generate increased amounts of ROI is a consistent biochemical marker of metabolic activity. Since, phagocytosis by Mø is usually accompanied by an increase in the production of superoxide ions, the change in RB correlates strongly with phagocytic activity.

Among the major advantages of measuring the RB by chemiluminescence, is that the sensitivity of this method is extremely high and can exceed 10^{-12} M (8). Possibly, owing to the extreme sensitivity of the assay, we obtained an increase in the RB using lower quantities of cocaine (1.25 mg/kg). In other experiments, (to be reported elsewhere) measuring both phagocytic activity and macrophage-mediated cytotoxicity, differences were obtained only at higher doses of cocaine (5-25 mg/kg).

We observed an increase in the RB using various routes of cocaine administration. It did not matter whether the exposure to cocaine was via the i.m., i.v, or i.p. route. The increase in the RB was measured within one hour after cocaine exposure and persisted for up to 48 hrs.

Alveolar Mø produced less ROI than peritoneal Mø. It should be noted, however, that we used fewer alveolar Mø (2.5×10^4) than peritoneal Mø (1×10^5). This was necessary because of the 10 fold lower yields of alveolar Mø per mouse. Taking into account the differences in numbers of Mø used, the alveolar Mø still required a higher level of cocaine (10 mg/kg) to induce the same luminescence compared with peritoneal Mø.

The next question addressed was whether the metabolites of cocaine could cause a change in the RB similar to that obtained with cocaine. The metabolites ecgonine HCl and ecgonine methyl ester HCl which are formed from ester hydrolysis of cocaine, were used in these studies. These are generally inactive and nontoxic. These metabolites did not affect the RB. The effect of cocaine metabolites, which are produced from oxidation of the tropane nitrogen (i.e., norcocaine and N-hydroxynorcocaine) were not studied at this time. These metabolites are known to cause increased hepatotoxicity (9).

Lastly, we investigated whether cocaine would have a direct effect on murine Mø *in vitro*. We were not able to detect any changes in the RB when cocaine was incubated directly with Mø. This finding seems to suggest that cocaine may either act through its "active" metabolites or it may act secondarily through the induction of other pharmacologically active compounds. Since our data indicate that the ester hydrolytic metabolites do not have an effect *in vivo*, it is possible that the N-oxidative metabolites norcocaine and N-hydroxynorcocaine may be involved.

Acknowledgement

This study was supported by a grant from the Southwest Institute for Addictive Diseases, Lubbock, Texas 79430.

REFERENCES

1. J. M. VanDette and L. A. Cornish, Medical complications of illicit cocaine use, *Clin. Pharmacol.* 8:401 (1989).
2. B. Watzl and R. R. Watson, Immunomodulation by cocaine-A neuroendocrine mediated response, *Life Sciences* 46:1319 (1990).
3. R. C. Allen, R. L. Stjernholm and R. H. Steel, Evidence for generation of (an) electronic excitation state(s) in human polymorphonuclear leukocytes and its participation in bactericidal activity. *Biochem. Biophys. Res. Commun.* 47:679 (1972).
4. R. C. Allen, Biochemiexcitation: Chemiluminescence and the study of biological oxygenation reactions, *in*: "Chemical and Biological Generation of Excited States", W. Adams and G. Cliento, eds. p 309, Academic Press, NY (1982).
5. D. L. Lefkowitz, K. Mills, D. Morgan and S. S. Lefkowitz, Macrophage activation and Immunomodulation by Myeloperoxidase, *Proc. Soc. Exptl. Biol. Med.* 199:204 (1992).
6. P. G. Holt, Alveolar macrophages: I. A simple technique for the preparation of high numbers of viable alveolar macrophages from small laboratory animals, *J. Immunol. Methods.* 27:189 (1979).
7. D. L. Lefkowitz, S. S. Lefkowitz, Ru-Qi Wei and J. Everse, Activation of macrophages with oxidative enzymes, *in*: "Methods in Enzymol." G. Di Sabato and J. Everse, eds., Academic Press, Orlando, FL 132:537 (1986).
8. T. P. Whitehead, L. J. Kricka, T. J. N. Carter, and G. H. G. Thorpe, Analytical luminescence: its potential in the clinical laboratory, *Clin. Chem.* 25:1531 (1979).
9. M. L.Thompson, L. Shuster, and K. Shaw, Cocaine-induced hepatic necrosis in mice: the role of cocaine metabolism, *Biochem. Pharmacol.* 28:2389 (1979).

COCAINE FACILITATION OF CRYPTOSPORIDIOSIS BY MURINE AIDS IN MALE AD FEMALE C_{57}/BL/6 MICE

H. Darban, R.R. Watson, J. Alak, and N. Thomas

Department of Family and Community Medicine
NIAAA Specialized Alcohol Research Center
Tucson, AZ 85724

ABSTRACT

As cocaine may affect progression of the Human Immunodeficiency Virus (HIV) infection to Acquired Immune Deficiency Syndrome (AIDS), we used a murine model of AIDS (MAIDS) induced by LP-BM5 murine leukemia virus to examine cocaine's possible role as a cofactor for secondary parasitic infections. Dissimilarities between the sexes were observed both in the absence and presence of the cocaine. The retrovirus-infected female mice had a much higher rate of Cryptosporidiosis than the retrovirus-infected male mice. Female, but not male, retrovirus-infected mice showed approximately 20-fold more *Cryptosporidium* per villus section than controls. Compared to respective gender controls, male and female animals infected with the retrovirus infection manifested a heightened *Cryptosporidium* oocysts count regardless of cocaine treatment. Overall, female groups incurred a higher incidence of infection compared to respective male groups. To determine the role of cocaine, groups of male and female C57BL-6 mice of similar age were treated with cocaine for 4 weeks followed by termination. Cocaine synergized with retrovirus infection in female mice to cause a 30-fold increase in the number of oocyst present. The spleen size and weight of female mice was significantly greater than uninfected controls or male mice. However, due to the very slow progression to murine AIDS in the males, parasite resistance was retained, including in cocaine treated C57BL-6 mice. Thymus cell number in the retrovirus-infected female mice decreased significantly in comparison to uninfected female controls. Continued resistance to the parasite in male mice and its loss in female mice was due to the rate of immunosuppression and thus development of retrovirus-induced murine AIDS.

INTRODUCTION

Although cryposporidiosis was recognized in 1907 (1), self-limitation by immunocompetent individuals (2) caused its study to be neglected for 70 years. Immunocompromised and immunodeficient individuals developed life threatening

Drugs of Abuse, Immunity, and AIDS, Edited by
H Friedman *et al*, Plenum Press, New York, 1993

Cryptosporidium infections (3-5). Recently, its high incidence in patients with AIDS has set off an intensive study (3,6,7). Where a severe to life-threatening diarrhea may persist for many months. As AIDS progresses with increasing immunosuppression, parasite infection becomes worse (7). Animals rendered immunodeficient congenitally, as well as AIDS patients, develop persistent *Cryptosporidium* infections. The study of Cryptosporidium infection in AIDS patients has been hampered by the lack of an adult animal model with immunosuppression. *Cryptosporidium* has been detected on intestinal mucous of mammals, including cattle, sheep, and humans (3). As it is not a host-specific pathogen (8), animal models of AIDS to study the cryptosporidiosis (5,9) have been sought. Mice infected by LP-BM5 murine leukemia retrovirus infection develop many similar immunodeficiencies and symptoms (10-18) caused by HIV infection in humans. *Cryptosporidium* persists in mice immunosuppressed by LP-BM5 retrovirus infection which had progressed to AIDS (19), but not immunocompetent animals.

A variety of cofactors have been suggested which could modulate retrovirally induced immunosuppression and further reduce resistance to opportunistic pathogens (20). Immunosuppression might be expanded by use of drugs of abuse (21,22). In particular, intravenous use of cocaine has strong association with risk of retroviral infection and may increase risk of retroviral proliferation (23). Recently LP-BM5 murine leukemia infection in adult mice allowed *Cryptosporidium* to persist (24), as the first model of retroviral infection permitting persistent parasite colonization. This model allows the investigation of the combined effects of the immunosuppressive factors of drug abuse and retrovirus infection upon *Cryptosporidium* resistance.

MATERIALS AND METHODS

Mice

Female C57BL/6 mice at 3-4 wks of age were obtained from the Charles River Laboratories, Inc. (Boston, MA.). They weighed approximately 15 g and were randomly assigned to different groups. Five mice per cage were housed in transparent lastic cages with a stainless steel wire lid in a room at 20-22°C with constant humidity and 12:12 hour light-dark cycle.

LP-BM5 Murine Leukemia Virus Infection

The mice assigned to the virus infected groups were injected intraperitoneally with 0.1 ml of an LP-BM5 (a gift from Dr. Robert Yetter) inoculum which had ectopic titer (xc) of 4.5 log 10 and PFU/ml and induced disease with a time course comparable to that published (25). Infection of adult female C57BL/6 mice with the retrovirus LP-BM5 leads to the rapid induction of clinical symptomology with virtually no latent phase (11-14). All mice were infected as shown by enlarged lymph nodes and spleens at 3-5 months post-infection indicating lymphoid cell proliferation.

Oocyst Suspension

Cryptosporidium oocysts originally obtained from Dr. H. Moon and were isolated from a calf. Feces were suspended in 2 volumes of 2.5 % potassium dichromate solution. This suspension was passed through a graded series of sieves to exclude particles larger than 63 μm, then subjected to discontinuous sucrose and isopycnic percoll centrifugation procedures and isolated oocysts were stored at 4°C (26). Before the mice were inoculated, the oocysts preparations (less than 2 wks old) were washed with 0.025 M phosphate-buffered saline (pH 7.2) to remove the potassium dichromate and counted with a hemacytometer by phase-contrast microscopy. Mice were inoculated via a stomach tube with 100 μl of concentrated material containing 1 x 10^5 oocysts after 4 wks of drugs injection.

Drug Treatment

One month after infection with LP-BM5 murine leukemia virus, the mice received interperitoneal cocaine injections daily. The dosages were as follows: 20 mg of cocaine HCl/kg body weight (BW)/day (first wk), 30 mg of cocaine HCl/kg BW/day (second week), and 40 mg of cocaine HCl/kg BW/day (third week). All mice after the third week received the highest dosage until termination.

RESULTS

Retrovirus Modification of Animal and Spleen Weight

No significant changes were observed in the body weights of the different groups of female and male mice (Table 1). However, spleen weights (Table 1) and spleen cell numbers of the retroviral infected female groups increased significantly ($P < .05$) compared to similarly treated non-retroviral infected mice (2.9 ± 0.8 versus 4.9 ± 2.8). This was also true with cocaine injected retroviral infected mice versus non-treated retrovirus infected mice (3.0 ± 0.9 versus 5.4 ± 1.4).

Cryptosporidium Detection in Feces and Villi of Retrovirally-Infected Mice

Feces isolated from the retrovirally infected female mice were collected from a 2 cm posterior portion of intestine. They showed a higher number of oocysts than from non-retrovirally infected controls (Table 2). The percentage of retrovirally infected female mice infected with *Cryptosporidium* also was higher than controls (Table 2). There was a significant ($P < .05$) increase in the number of parasites per villus section of the retrovirally infected female mice compared to controls infected simultaneously with *Cryptosporidium* (Table 3).

As a group, more animals with MAIDS were infected with oocysts if treated with cocaine than the saline injected mice. These changes were not seen in non-retrovirally infected animals. The drug treated non-retrovirally infected mice, when evaluated as a single group, were not different from saline injected mice in the non-retrovirally infected groups. In the male mice, parasite resistance was retained including in cocaine treated C57BL6 mice (Table 3).

DISCUSSION

Cryptosporidiosis is a common infection in immunosuppressed and immunocompromised individuals. In mice, exposure to the parasite does not appear to be necessary for the development of resistance to infection (27). Mice older than 3 weeks of age are resistant to Cryptosporidium, even in the absence of previous exposure (28,29). In the LP-BM5 induced murine AIDS model, mice are more susceptible to opportunistic infection (10) including *Cryptosporidium* (19). This was reconfirmed here as retrovirus infected mice had greater parasite colonization. Diarrhea, intestinal injury, and Animal weight and spleen weight of female and male mice infected with LP-BM5 and injected with cocaine.malnutrition are very common among patients with AIDS (30).

Table 1. Animal weight and spleen weight of female and male mice infected with LP-BM5 and injected with cocaine.

Treatment Retrovirus	Injection	Animal Weight (g) (Female)	Spleen Weight (g) (Male)	Animal Weight (g) (Male)	Spleen Weight (g) (Male)
-	Saline	24.0 ± 0.8	0.09 ± 0.0	29.8 ± 2.7	0.08 ± 0.02
-	Cocaine	22.4 ± 1.2	0.07 ± 0.0	31.1 ± 2.6	0.13 ± 0.03
+	Saline	24.4 ± 1.3	0.52 ± 0.4*	30.5 ± 1.5	0.15 ± 0.06*
+	Cocaine	24.4 ± 1.3	0.37 ± 0.1*	28.5 ± 1.5	0.17 ± 0.06*

*Significantly different at the $p < .05$ level from saline treated non-retrovirus infected mice.
N = Number of mice per group as shown on Table 2.

Table 2. Number of *Cryptosporidium* oocysts present in feces of retrovirus infected female and male mice.

Treatment Retrovirus	Injection	Number of Oocysts in Feces (Female)	Positive Mice (%) (Female)	Number of Oocysts in Feces (Male)	Positive Mice (%) (Male)
-	Saline	1.5 ± 4.5	25 (8)	0.0 ± 0.0	0 (4)
-	Cocaine	0.6 ± 1.7	13 (8)	0.1 ± 0.0	0 (5)
+	Saline	32 ± 38*	86* (7)	0.11 ± 0.03	20* (5)
+	Cocaine	20 ± 24*	100* (7)	0.05 ± 0.04	25* (4)

*Significantly different at the $p < 0.05$ level from saline treated non-retrovirally infected mice.
( ) = Number of mice per group.

Table 3. Number of *Cryptosporidium* present on villi of female and male mice infected with LP-BM5 and injected with cocaine

Treatment		*Cryptosporidium*/ Villus Section	*Cryptosporidium*/ Villus Section
Retrovirus	Injection	(Female)	(Male)
-	Saline	0.15 ± 0.17	0.00 ± 0.00
-	Cocaine	0.17 ± 0.18	0.00 ± 0.00*
+	Saline	2.30 ± 1.40*	0.11 ± 0.10*
+	Cocaine	6.80 ± 5.60*+	0.27 ± 0.20*

*Significantly different at the $p < 0.05$ level from saline treated non-retrovirus infected mice.
+Significantly different at the $p < 0.05$ level from saline treated retrovirus infected mice.
N = Number of mice per group as shown on Table 2. Controls were age matched but not retrovially infected. Data are parasites per villus section (mean ± SE) as determined by histologic sections of terminal ileum (at least 25 sections per villus).

Damage to the mucous membranes in the gastrointestinal tract caused by protozoan infection may impair the intestinal tract's ability to maintain its integrity as a barrier against the external environment. *Cryptosporidium*, the most common enteric disease in AIDS patients, causes a chronic debilitating diarrheal illness (31). Diarrhea in patients with AIDS is associated with enhanced immunosuppression, morbidity and mortality (31).

In non-retrovirally infected mice, cocaine injection caused no significant differences in the number of oocysts in feces or villus section, nor in the percentage of mice infected with *Cryptosporidium*. However, there were significant differences in parasite infection of retrovirally infected male and female mice. Murine retroviral infection facilitated *Cryptosporidium* growth in adult mice which was aggravated by cocaine injection. This suggests that cocaine may be a co-factor in retrovirally induced suppression of the immune system. Several recent reviews suggest that cocaine's damage to the immune system should accelerate immunosuppression due to AIDS (32-34).

The above observation of a sex difference in murine AIDS may be relevant to human AIDS. While epidemiological research has not revealed a difference in the progression of AIDS between male and female humans (35), nevertheless, there may exist gender-related factors which have not been discerned in humans. One factor could be the effect of sex hormones upon autoimmunity, which may be an important aspect of AIDS (36-40). LP-BM5, as well as HIV, contain superantigenic components (41-42), which are believed to be important causative factors of autoimmunity (43). Autoimmune conditions are manifest with greater severity and incidence in females of human and animal species (44-48). Male C57BL6 mice are more resistant to LP-BM5 infection. It is definitely a Y-linked effect which seems to be, at least in part, a result of slower increase in LP-BM5 MuLV burden. They appear not to replicate the retrovirus as well as females (personal communication with Dr. Robert Yetter). Male and female hormones may contribute to these differences, as androgens down regulate autoimmune conditions whereas estrogens exert an upregulatory effect (49-51). Interestingly, tamoxifen, an estrogen blocker, inhibits induction of HIV replication (40). Whether this effect is exerted upon LP-BM5 remains to be determined.

Murine retroviral infection in mice functions as a model to study *Cryptosporidium* disease in AIDS patients. Our findings suggest that use of cocaine is a cofactor for *Cryptosporidium* infection in AIDS patients.

Acknowledgement

This project supported by NIH grants AAO8037. A special thanks to Mrs. Gail Crawford for her contributions to this project. Appreciation to B. Issel for his comments to the Discussion section.

REFERENCES

1. E. E. Tyzzer, A sporozoan found in the peptic glands of the common mous, *Proc. Soc. Exp. Biol. Med.* 5:12 (1907).
2. M. H. Hart, R. Kruger, S. Nielson, and S.S. Kaufman. Acute self-limited colitis associated with Cryptosporidium in an immunocompetent patient, *J. Pediatr. Gastroenterol. Nutr.* 8:401(1989).
3. R. Fayer, and B.L.P. Unger, Cryptosporidium SPP and Cryptosporidiosis, *Microbiol. Rev.* 50:458 (1986).
4. R. M.D. Dias, A.C.S. Mangini, D.M.G.V. Torres, M.O.A. Corra, N. Lupetti, F.M.A. Corra, and P.P. Chieffi, Cryptosporidiosis among patients with acquired immunodeficiency syndrome (AIDS) in the country of Sao Paulo, Brazil, *Rev. Inst. med. Trop. Sao Paulo* 30:310 (1988).
5. B. L.P. Nuger, J.A. Burris, C.A. Quinn, and F. Finkelman, New mouse models for chronic Cryptosporidium infection in immunodeficient hosts, *Infect. Immun.* 58:961 (1990).
6. M. Armstrong, Cryptosporidiosis, *Med. Lab. Sci.* 44:280 (1987).

7. W. L. Current, N.R. Reese, J.V. Ernst, W.S. Bailey, M.B. Heyman, and W.M. Weinstein, Human cryptosporidiosis in immunocompetent and immunodeficient persons, Studies of an outbreak and experimental transmission, *N. Eng. J. Med.* 308:1252 (1983).
8. R. Soave, and D. Armstrong, Cryptosporidium and cryptosporidiosis, *Rev. Infect. Dis.* 8:1012 (1986).
9. C. Chrisp, W.C. Reid, H.G. Rush, M.A. Sucknow, A. Bush, and M.J. Thomann, Cryptosporidiosis in Guinea pigs: An animal model, *Infect. Immun.* 58:647 (1990).
10. S. K. Chattopadhyay, M. Makino, J.W. Harlety, and H.C. Morse III, Pathogenesis of MAIDS: a retrovirus-induced immunodeficiency disease of mice, *in*: "Immune-deficient anlmal in experimental medicine, Sixth International Workshop on Immune-Deficient Animals, B-Q. Wu, and J. Zeng, eds., Basel Karger, p. 12 (1989.(1988).
11. R. R. Watson, Murine models for acquired immune deficiency syndrome, *Life Sci.* 44:1-xiii (1989).
12. L. A. Salzman, ed. "Animal Models of Retrovirus Infection and their Relationship to AIDS", Academic Press, Orlando, FL, (1986).
13. D. E. Mosier, R.A. Yetter, and H.C. Morse III, Retroviral induction of acute lymphoproliferative disease and profound immunosuppression in adult C47BL/6 mice, *J. Exp. Med.* 161:766 (1985).
14. S. P. Ninken, T.N. Fredrickson, J.W. Hartley, R.A. Yetter, and H.C. Morse III., Evaluation of B-cell lineage lymphomas in mice with retrovirus-induced immunodeficiency syndromes, MAIDS, *J. Immunol.* 140:1123 (1988).
15. R. M.L. Buller, R.A. Yetter, T.N. Fredrickson, and H.C. Morse III, Abrogation of resistance to severe mouse pox in C57BL/6 mice infected with LP-BM5 murine leukemia viruses, *J. Virol.* 61:383 (1987).
16. D. E. Mosier, Animal models for retrovirus-induced immunodeficiency disease, *Immunol. Invest.* 15:233 (1986).
17. D. E. Mosier, R.A. Yetter, and H.C. Morse III, Functional T-lymphocytes are required for a murine retrovirus-induced immunodeficiency disease (MAIDS), *J. Exp. Med.* 165:1737 (1987).
18. A. Cerny, A.W. Hugin, R.R. Hardy, K. Hayakawa, R.M. Zinkernagel, M. Makino, and H.C. Morse III, B cells are required for induction of T-cell abnormalities in murine retrovirus-induced immunodeficiency model, *J. Exp. Med.* 171:315 (1990).
19. H. Darban, J. Enriquez, C.R. Sterling, M.C. Lopez, G. Chen, R.R. Watson, and M. Abaszadegan, Cryptosporidiosis facilitated by murine retroviral infection with LP-BM5, *J. Infect. Dis.* 164:741 (1991).
20. R. Taghi-Kilani, L. Sekla, and K.T. Hayglass, The role of humoral immunity in Cryptosporidium SPP infection studies with B cell-depleted mice, *J. Immunol.* 145:1571 (1990).
21. B. Watzl, and R.R. Watson, Immunomodulation by cocaine -- A neuroendocrine mediated response, *Life Sci* 46:1319 (1990).
22. M. Holsapple, and A. Munson, Immunotoxicology of abused drugs, *in:* "Immunotoxicol. and Immunopharmacol." J. Dean, ed.,Raven Press, NY, pp. 381-392 (1985).
23. D. W. Ou, M. Shen, and Y-D Luo, Effect of cocaine on the immune system of BALB/c mice, *Clin. Immunol. Immunopathol.* 52:305 (1989).
24. G. Chen, and R.R. Watson, Modulation of tumor necrosis factor and gamma interferon production by cocaine and morphine in aging mice infected with LP-BMS, a murine retrovirus, *J. Leuk. Biol.* 50:349 (1991).
25. S. Chattopadhyay, K. Sisio, M. Makino, J.W. Hartley, and H.C. Morse III, Pathogenesis of MAIDS, a retrovirus-induced immunodeficiency disease of mice, *Immunodeficient Animals in Experimental Med.* 12:18 (1989).
26. M. J. Arrowood, J.R. Mead, J.L. Mahrt, and C.R. Sterling, Effects of immune colostrum and orally administered anti-sporozoite monoclonal antibodies on the outcome of Cryptosporidium parvum infections in neonatal mice, *Infect. Immun.* 57:2283 (1989).
27. J. A. Harp, and H.W. Moon, Susceptibility of mast cell-deficient w/wV mice to *Cryptosporidium parvum*, *Infect. Immun.* 59:718 (1991).
28. J. A. Ernest, B.L. Balgburn, D.L. Lindsey, and W.L. Current, Infection dynamics of *Cryptosporidium parvum* in neonatal mice, *J. Parasitol.* 72:796-98 (1986).
29. J. A. Harp, M.W. Wannemuehler, D.B. Woodmansee, andH.W. Moon, Susceptibility of germ free or antibiotic-treated adult mice to *Cryptosporidium parvum*, *Infect. Immun.* 56:2006 (1988).
30. D. P. Kotler, H.P. Gaetz, M. Lange, and P.R. Holf, Enteropathy associated with the acquired immunodeficiency syndrome, *Ann. Intern. Med.* 101:421(1984).
31. T. J. Quinn, Protozoan infections, *in*: "Gastrointestinal infections in AIDS" Smith PD, moderator, *Ann. Intern. Med.* 116:63 (1992).p 66-68.
32. R. M. Pillai, and R.R. Watson, AIDS: Disease progression and immunomodulation by drugs of abuse and alcohol, *AIDS Med Report* 4:25 (1991).
33. R. M. Pillai, and R.R. Watson, *In vitro* immunotoxico}ogy and immunopharmacology: Studies on drugs of abuse, *Toxicol. Letters* 53:269 (1990).

34. R. R. Watson, Cofactors in HIV infection: Progression to AIDS and increased susceptibility to disease, *AIDS Med Report* 4:74 (1991).
35. T. V. Ellerbrock, T.J. Bush, M.E. Chamberland, and M.J. Oxtoby, Epidemiology of women with AIDS in the United States, 1981, through 1990. A comparison with heterosexual men with AIDS, *JAMA* 265:2971 (1991).
36. T. Beardsley, Cross reaction, Could AIDS really be an autoimmune disease? *Sci. Am.* 265:56 (1991).
37. G. W. Hoffman, T.A. Kion, and M.D. Grant, An idiotypic network model of AIDS immunopathogenesis, *Proc. of the Nat. Acad. Sci.* 88:3060 (1991).
38. W. J. Morrow, D.A. Isenberg, R.E. Sobol, R.B. Stricker, and T. Kieber-Emmons, AIDS virus infection and autoimmunity: a perspective of the clinical, immunological, and molecular origins of the autoallergic pathologies associated with HIV disease, Clin *Immun. and Immunopath.* 58:163 (1991).
39. A. M. Solinger, and E.V. Hess, Induction of autoantibodies by human immunodeficiency virus infection and their significance, *Rheum. Dis. Clin. of NAm.* 17:157 (1991).
40. A. W. Hugin, M.S. Vaccio, and H.C. Morse III, A virus encoded "superantigen" in a retrovirus-induced immunodeficiency syndrome of mice, *Sci.* 252:424 (1991).
41. J. Laurence, H. Cooke, and S.K. Sikder, Effects of tamoxifen on regulation of viral replication and human immunodeficiency virus (HIV) long terminal repeat-directed transcription cells chronically infected with HIV-1, *Blood* 75:696 (1990).
42. L. Imberti, A. Sottini, A. Bettinardi, M. Puoti, and D. Primi, Selective depletion in HIV infection of T cells that bear specific T cell receptor V beta sequences, *Sci.* 254:860 (1991).
43. C. G. Drake, and B.L. Kotzin, Superantigens: Biology, immunology, and potential role in disease, *J. Clin. Immunol.* 12:149 (1992).
44. F. Homo-Delarche, F. Fitzpatrick, N. Christeff, E.A. Nunez, J.F. Bach, and M. Dardenne, Sex steroids, glucocorticoids, stress and autoimmunity, *J. Ster. Biochem. Mol. Biol.* 9:619 (1991).
45. C. J. Grossman, G.A. Roselle, and C.L. Mendenhall, Sex steroid regulation of autoimmunity, *J. Ster. Biochem. Mol. Biol.* 11:649 (1991).
46. A. H. Schuurs, and H.A. Verheul, Sex hormones and autoimmune disease, *Brit. J. Rheum.* 28:59 (1989).
47. N. Talal, Autoimmunity and sex revisited, *Clin. Immunol. Immunopath.* 53:355 (1989).
48. N. Talal, and S.A. Ahmed, Sex hormones, CD5+ (Lyl+) B- cells, and autoimmune diseases, *Israel J. Med. Sci.* 24:725 (1988).
49. S. A. Ahmed, and N. Talal, Sex hormones and the immune system--Part 2, Animal data, *Baillieres Clin. Rheumat.* 4:13 (1990).
50. A. H. Schuurs, and H.A. Verheul, Effects of gender and sex steroids on the immune response, *J. of Ster. Biochem.* 35:157 (1990).
51. H. Carlsten, R. Holmdahl, A. Tarkowski, and L.A. Nilsson, Oestradiol-and testosterone-mediated effects on the immune system in normal and autoimmune mice are genetically linked and inherited as dominant traits, *Immunol.* 68:209 (1989).

ETHANOL-INDUCED SUPPRESSION OF *IN VIVO* HOST DEFENSE MECHANISMS TO BACTERIAL INFECTION

Thomas R. Jerrells,[1] A. Joe Saad,[2] and Thomas E. Kruger [1]

[1]Department of Cellular Biology and Anatomy, Louisiana State Univ. Med. Center, Shreveport, LA 71130
[2]Department of Pathology, Baylor College of Medicine, One Baylor Plaza, Houston, Texas 77030

Study findings have shown that chronic ethanol (ETOH) abuse causes individuals to have an increased incidence of infections related to opportunistic and pathogenic organisms (1-3). This is particularly true for bacterial pneumonias, which cause greater mortality in alcoholics as compared with nonalcoholics. Alcoholics also have an increased incidence of tumors of the head, neck, and gastrointestinal tract (4,5). Individuals with alcohol-induced liver cirrhosis have circulating lymphocytes that are cytotoxic to hepatocytes, suggesting that ETOH may induce an immune dysfunction that leads to autoimmunity (6-8). Although the exact role of ETOH in these diseases is not well understood, its effects on both specific and nonspecific aspects of immune function are thought to be involved. With ETOH consumption, many of the nonspecific aspects of immune function are altered. For example, consumption of ETOH by mice leads to depressed natural killer cell activity (9). Ethanol consumption also results in diminished granulocyte function such as decreased phagocytosis and altered migration to chemotactic factors by polymorphonuclear leukocytes (10,11). Ethanol directly alters monocyte and macrophage functions in human beings and experimental animals. For example, exposure of human macrophages to ETOH *in vitro* reduces the production and release of lysozyme, as well as the total number of macrophages containing lysozyme (12). Furthermore, study findings have shown that ETOH impairs phagocytosis in human monocytes and macrophages (13). Similar results have been obtained by investigators examining the effects of ETOH on rat peritoneal, alveolar, and splenic macrophages (14,15). Additionally, ETOH suppresses the production of tumor necrosis factor-alpha by rat alveolar macrophages and interferon gamma by mouse splenocytes (16,17), two important cytokines involved in the activation of macrophages.

The effects of ETOH on nonspecific aspects of immune function after ETOH consumption have also been demonstrated. With the use of a murine model, in which half the mice are maintained on an ETOH-containing (7% v\v) Leiber-DeCarli liquid diet and the other half (control group) are pair-fed an isocaloric Leiber-DeCarli diet without ETOH, ETOH consumption results in drastic alterations in the cellularity of the

Drugs of Abuse, Immunity, and AIDS, Edited by
H. Friedman *et al.*, Plenum Press, New York, 1993

peripheral lymphoid organs, such as the thymus and spleen. When compared with the numbers of thymocytes found in the pair-fed control diet animals, mice receiving ETOH diet for 7 days lost approximately 72% of the thymocytes that make up this tissue (18,19). After 14 days when the loss of thymocytes increased to 93.8%, as compared to that observed in control animals. Interestingly, with the absolute numbers of mature thymocytes were diminished, the greatest numbers of cells lost from this tissue although seemed to be immature thymocytes, as determined by flow cytometric analysis of CD4+/CD8+, peanut agglutinin+ (PNA+) (immature), and CD4+/CD8-, CD4-/-CD8+ (mature) henotypes (19). Of the mature thymocytes lost from this tissue, the CD4-/CD8+ thymocytes were depleted in the greatest numbers. The cell loss from this tissue after 14 days of ETOH consumption was so great that, in sections of the extricated thymus stained with hematoxylin-eosin, the medullary and cortical regions were almost indistinguishable.

The effects of ETOH after consumption of ETOH were evident in the spleens of mice. The number of splenocytes isolated from mice maintained on ETOH-containing diet for 14 days was 64% less than the total number of splenocytes isolated from control animals. Although the percentage of Thy 1.2+ cells in the spleen increased, their absolute number was reduced after ETOH consumption. The greatest ETOH effect after 14 days of ETOH consumption was on the number of B cells in the spleen. In comparing the total number of surface IgM+ splenocytes isolated from control and ETOH-treated animals, the total number of B cells was reduced from 38.5 million per spleen in the control group to 8.2 million per spleen in the ETOH-consuming group. This represents approximately a fivefold reduction in the number of splenic B cells after 14 days of ETOH consumption. Taken together the findings from this work (18,19) support the suggestion that ETOH consumption results in numerous adverse effects on many nonspecific aspects of immunity, including a reduction in the cellularity of lymphoid tissues. Ethanol consumption also may alter specific aspects of the immune response, in particular those mediated by T cells. In examining the proliferative responses of splenocytes isolated from control animals and animals consuming ETOH diets, it was found that an ETOH-induced inhibition in the ability of T cells to proliferate in response to both mitogenic (concanavalin A) and antigenic (mixed lymphocyte reaction) stimuli existed (18). Although there was no difference in the lipopolysaccharide response of splenic B cells in control and ETOH-treated animals, splenic B cells from ETOH consuming animals were impaired in their ability to produce antibody to a T-cell-dependent antigen (sheep red blood cells). These cells were, however, able to respond to a T-cell-independent antigen (TNP-ficoll) (18). Similar results have been observed in a rat model, demonstrating a lack of ETOH effects on the T-cell-independent antibody response to pneumococcal polysaccharide (20). Thus the findings support the suggestion that animals that consume ETOH have defective T-cell-dependent immune function but at least some aspects of normal B-cell function.

One possible explanation for T-cell dysfunction after ETOH consumption is that these cells may be unable to use or respond to various cytokines. Results of studies, examining splenic T cells from rats given ETOH (by gastric intubation) for 4 days, revealed a defect in the ability of concanavalin A-induced T-cell blasts to proliferate in response to recombinant interleukin-2 (rIL-2), whereas the T-cell blasts generated from the control animals responded normally. The T-cell blasts from both groups bound similar amounts of iodinated rIL-2 by the high-affinity IL-2 receptor (21). Other investigators have demonstrated ETOH-induced impairments in the ability of cells of the immune system to produce and respond to various cytokines. For example, ETOH has been shown to suppress macrophage production of tumor necrosis factor-alpha (17) and T-cell production of interferon-gamma (16). Results of recent studies suggest that ETOH inhibits the production of interferon alpha or interferon-beta (or both) by mouse splenocytes (16). An extension of these observations is that human macrophages and Kupffer cells are impaired in their ability to respond to tumor necrosis factor-alpha and granulocyte-macrophage colony-stimulating factor after ETOH exposure *in vitro* (22). These findings support the suggestion that observed defects in nonspecific and specific aspects of immunity after ingestion of ETOH may be due in part to an inability of cells of the immune system to produce or respond to appropriate cytokines during an immune response.

The effects of ETOH consumption on the *in vivo* murine host response to the obligate intracellular bacteria *Listeria monocytogenes* have been examined (23). Mice received a Leiber DeCarli diet, with or without ETOH, for 7 days and then were infected intravenously with Listeria at 0.5 median lethal dose (LD_{50}; 2.5 x 10^4 bacteria). At 2 and 5 days after infection, the host response in the liver was assessed by (1) using immunohistochemical studies and (2) determining the serum levels of liver enzymes released from lysed parenchymal cells and Listeria colony counts from isolated liver tissue.

Examination of hematoxylin-eosin stained sections of liver 2 days after infection revealed similar sized lesions in both ETOH and control diet groups. Although similar numbers of acute inflammatory cells found in the liver abscesses suggests no impairment in the ability of these animals to mount an acute inflammatory response to Listeria, ETOH-consuming animals had elevated serum levels of aspartate aminotransferase (AST) and alanine aminotransferase (ALT), suggesting greater pathologic changes occurred in the ETOH diet group. Additionally, Listeria colony counts from liver isolates were clearly higher in the ETOH diet group when compared with those observed in control diet animals. At 5 days after infection, distinct differences were noted in the liver lesions in comparisons of ETOH and control diet groups. In the control diet group, lesions appeared as small granulomas. In contrast, the ETOH diet group had large liver lesions that contained large numbers of acute and chronic inflammatory cells. No granuloma formation was observed in hematoxylin-eosin stained liver sections from the ETOH diet group 5 days after infection. Additionally, liver enzymes remained higher in the ETOH diet group than in control diet animals, suggesting that the clearance of Listeria from the livers of ETOH-consuming animals was impaired. These results are most likely not due to impaired Kupffer cell activity because both ETOH and control diet animals were able to clear (within the first 18 hrs after infection) 90% of an initial intravenous injection of Listeria that reached the liver. These findings further show that ETOH consumption does not impair the influx of inflammatory cells into the liver, but does reduce the ability of the host to inhibit Listeria growth resulting in greater liver pathogenesis.

Because protection against Listeria depends completely on antigen-specific T cells, particularly the production of interferon-gamma by the T cell, the effect of ETOH consumption on the anti-Listeria immune response in Listeria-immune mice was examined. Mice were given an immunizing dose of Listeria (2.5 x 10^3 bacteria) and maintained for 9 days on laboratory chow and water. After this 9-day period, they were assigned randomly to either a treatment (Leiber-DeCarli diet with ETOH) or control (Leiber-DeCarli diet without ETOH) group and maintained for 7 days. After this time, they were challenged with a lethal dose (5 LD_{50} or 2.5 x 10^5 bacteria) of Listeria. Five days after infection, the host response in the liver was assessed as described earlier. Animals consuming ETOH diet had lesions containing numerous polymorphonuclear lymphocytes and mononuclear inflammatory cells surrounded by regions of hepatic necrosis. Control animals had numerous granulomatous lesions, which were much smaller than the lesions in ETOH-consuming animals. No granuloma formation was found in hematoxylin-eosin stained liver sections from the ETOH-consuming animals. Although liver enzyme (AST and ALT) levels were elevated in the control diet animals, the levels observed in ETOH consuming animals were approximately five times those of control animals. Listeria colony counts from liver homogenates demonstrated approximately 100-fold more Listeria in the ETOH diet animals as compared with the numbers of bacteria in control diet immune animals. Finally, although the mortality rate in the ETOH-consuming Listeria immune mice was approximately 10% to 43%, none of the control diet immune mice died.

These findings show that ETOH increases the susceptibility of mice to infection with the intracellular bacterium, *L. monocytogenes*. Although ETOH consumption did not appear to impair the acute and chronic inflammatory response to this bacteria, ETOH-consumption did impair the ability of immune and nonimmune animals to clear Listeria from the infective foci in the liver. These results demonstrated that ETOH-consumption results in an impairment of immune function during an ongoing infection with the intracellular bacteria *L. monocytogenes*.

Acknowledgement

This research was supported by National Institute on Alcoholism and Alcohol Abuse Grants AA 07731 and AA 00129. We thank Janice Jerrells for professional editorial assistance.

REFERENCES

1. H. G. Adams, and C. Jordan, Infections in the alcoholic, *Med. Clin. North Am.* 68:179 (1984).
2. R. R. MacGregor, Alcohol and immune defense, *J. Am.Med. Assoc.* 256:1474 (1986).
3. F. E. Smith, and D.L. Palmer, Alcoholism, infection and altered host defenses - review of clinical and experimental observations, *J. Chronic Dis.* 29:35 (1976).
4. J. H. Breeden, Alcohol, alcoholism, and cancer, *Med. Clin. North Am.* 68:163 (1984).
5. I. Martinez, Retrospective and prospective study of carcinoma of the esophagus, mouth, and pharynx in Puerto Rico, *Bol. Assoc. Med. PR.* 62:170 (1970).
6. A. M. Cochrane, A. Moussouros, B. Portman, et al., Lymphocyte cytotoxicity for isolated hepatocytes in alcoholic liver disease, *Gastroenterol.* 72:918 (1977).
7. S. Kakumu, and C.M. Leevy, Lymphocyte cytotoxicity in alcoholic hepatitis, *Gastroenterol.* 72:594 (1977).
8. M. G. Mutchnick, A. Missirian, and A.G. Johnson, Lymphocyte cytotoxicity in human liver disease using rat hepatocyte monolayer cultures, *Clin. Immunol. Immunopathol.* 16:423 (1980).
9. G. G. Meadows, S.E. Blank, and D.D. Duncan, Influence of ethanol consumption on natural killer cell activity in mice, *Alcohol Clin. Exp. Res.* 13:476 (1989).
10. R. G. Brayton, P.E. Stokes, M.S. Schwartz, and D.B. Louria, Effect of alcohol and various diseases on leukocyte mobilization, phagocytosis and intracellular bacterial killing, *N. Engl. J. Med.* 282:123 (1970).
11. P. J. Spagnuolo and R.R. MacGregor, Acute ethanol effect of chemotaxis and other components of host defense, *J. Lab. Clin. Med.* 86:24 (1975).
12. S. P. McCarthy, C.E. Lewis, and J.O. McGee, Effects of ethanol on human monocyte/macrophage lysozyme storage and release. Implications for the pathobiology of alcoholic liver disease, *J. Hepatol.* 10:90 (1990).
13. N. E. Gilhus, and R. Matre, *In vitro* effect of ethanol on subpopulations of human blood mononuclear cells, *Int. Arch. Allergy Appl. Immunol.* 68:382 (1982).
14. O. Bagasra, A. Howeedy, and A. Kajdacsy-Balla, Macrophage function in chronic experimental alcoholism. I. Modulation of surface receptors and phagocytosis, *Immunol.* 65:405 (1988).
15. B. Morland, and J. Morland, Effects of long-term ethanol consumption on rat peritoneal macrophages, *ACTA Pharmacol. Toxicol.* (Copenh) 50:221 (1982).
16. K. C.Chadha, I. Stadler, B. Albini, S.M. Nakeeb, and H.R. Thacore, Effect of alcohol on spleen cells and their functions in C57BL/6 mice, *Alcohol* 8:481 (1991).
17. S. Nelson, G.J. Bagby, and W.R. Summer, Alcohol-induced suppression of tumor necrosis factor - a potential risk factor for secondary infection in the acquired immunodeficiency syndrome, *in*: "Alcohol, Immunomodulation, and AIDS", D. Seminara, R.R. Watson, and A. Pawlowski, eds., Alan R. Liss, Inc., New York pp 211-220, (1990).
18. T. R. Jerrells, W. Smith, and M.J. Eckardt, Murine model of ethanol-induced immunosuppression, *Alcohol Clin. Exp. Res.* 14:546 (1990).

19. A. J. Saad, and T.R. Jerrells, Flow cytometric and immunohistochemical evaluation of ethanol-induced changes in splenic and thymic lymphoid cell populations, *Alcohol Clin. Exp. Res.* 15:796 (1991).
20. O. Bagasra, A. Howeedy, R. Dorio, and A. Kajdacsy-Balla, Functional analysis of T-cell subsets in chronic experimental alcoholism, *Immunol.* 61:63 (1987).
21. T. R. Jerrells, D. Peritt, M.J. Eckardt, and C. Marietta, Alterations in interleukin-2 utilization by T-cells from rats treated with an ethanol-containing diet, *Alcohol Clin. Exp. Res.* 14:245 (1990).
22. L. E. Bermudez, and L.S. Young, Ethanol augments intracellular survival of *Mycobacterium avium* complex and impairs macrophage responses to cytokines, *J. Infect. Dis.* 163:1286 (1991).
23. A. J. Saad, and T.R. Jerrells, Ethanol ingestion increases susceptibility of mice to *Listeria monocytogenes*, *Alcohol Clin. Exp. Res* (in press) (1992).

ALCOHOL, CYTOKINES AND IMMUNODEFICIENCY

John J. Spitzer and Abraham P. Bautista

Department of Physiology, Louisiana State University Medical Center
New Orleans, LA 70112

Ethanol has a multiplicity of actions in the body affecting a variety of organs. In this brief review we will concentrate on some of the effects of ethanol in the liver. Ethanol is a well-known hepatotoxic agent and it also increases susceptibility to microbial infections. The liver is in a strategic position to be affected by ethanol intake, both because it is a major site of alcohol metabolism and also because it is the first major organ that encounters the absorbed alcohol via the portal vein.

One of the common denominators between the hepatotoxic affects of ethanol and its actions in impairing the immune defense system is the alteration of free radical production following ethanol administration. Thus, this presentation will deal with two series of studies involving oxygen free radical formation in the liver: a) the release of superoxide anions by the rat liver following ethanol administration; and b) the attenuation of superoxide anion release by alcohol in hepatic phagocytes in endotoxemic rats.

THE EFFECTS OF ETHANOL ON SUPEROXIDE ANION PRODUCTION IN THE LIVER

Oxygen-derived free radicals have long been implicated in the pathogenesis of alcohol-induced tissue injury (1-4). Since the liver is a major site of alcohol metabolism, it is likely to be directly exposed to the potentially deleterious affects of oxygen-derived toxic radicals. However, the exact site and mechanism of such radical formation in the liver remains to be elucidated. Although the Kupffer cells, the resident macrophages of the liver, only represent approximately 9% of the total cell population and even a smaller fraction of the total hepatic protein content, our previous work has shown that the Kupffer cells are the major sources of hepatic superoxide anion release following either endotoxin or TNF administration (5-7). Based on this information and other available data, we postulated that the Kupffer cells are the primary sources of free radicals following alcoholic liver injury. We therefore investigated the effect of a primed-constant infusion of ethanol on the release of superoxide anions both in the isolated, *in situ* perfused whole liver and in freshly isolated hepatic cells. Conscious,

Drugs of Abuse, Immunity, and AIDS, Edited by
H. Friedman *et al.*, Plenum Press, New York, 1993

fasted male rats with indwelling arterial and venous catheters were used in these studies, as described earlier (7,8). The animals were given a primed continuous infusion of ethanol that resulted in an arterial concentration of 170 mg/dl. After one to seven hours of infusion, the livers were either perfused *in situ* with an artificial perfusate containing ferricytochrome c, or were subjected to enzymatic digestion and centrifugal elutriation in order to separate parenchymal, sinusoidal endothelial cells and Kupffer cells. The details of these procedures have been described earlier (7, 8).

It can be observed in Fig. 1 that infusion of ethanol for one, three or five hours stimulated hepatic output of superoxide anions even in the absence of the tumor promoter, PMA. The peak of superoxide release occurred around three hours of ethanol infusion, and by seven hours of continuous ethanol infusion the stimulatory effect on hepatic superoxide anion production was virtually absent. Fig. 1 also demonstrates that adding PMA directly into the perfusate had only a very slight additional effect on superoxide release.

Since many of the metabolic effects of ethanol are known to be exerted through its metabolic product, acetaldehyde, in a separate group of experiments the metabolism of ethanol moiety was inhibited by the administration of 4-methylpyrazole, a competitive inhibitor of alcohol dehydrogenase. No attenuation of the alcohol effect was noted due to the pretreatment with 4-methylpyrazole, indicating that the metabolism of the alcohol moiety is not necessary for this effect.

In previous studies we have observed that the influence of immunomodulatory agents on hepatic superoxide anion release was dependent on cyclooxygenase products. Therefore in another series of experiments, we administered ibuprofen into the perfused liver which completely inhibited the ethanol-induced superoxide production 8 indicating that cyclooxygenase products play an important role in the alcohol-induced effect. In the next series of experiments, we isolated parenchymal, sinusoidal endothelial cells

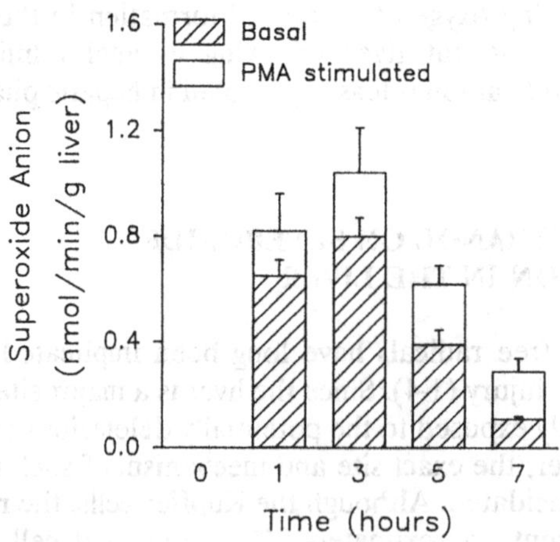

Fig. 1. Superoxide anion release by *in situ* perfused liver after ethanol intoxication. Rats received an i.v. injection of ethanol (1.75 gm/kg body weight) followed by continuous infusion (250-300 mg/kg/hr) for up to 7 hr. The experimental animals were anesthetized at appropriate intervals indicated above. The livers were perfused with ferricytochrome c, the substrate for superoxide anion as described earlier (7,8). Superoxide anion was measured based on the molecular extinction coefficient of 21.1 μmol/1 cm. Final PMA concentration was 0.1 μM.

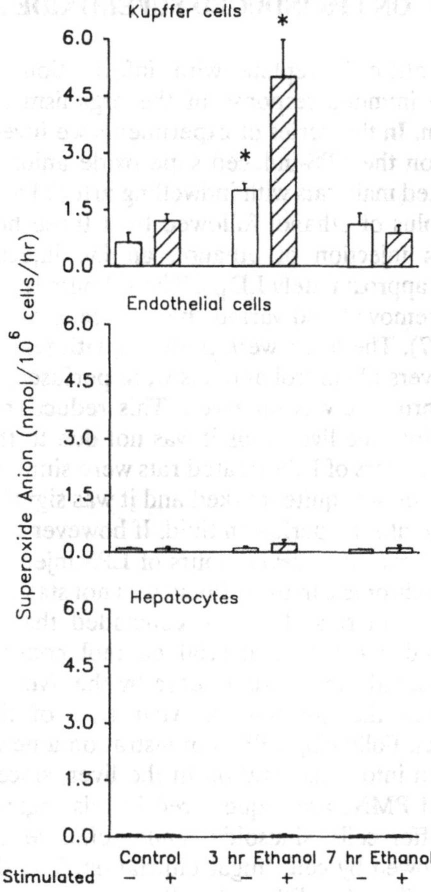

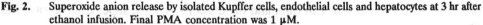

Fig. 2. Superoxide anion release by isolated Kupffer cells, endothelial cells and hepatocytes at 3 hr after ethanol infusion. Final PMA concentration was 1 μM.

with an infusion of ethanol for three hours. Following cell isolation, these cell groups were incubated in the presence of ferricytochrome c and the release of SOD-inhibitable superoxide anion was determined. Fig. 2 indicates that Kupffer cells isolated from rats treated with ethanol for three hours released significantly more superoxide anions than did cells isolated from control rats. The *in vitro* addition of PMA further stimulated the release of superoxide anions. Kupffer cells from animals treated with ethanol for seven hours did not release significantly higher amounts of superoxide anions than did cells that originated from control rats. Fig. 2 shows that the superoxide anion release was barely detectable from endothelial cells and that ethanol treatment had no affect in these cells. Parenchymal cells also failed to release significant quantities of superoxide anions following ethanol stimulation (Fig. 2). The conclusion from these experiments is that acute administration of ethanol causes prostanoid-mediated superoxide anion production in the liver. Kupffer cells are responsible for this effect. The production of oxygen radicals following ethanol treatment may contribute to the hepatotoxic effects of ethanol both under acute and presumably also chronic conditions.

EFFECT OF ETHANOL ON LPS-INDUCED SUPEROXIDE ANION PRODUCTION

The existing literature is replete with information indicating that ethanol intoxication impairs the immune response of the organism and causes an increased susceptibility to infection. In this series of experiments we investigated the influence of ethanol administration on the LPS-induced superoxide anion production in the liver. Conscious overnight fasted male rats with indwelling arterial and venous catheters were given an intravenous bolus of ethanol followed by a three hour continuous infusion. Shortly after the bolus injection of ethanol, an i.v. injection of LPS was given (equivalent to a dose of approximately LD_{10}). Three hours later, the liver was perfused *in situ* or the liver was removed and various hepatic cells were isolated by techniques previously described (5-7). The livers were perfused with ferricytochrome c containing perfusion fluid. When livers of control animals were perfused, a small reduction of the effluent fluid ferricytochrome c was observed. This reduction was not altered by the direct addition of SOD into the liver, thus it was not due to the release of superoxide anions (Fig. 3). When the livers of LPS-treated rats were similarly perfused, the effluent ferricytochrome c reduction was quite marked and it was significantly attenuated by the addition of SOD directly into the perfusion fluid. If however the livers were taken from LPS plus ethanol treated rats after seven hours of LPS injection and ethanol infusion, the reduction of ferricytochrome c in the effluent was not statistically different from that observed in livers of control rats. Thus we concluded that seven hours of ethanol infusion (which produced a constant arterial ethanol concentration of 170 mg/dl) abolished the LPS stimulated superoxide release by the liver.

Next we considered the question of what type of liver cells are primarily responsible for this effect. Following LPS administration a new group of nonparenchymal cells has to be taken into consideration in the liver, since under such conditions, considerable numbers of PMNs are sequestered in this organ. Therefore we isolated parenchymal cells, Kupffer cells, sinusoidal endothelial cells and hepatic PMNs by enzymatic digestion followed by centrifugal elutriation. The details of these methods were described earlier (7). The different cell groups were then incubated in the presence of ferricytochrome c *in vitro,* and the SOD-inhibitable superoxide release was determined.

No significant superoxide release was detected by either the parenchymal cells, or the sinusoidal endothelial cells. Kupffer cells from control (saline-infused) rats showed little spontaneous superoxide production. However, addition of PMA increased the release of superoxides by these cells (Table 1). Ethanol alone had no effect. LPS *in vivo* markedly stimulated the spontaneous release *in vitro,* and this was even more noticeable in the presence of PMA. When cells were isolated from rats that had been treated with both LPS and ethanol, a marked attenuation of the LPS effect was noted.

Table 1 also indicates the production of superoxide anions by hepatic PMNs. No spontaneous superoxide release was noted even in the presence of PMN. However, LPS stimulated markedly the superoxide anion release which was significantly attenuated in cells isolated from animals that received both LPS and ethanol treatments.

We concluded from these experiments that the immunomodulation by LPS includes elevated glucose utilization by macrophages (shown previously) and enhanced ability of these cells to produce toxic oxygen metabolites. Alcohol attenuates these changes, thus potentially causing an impaired immune response. Although the exact mechanism(s) of action of ethanol in counteracting the immunomodulatory effects of LPS is incompletely understood, it appears that TNF plays a role in this response, as our earlier investigations indicated that the LPS-induced TNF elevation in the blood is markedly ameliorated when the animals had been treated with alcohol (9). This attenuation of the LPS effect was proportional to the concentration of ethanol in the blood.

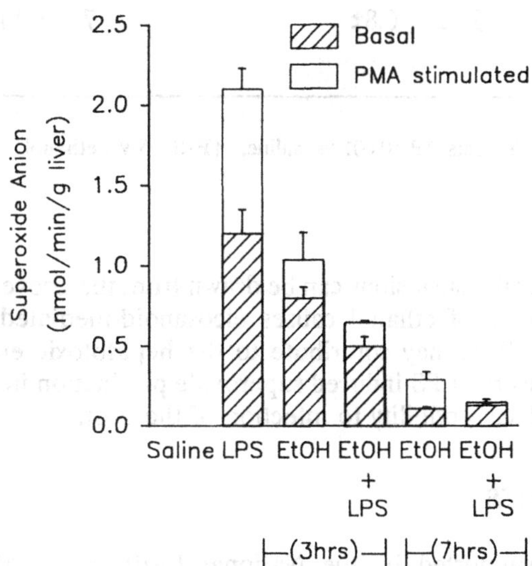

Fig. 3. **Superoxide anion release by *in situ* perfused liver after ethanol and LPS treatments. Rats received an i.v. injection of ethanol (1.75 gm/kg body weight) followed by a continuous infusion (250-300 mg/kg/hr) for 3-7 hr. *Escherichia coli* LPS (1 mg/kg body weight) was given at 0 or 4 hr after the i.v. injection of ethanol. Infusion was continued for 3-7 hr. Rats were sacrificed at 3 hr after LPS treatment. Final PMA concentration was 0.1 μM.**

Table 1. Phorbol myristate acetate-induced generation of superoxide anion by Kupffer cells and hepatic neutrophils.

Treatment	0_2^-, nmol/10^6 cells	
Group	KC2	PMN
Saline	1.2 ± 0.2	NT
Ethanol	1.1 ± 0.2	NT
Saline + LPS	12 ± 1.3*,†	13 ±1.3†
Ethanol + LPS	5 ± 0.8‡	7 ±0.14

Values are means ± SE; = 5-8 rats. *P<0.001 vs. saline. †P<0.05 vs. ethanol + LPS. ‡ P<0.001 vs. ethanol.

The following overall conclusions can be drawn from the above data: 1) Relatively short acute administration of ethanol causes eicosanoid-mediated superoxide anion production in the liver. This may contribute to the hepatotoxic effect of ethanol. 2) Ethanol also ameliorates the LPS-induced superoxide production in the liver. This may contribute to increased susceptibility to infection of the host.

ACKNOWLEDGEMENTS

This work was supported by the National Institute on Alcohol Abuse and Alcoholism Grants AA07287 (JJS) and AA08846 (APB).

REFERENCES

1. M. Comporti, Lipid peroxidation and cellular damage in toxic liver disease, *Lab. Invest.* 53:599 (1985).
2. M. Younes, O. Strubelt, Alcohol-induced hepatotoxicity: a role for oxygen-free radicals, *Free Radic. Res.* Comnun. 3:1(1987).
3. A. I. Cederbaum, Role of lipid peroxidation and oxidative stress in alcohol toxicity, *Free. Rad. Biol. Med.* 7:537 (1989).
4. E. R. Rosenblum, J.S. Gavalier, D. Van Thiel, Lipid peroxidation: a mechanism for alcohol-induced testicular injury, *Free Radic. Biol. Med* 7:569 (1989).
5. A. B. Bautista, K. Meszaros, J. Bojta, and J.J. Spitzer, Superoxide anion generation in the liver during the early stage of endotoxemia in rats, *J. Leuk. Biol.* 48:123 (1990).
6. A. P. Bautista, N.B. D'Souza, C.H. Lang, J. Bagwell, J.J. Spitzer, Alcohol-induced downregulation of superoxide anion production by hepatic phagocytes in endotoxemic rats, *Am. J. Physiol.* 260: R969 (1991).
7. A. P. Bautista, A. Schuler, Z. Spolarics, J.J. Spitzer, Tumor necrosis factor stimulates superoxide anion production by the perfused liver and Kupffer cells, *Am. J. Physiol.* 261:G891 (1991).
8. A. P. Bautista, J.J. Spitzer, Acute ethanol intoxication stimulates superoxide anion production by in situ perfused rat liver, *Hepatol.* 15:892 (1992).
9. N. B. D'Souza, G.J. Bagby, S. Nelson, C.H. Lang, and J.J. Spitzer, Acute alcohol infusion suppresses-endotoxin-induced serum tumor necrosis factor, *Alcohol. Clin. Exp. Res.* 13:295 (1989).

HUMAN POLYMORPHONUCLEAR LEUKOCYTE (PMN)

PRIMING/ACTIVATION BY ACUTE ETHANOL INTOXICATION

André K. Balla[1], Elvira M. Doi, Paulo R. Wunder,
James D. Ogle[2], and Lawrence E. DeBault

[1]Dept. of Pathology, University of Oklahoma Health Science Center, Oklahoma City, OK, and [2]Dept. of Biochemistry and Molecular Biology, University of Cincinnati Medical Center, Cincinnati, OH

The effects of chronic alcoholism on susceptibility to infections are well documented. Less is known on the effect of sporadic acute ingestion of ethanol on the immune system. One should not assume that it induces neutrophil function deficiency *in vivo*. One example of upregulation caused by ethanol treatment was described by Dorio (1): *in vitro* ethanol treatment of rat macrophages causes an acute rise in intracellular calcium, stimulates a small amount of superoxide production, but it also inhibits concanavalin A- and phorbol ester-induced superoxide formation. Acute ingestion of ethanol has been shown to affect some, but not all PMN functions: decreased adherence to surfaces, decreased delivery to inflammation sites, but no abnormality of chemotaxis, superoxide generation, bacterial killing, or intracellular cAMP and cGMP levels (2,3). In other experimental studies in mice, both low dose (1 mg/Kg) and high dose (4 mg/Kg of body weight) of ethanol increased the number of sticking or plugging PMNs in sinusoids of the liver (4). A small decrease in phagocytosis has been detected by some (3), but not by others (2).

While chronic alcoholism is associated with immune dysfunctions that may be related to nutritional abnormalities, sleep disorders, hepatic and neuropathologic disorders, etc., acute alcoholism has fewer interfering variables, thus offering a better model to study abnormalities of PMN function. The purpose of this study is to determine whether social drinking has any effect on various PMN functions.

METHODS

Normal Subjects and Study Protocol

Ten normal healthy volunteers, non-habitual drinkers were asked to abstain from alcoholic beverages and medications for a period of at least one week before the study. Urine was screened for drugs of abuse and alcohol before ethanol ingestion. Blood samples were collected on Day 1 and on Day 2 at the same time of the day. On Day 2, the subjects drank approximately 90 ml of grain alcohol (Ever Clear) mixed with fruit juice within a period of approximately 15 min. Between 45 and 60 min their blood alcohol level reached peak values (as monitored by breath analysis), when the second

Drugs of Abuse, Immunity, and AIDS, Edited by
H. Friedman *et al.*, Plenum Press, New York, 1993

blood sample was collected (blood alcohol concentration was 106 + 12 mg/dL, gas chromatographic assay). Samples were processed immediately. All assays were done on a FACscan flow cytometer. Standardized fluorescent beads were used for comparison of values obtained on Day 1 vs. Day 2. The two blood samples of each individual were paired for Wilcoxon rank sum test statistical analysis.

Separation of Cells

Except for the phagocytosis assays, where Ficoll-Hypaque separation was necessary, leukocytes were obtained by hypotonic lysis of red blood cells.

PMN Expression of FcR II (CD32), FcR III (CD16), CR1 (CD35 and CR3 (CDllb/CD18)

Cells were labeled with fluorochrome- conjugated mouse monoclonal antibodies (CR3, Becton and Dickinson), or by indirect fluorescence with unlabeled mouse monoclonal antibodies (CR1, AMAC Inc.; FcR II and FcR III, Medarex,Inc.) followed by fluorochrome-labeled anti-murine antibodies (TAGO Corp.). FcR assays required previous blocking of receptors with excess heat-aggregated human IgG. All these receptor studies were done in an ice-bath in the presence of sodium azide and saturating concentrations of primary antibodies.

Immunoadherence and Phagocytosis of IgG and C3b-opsonized Fluorescent Microspheres (5)

Polystyrene fluorescent (coumarin) microspheres of approximately the size of bacteria were coated with purified IgG and C3b or with bovine serum albumin controls. These microspheres were incubated with PMNs at a ratio of 150 particles/cell. Phagocytosis was stopped by placing the tube in an ice-bath. After washing the cells, bound but not ingested microspheres were double-labeled with rabbit anti-human C3c and later with phycoerythrin-labeled goat-anti-rabbit $F(ab')_2$ antibody. This quantitative technique discriminates between simple adherence and phagocytosis (5).

Generation of Oxidative Products (6)

Cells were incubated with 2',7'-dicholorofluorescin diacetate (DCFH-DA) in an 37°C water-bath. Cellular fluorescence was determined at this point to evaluate spontaneous generation of oxidative products. Cells were then stimulated with phorbol myristate acetate (PMA) and the generation of oxidative products was assessed by increase of green fluorescence (dichlorofluorescein, DCF) at 24 min. of incubation at 37°C.

RESULTS

The results are summarized in Table 1. The amount of alcoholic beverages ingested induced mild to moderate intoxication, reaching peak blood alcohol levels at approximately 45 to 60 min after ingestion. PMNs collected at that point showed signs of mild activation and/or priming: a) Up-regulation of CR3 (CD11b/CD18) and CR1 (CD35) expression, b) priming for increased generation of oxygen reactive products, and c) increased binding of foreign particles coated with purified IgG and the C3b fragment of complement.

Table 1. Effects of acute ethanol intoxication on human PMNs

Parameter	% Change		P value
CR1[b]	+	9.5%	0.030[a]
CR3[b]	+	26.0%	0.016[a]
FcR II[b]		3.5%	0.361
FcR III[b]		1.6%	0.399
Oxidative Products[c]	+	185.0%	0.025[a]
Immunophagocytosis[d]		234.1%	0.221
Immunoadherence[d]	+	493.2%	0.033[a]

[a]Statistically significant difference ($P < 0.05$) between values before and after ingestion of alcoholic beverages.
[b]Surface expression of antigen as expressed by flow cytometry.
[c]DCFH-DA conversion to DCF, a measure of generation of oxygen reactive products after stimulus with PMA. There was no change in spontaneous, unstimulated. DCFH-DA conversion after ethanol ingestion.
[e]Even though there was marked increase in adherence of opsonized particles to the external surface of PMNs, there was no increase in particle ingestion (phagocytosis).

There were, however, no statistical differences in phagocytosis, or in membrane expression of FcR II tCD32) and FcR III (CD 16). Interestingly, six individuals showed marked decrease in phagocytosis after drinking alcoholic beverage while the other four showed a several-fold increase. In none of the 10 subjects did the values remain close to pre-ethanol levels.

DISCUSSION

Priming of neutrophils is defined as an enhanced response to an agonist after these cells interact with a first stimulus which does not activate them. Small doses of endotoxin, for example, injected into rats do not activate PMNs to generate oxygen reactive products, but when these cells are subjected to a second stimulus, PMA, they respond with up to fourfold more DCFH-DA conversion than control PMNs that were not exposed to endotoxin (7). Increased immunoadherence and PMN-induced oxidative product generation are signs of PMN priming by ethanol. The increase in CD11b/CD18 expression could be interpreted as an evidence of either priming or activation of PMNs. Our data on phagocytosis showed profound individual variations of either marked decrease or marked increase. Other investigators (2,3), found no decrease in phagocytosis of opsonized particles when the blood alcohol concentration reached peak values at 45 to 60 min., but Corberrand et al., (3), found a small decrease that occurred several hours after alcohol ingestion.

These results should be compared with those we found in a previous study of another phagocytic cell, the tissue macrophage, in chronic alcoholic rats: increased adherence of sheep red blood cells through C3b or IgG receptors, decreased phagocytic ability, and decreased oxygen free radicals production (8).

We conclude that ethanol acts as a weak activator/priming agent of PMNs. Prolonged stimulation of these cells by ethanol would theoretically lead to depletion, a cross-deactivation that would explain some of the PMN deficiencies found later in chronic alcoholism.

REFERENCES

1. R. Dorio, The effect of ethanol on signal transduction in the rat alveolar macrophage, in "Alcohol, Immunomodulation, and AIDS, D. Seminara, R. R. Watson, A. Pawlowski, eds., Alan R. Liss, Inc, N. York (1989).
2. R. R. MacGregor, Alcohol and immune defense, *JAMA*, 256:74 (1986).
3. J. X. Corberrand, P. F. Laharrague, G. Fillola, Human neutrophils are not severely injured in conditions that mimic social drinking, Alcoholism, *Clin. Exp. Res.* 13:542 (1989).
4. H. Eguchi, P. McCuskey, R. McCuskey, Kupffer cell activity and hepatic microvascular events after acute ethanol ingestion in mice, *Hepatology* 13:751 (1991).
5. J. D. Ogle, J. Q. Noel, R. M. Sramkoski, C. K. Ogle, J. W. Alexander, Phagocytosis of opsonized fluorescent microspheres by human neutrophils. A two-color flow cytometric method for the determination of attachment and ingestion, *J. Immunol. Methods* 115:17 (1989).
6. D. A. Bass, P. Olbrantz, P. Szejda, M. Seeds, C. E. McCall, Subpopulations of neutrophils with increased oxidative product formation of patients with infection, *J. Immunol.* 136:860 (1986).
7. A. K. Balla, D. J. Brackett, E. M. Doi, M. R. Lerner, W.D. Bales, L.T. Archer, P. R. Wunder, M. F. Wilson, Dose-response effect of *in vivo* endotoxin on polymorphonuclear leukocytes oxidative burst, *J. Leuk. Biol. Suppl.* 1:20 (1990).
8. O. Bagasra, A. Howeedy, A. Kajdacsy-Balla, Macrophage function in chronic experimental alcoholism: I. Modulation of surface receptors and phagocytosis, *Immunol.* 65:405 (1988).

ETHANOL AFFECTS MACROPHAGE PRODUCTION OF IL-6 AND SUSCEPTIBILITY TO INFECTION BY *LEGIONELLA PNEUMOPHILA*

Yoshimasa Yamamoto, Thomas W. Klein, and Herman Friedman

Department of Medical Microbiology and Immunology
University of South Florida College of Medicine
Tampa, FL 33612

A number of investigators have reported that prolonged and excessive consumption of alcohol results in alterations of host immunity (1). Such alterations are believed to lead to increased susceptibility to infections (2). In fact, it has been pointed out in many reports that infections in alcoholics are serious problems (3). For example, bacterial pneumonia occurs frequently and is a more serious problem in alcoholics. In this regard, various experimental studies have shown deleterious effects of alcohol on host immune cells such as lymphocytes (4,5), natural killer cells (6), polymorphonuclear cells (7) and macrophages (8). All of these cells have critical roles in defense mechanisms against not only microbial infections but also development of malignant cells. Furthermore, recent studies have shown that when macrophages are treated with alcohol, there is a significant increase in susceptibility of the cells to *Mycobacteria* (9). Such reports suggest that alcohol treatment *in vitro* and *in vivo* induces disturbance of a host's immune system and also impairs effector cells such as macrophages. However, there is only limited information about how such deleterious effects of alcohol impact on the immune defense mechanism against infections. For example, it has not yet been elucidated what type of infections are serious in experimental alcoholism, whether direct or indirect effects of alcohol on effector cells are more crucial, how cytokine production is modulated by alcohol and how these effects, if any, correlate with susceptibility to infection. In this regard, we examined the direct effect of ethanol on susceptibility of macrophages to *Legionella pneumophila* infection, since this bacteria is a typical intracellular gram-negative bacillus and causes pulmonary infection in immunocompromised hosts (10).

ETHANOL AFFECTS *LEGIONELLA PNEUMOPHILA* GROWTH IN MACROPHAGES

L. pneumophila can multiply in A/J mice macrophages as well as guinea pig and

Drugs of Abuse, Immunity, and AIDS, Edited by
H. Friedman *et al.*, Plenum Press, New York, 1993

human macrophages/monocytes (11). However, macrophages from most mouse strains such as BALB/c, C3H/HeN, C57BL/6, DBA/2 and BDF1 are not permissive for growth of *L. pneumophila* (11-13). The multiplication of *L. pneumophila* in macrophage cultures seems to reflect the resistance of the cells to infection by opportunistic microorganisms. This bacterium is not able to grow either in tissue culture medium or conditioned medium without macrophages being present (14,15). Furthermore, activation of macrophages by bacterial lipopolysaccharide or interferon gamma converts the permissiveness of the cells to resistance to *Legionella* growth (16,17). Therefore, if ethanol has modulatory effect on macrophage function involved in anti-*Legionella* activity, growth of these bacteria in the cells should be modulated by the treatment with ethanol.

As apparent in Fig. 1, *L. pneumophila* grow vigorously in cultures of A/J mouse macrophages. From an initial number of approximately 8 x 10^4 bacteria per culture, there was a rapid increase so that by 48 hrs the number of bacteria reached nearly 1 x 10^7. In contrast, BALB/c mouse macrophage cultures evinced nonpermissiveness for *Legionella* growth. There was only a 4 to 5 fold increase in the number of bacteria in the BALB/c mouse macrophage cultures after 48 hrs of infection. However, when such nonpermissive BALB/c mouse macrophages were treated with ethanol, there was a marked increase in *L. pneumophila* growth 24 and 48 hrs after infection (Table 1). However, such an effect of ethanol on the growth of *Legionella* required a relatively long incubation period with ethanol, such as 7 days. A shorter period of incubation with ethanol, such as 2 days, did not result in any significant changes in the number of bacteria.

The concentrations of ethanol which resulted in this enhancement of bacterial growth were 0.5 and 0.1% (v/v). A lower concentration such as 0.02%, did not have any detrimental effect on *Legionella* growth, even when preincubated with alcohol for 7 days (data not shown). There was essentially no difference in the uptake of bacteria by macrophages treated with alcohol at any dose tested and there was also no significant effect of the ethanol treatment on the viability of the macrophages as determined by the trypan blue dye exclusion assay (data not shown). Similary, there was no effect by these concentrations of ethanol on the viability of *L. pneumophila* (data not shown). It seems clear from this study that ethanol, at relatively low doses, can modulate the ability of nonpermissive mouse macrophages to replicate *L. pneumophila*, an opportunistic intracellular bacterium. These observations are essentially similar to a previous report by Bermudez and Young, which showed a deleterious effect of ethanol on macrophages (9). That is, cultured human monocyte-derived macrophages exposed to ethanol *in vitro*, showed significantly greater *Mycobacterium avium* growth as compared to growth in nontreated control cells. These data indicate that ethanol may directely affect anti-*Legionella* and anti-*Mycobacterium* activities of macrophages. However, the required incubation periods with ethanol for modulation of anti-microbial activity of macrophages appears to be different for the two microorganisms. Such difference may be related to the nature or mechanism of anti-microbial activities against these different microorganisms.

ETHANOL MODULATES IL-6 PRODUCTION

Interleukin 6 (IL-6) is an important acute phase inflammatory cytokine produced by a wide variety of cells, including macrophages. Recent studies on IL-6 included by bacterial invasion and other noxious stimuli show that this cytokine is involved in

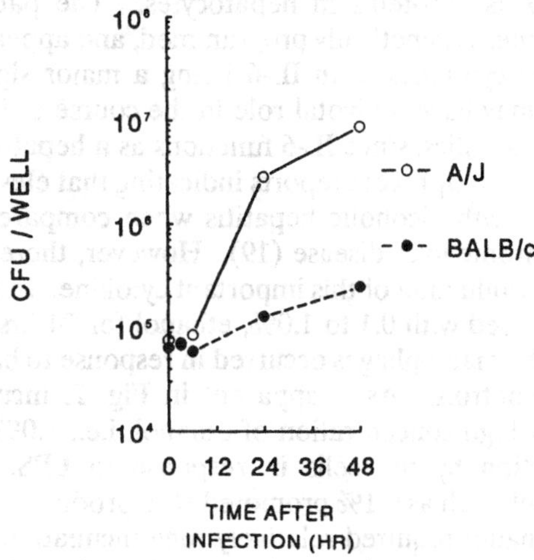

Fig. 1. Growth of *L. pneumophila* in A/J vs. BALB/c mouse macrophages. Thioglycolate-elicited peritoneal macrophages obtained from either A/J or BALB/c female mice were allowed to adhere to 24-well tissue culture plates for 2 hrs and then washed to remove non-adherent cells. Macrophage monolayers (approximately 1 x 10^6 cells per well) were infected with 1 x 10^7 *L. pneumophila* for 30 min at 37°C in 5% CO_2, washed to remove non-phagocytized bacteria and then incubated further for 48 hrs in 10% FCS-RPMI 1640 medium. The number of viable bacteria (CFU) in macrophage lysates were determined on BCYE agar plates. Each point represents the mean ± S.D. for triplicate macrophage cultures.

Table 1. Effect of ethanol on the growth of *L. pneumophila* in BALB/c mouse macrophage cultures[a]

Preincubation with ethanol		Hrs After Infection 24 hrs	(CFU x 10^4/well)[b] 48 hrs
2 Days			
None (control)		36.6 ± 3.3	28.3 ± 9.0
ethanol	0.5%	36.2 ± 11.7	33.0 ± 4.2
	0.1%	43.3 ± 10.1	37.5 ± 12.0
	0.02%	49.1 ± 12.2	36.6 ± 5.0
7 Days			
None (Control)		6.5 ± 0.4	7.1 ± 0.3
ethanol	1.0%	10.5 ± 1.2*	32.0 ± 12.2*
0.5%		11.9 ± 1.9*	14.4 ± 2.5*
	0.1%	12.5 ± 1.9*	15.3 ± 3.0*

[a]Macrophage monolayers (1 x 10^6 cells/well) preincubated with indicated concentrations of ethanol for 2 to 7 days, culture medium with ethanol changed every 24 hrs, and then infected with *L. pneumophila*; infectivity ratio 10 bacteria per macrophage and number of viable bacteria in macrophage lysates determined at 24 and 48 hrs after infection by plate count method.
[b]Mean ± S.D. for triplicate macrophage cultures. *; $p<0.05$.

production of acute phase proteins in hepatocytes. The pattern of these proteins synthesized by hepatocytes is genetically programmed, and appears related to the action of variou inflammatory cytokines, with IL-6 being a major signal (18). Therefore, it seems likely that IL-6 may have a pivotal role in the course of inflammatory responses involving cirrhosis in alcoholics, since IL-6 functions as a hepatocyte stimulating factor. This possibility is supported by recent reports indicating that elevated plasma IL-6 levels are evident in patients with alcoholic hepatitis when compared with control groups, including those with chronic liver disease (19). However, there is little information as to how ethanol affects production of this important cytokine. In the present study, when macrophages were cultured with 0.1 to 1.0%, ethanol for 24 hrs, a marked modulation of IL-6 production by the macrophages occurred in response to bacterial lipopolysaccharide as compared to controls. As is apparent in Fig. 2, incubation of macrophage cultures with relatively high concentration of ethanol, i.e., 1.0%, for 24 hrs resulted in inhibited IL-6 production by the cells in response to LPS. In contrast, a lower concentration of ethanol, such as 0.1% promoted IL-6 production rather than inhibition. This modulation by ethanol required relatively long incubation periods such as 24 hrs or more. A short incubation period with ethanol, such as 3 hrs, did not result in modulation of IL-6 production (data not shown). Furthermore, ethanol itself did not have any IL-6 induction activity for the macrophages when similar concentrations were used (up to 1.0%). However, the mechanisms of modulation by ethanol on IL-6 production is not clear. Nevertheless, these data cleary indicate the possibility that ethanol may affect the early phase of inflammatory responses involving IL-6 production.

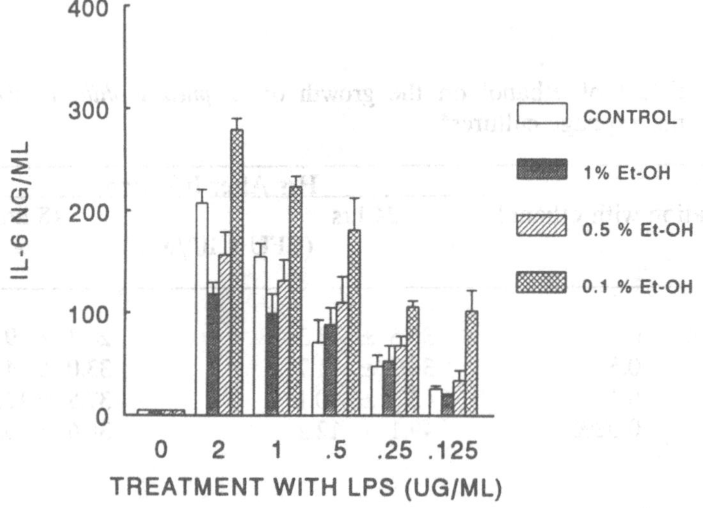

Fig. 2. Effect of ethanol on macrophage production of IL-6 in response to LPS. Thioglycolate-elicited BALB/c mouse macrophage monolayers (1 x 10^6 cells/well) pretreated with indicated concentrations of ethanol in 10% FCS-RPMI 1640 medium for 24 hrs and then stimulated with various concentrations of E. coli LPS in the presence of ethanol for 24 hrs. The IL-6 contents in the culture supernatants determined by enzyme immunoassay using monoclonal anti-IL-6 antibody. Each bar represents the mean ± S.D. for triplicate macrophage cultures.

ACKNOWLEGEMENT

The authors thank Peijun He for technical assistance. This work was supported in part by grant AI16618 from the National Institute of Allergy and Infectious Diseases.

REFERENCES

1. R. R.MacGregor, Alcohol and immune defense, *J. Amer. Med. Assoc.* 256:1474 (1986).
2. H. G. Adams and C. Jordan, Infections in the alcoholic, *Med. Clin. North Am.* 68:179 (1984).
3. F. Smith, and D. Palmer, Alcoholism, infection, and altered host defenses: a review of clinical and experimental observations, *J. Chronic Dis.* 29:35 (1976).
4. G. A. Roselle and Mendenhall. Ethanol-induced alterations in lymphocyte function in the guinea pig. *Alcoholism* 8:62 (1984).
5. G. P. Young, M.B. Van der Weyden, I. S.Rose, F. J. Dudley, Lymphopenia and lymphocyte transformation in alcoholics, *Experientia* 35:268 (1970).
6. S. E. Blank, D. A. Duncan, and G. G. Meadows, Suppression of natural killer cell activity by ethanol consumption and food restriction, *Alcoholism* 15:16-22, 1991.
7. E. Nilsson, P. Lindstrom, M. Patarroyo, B. Ringertz, R. Lerner, J. Rincon, and J. Palmblad, Ethanol impairs certain aspects of neutrophil adhesion in vitro: comparisons with inhibition of expression of the CD18 antigen, *J.Infect.Dis.* 163:591-597, 1991.
8. R. R. Watson , Prabhala RH, Abril E, and Smith TL, Changes in lymphocyte subsets and macrophage functions from high, short-term dietary ethanol in C57/BL6 mice, *Life Sci.* 43:865 (1988).
9. L. E. Bermudez , Young LS. Ethanol augments intracellular survival of *Mycobacterium avium* complex and impairs macrophage responses to cytokines, *J. Infect. Dis.* 163:1286 (1991).
10. M. H. Nguyen, J. E. Stout, and V. L. Yu, Legionellosis, *Infect. Dis. Clin. North Am.* 5:561 (1991).
11. Y. Yamamoto, T. W. Klein, C. A. Newton, R. Widen, and H. Friedman, Growth of *Legionella pneumophila* in thioglycolate-elicited peritoneal macrophages from A/J mice, *Infect. Immun.* 56:370 (1988).
12. Y. Yamamoto, T. W. Klein, C. A. Newton, R. Widen, and H. Friedman, Differential growth of Legionella pneumophila in guinea pig vs. mouse macrophage cultures, *Infect. Immun.* 55:1369 (1987).
13. S. Yoshida and Y. Mizuguchi, Multiplication of *Legionella pneumophila* Philadelphia-1 in cultured peritoneal macrophages and its correlation to susceptibility of animals, *Can. J. Microbiol.* 32:438 (1986).
14. J. A. Daisy, C. E. Benson, J. McKitrick, and H. M. Friedman, Intracellular replication of *Legionella pneumophila*, *J. Infect. Dis.* 143:460 (1981).
15. L. J. Oldham and F. G. Rodgers, Adhesion, penetration and intracellular replication of *Legionella pneumophila*: an *in vitro* model of pathogenesis, *J. Gen. Microbiol.* 131:697 (1985).
16. T. W. Klein, Y. Yamamoto, H. K. Brown, and H. Friedman, Interferon-γ induced resistance to *Legionella pneumophila* in susceptible A/J mouse macrophages, *J. Leuk. Biol.* 49:98 (1991).
17. K. Egawa, T. W. Klein, Y. Yamamoto, C. A. Newton, and H. Friedman, Enhanced growth restriction of *Legionella pneumophila* in endotoxin-treated macrophages, *Proc. Soc. Exp. Biol. Med.* 200:338 (1992).
18. A. Koj, The role of interleukin-6 as the hepatocyte stimulating factor in the network of inflammatory cytokines, *Ann. N. Y. Acad. Sci.* 557:1 (1989).
19. N. Sheron, G. Bird, J. Goka, G. Alexander, and R. Williams, Elevated plasma interleukin-6 and increased severity and mortality in alcoholic hepatitis, *Clin. Exp.Immunol.* 84:449 (1991).

SUPPRESSION BY DIETARY ALCOHOL OF RESISTANCE TO *CRYPTOSPORIDIUM* DURING MURINE ACQUIRED IMMUNE DEFICIENCY SYNDROME

John I. B. Alak[1], Masoud Shahbazian[2], Dennis Huang[2], Yuejian Wang[2], Hamid Darban, Ronald R. Watson[2], and Edward M. Jenkins [1]

[1]Tuskegee University, Tuskegee, AL and [2]University of Arizona, Tucson, AZ

Significant immunological changes occur following LP-BM5 murine leukemia retrovirus infection as well as chronic alcohol comsumption. Retrovirus infection which has proceeded to murine AIDS permitted persistent *Cryptosporidium* infection, while non-retrovirus infected mice were resistant. Dietary alcohol provided until the day before parasite challenge did not affect resistance in controls, but increased the numbers of oocysts in the feces of retrovirus suppressed mice. Mortality was significant in retrovirus infected mice, and exacerbated slightly by dietary ethanol, while all controls survived parasite challenge. The retrovirus infected mice had greatly reduced numbers of intestinal $CD4^+$ T helper cells and IgA^+ B cells, which may explain their loss of intestinal resistance. Clearly, the severely immunosuppressed animals with murine AIDS were more sensitive to alcohol consumption than uninfected controls. This suggests that alcohol can synergize with murine retrovirus infection to exacerbate loss of resistance to an opportunistic pathogen common in human AIDS patients.

INTRODUCTION

Cryptosporidium species parasitize enterocytes of the intestine with a wide host range (1) including man (2). Infections are characterized by self-limiting diarrhea in immunocompetent humans and could escalate to proliferative watery diarrhea and death due to loss of electrolytes in the immunodeficient with severe immune dysfunctions (2, 3, 4). Prevalence of Cryptosporidiosis is low (2 to 10%) in the general population but may range from 16 to 50% in AIDS patients (4, 5). About 30 to 35% of the U.S. and over 65% populations in developing countries show pre-exposure to *C. parvum* infection (5). The distal ilium is more frequently parasitized, however, severe immunosuppression can enhance parasite colonization of the entire gastrointestinal tract and other organs leading to generalized cryptosporidiosis (1). As chronic alcohol consumption and retrovirus infection reduce intestinal $CD4^+$, $CD8^+$, and IgA^+ cell numbers (6, 7), they could affect cytokine production required for immunoregulation and host defenses against *Cryptosporidium*. Thus, alcohol or retrovirus-induced damage of the intestine and

Drugs of Abuse, Immunity, and AIDS, Edited by
H. Friedman *et al.*, Plenum Press, New York, 1993

immune system could reduce resistance to various pathogens including intestinal parasites. Therefore, this study was initiated to determine the effects of LP-BM5 infection on resistance to *C. parvum* after chronic ethanol consumption.

MATERIALS AND METHODS

Mice and Ethanol Treatment - Female C57BL/6 mice 3 to 4 wks of age were obtained from the Charles River Laboratories, Inc. (Boston, MA). They were housed in transparent plastic cages having stainless steel wire lids in a housing facility with constant humidity and animals were exposed to a 12:12 hr light-dark cycle. Water and mouse chow (Tekland, Madison, WI) were provided ad libitum. Mice were then randomly assigned to the following treatments: control, ethanol (5% v/v) diet, retrovirus, and ethanol (5% v/v) diet plus retrovirus. Four months post-retrovirus infection, the mouse chow diet was replaced with Lieber-DeCarli liquid diets. All diets were made isocaloric by substituting 26% of the total calories with ethanol for the ethanol diet and dextrose for the control diet. Animals were fed the respective diets for 4 wks beginning 16 wks post-retrovirus inoculation. The day before parasite challenge, all animals were fed mouse chow and none received alcohol thereafter.

***C. parvum* Inoculation** - After 4 wks of alcohol consumption, the mice were then inoculated with purified oocysts of *C. parvum* within 48 hrs. Each animal was inoculated with approximately 2.0×10^5 *C. parvum* oocysts via stomach tube. This oocyst concentration has been previously shown to cause parasite growth in the gut epithelium of immunocompromised mice (1). Partially purified oocysts of *C. parvum* from calf feces were preserved in 2.5% potassium dichromate. Before the mice were inoculated, oocyst preparations were centrifuged to remove the potassium dichromate and then resuspended in phosphate buffered saline (PBS). Oocysts were counted using a hemocytometer under phase-contrast microscopy (O.M Systems BH2-Olympus).

Enumeration of *C. parvum* Oocysts in the Intestine and Feces - Two cm of the terminal ilium was surgically removed from each mouse. The fecal material from each section was removed and placed in a microcentrifuge tube. It was allowed to dry and then weighed. The fecal samples were used to enumerate *C. parvum* oocysts. Fecal specimens from each microcentrifuge plastic tube (National Scientific Supply Company, Inc., CA) was meshed with an applicator stick after adding 1.0 ml of 10% formalin to each sample. The tubes were vortexed vigorously on a vortex shaker and 500 μl of sample from each tube was stained with anti-*Cryptosporidium* monoclonal antibodies provided.

RESULTS

Oocysts Shedding into the Feces - *Cryptosporidium* shedding into the feces of untreated as well as ethanol fed animals was not observed at day 10 post parasite challenge. Persistent oocysts shedding into the feces was detected in all retrovirus infected mice (Table 1). There were significantly more oocysts found in feces of retrovirus-infected mice which had been fed alcohol prior to parasitge challenge (Table 1) although both retrovirus-infected groups continued to shed significant numbers of oocysts while non-retrovirus infected ones had previously cleared the infection. While survival approached approximately 100% for untreated mice as well as those fed the alcohol diets alone, retrovirus infected groups had 42.9 to 69.4% mortality at 20 weeks post infection.

***Cryptosporidium* Colonization of Intestinal Villae** - There was no significant difference ($p. < 0.05$) in the colonization of the intestinal mucosae by *Cryptosporidium* in non-retrovirus infected mice (Table 2). Parasites were rapidly cleared from non-retrovirus infected animals shortly after oocyst inoculation and were not detectable by 20 days post infection. However, persistent *Cryptosporidium* infection was established in all retrovirus infected animals (Table 2) with a heavy parasite colonization as shown by numbers on villus sections. Alcohol consumption by the retrovirus infected mice did not significantly alter parasite numbers on the villae (Table 2). Each intestinal piece was histologically stained with hematoxylin-eosin. The average number of oocysts colonization per villus section was counted using a hemocytometer under phase-contrast microscopy at 40X objective microscope lens. Oocysts from 25 intestinal villus sections per mouse were counted and expressed as oocysts/villus section.

DISCUSSION

Infection of C57BL/6 female mice with LP-BM5 murine leukemia virus induced a syndrome with many functional similarities to human AIDS due to human immunodeficiency virus (HIV). They included progressive splenomegaly, lymphadenopathy, reduced splenocyte responses to con-A stimulation but not LPS and enhanced susceptibility to *C. parvum* infection. However, adult C57BL/6 mice not inoculated with LP-BM5 were refractory to infection by the parasite. These findings agree with previous reports defining the murine retrovirus suppression of resistance to *Cryptosporidium* (1, 8, 9, 10). We found that loss of parasite resistance during murine AIDS and alcohol consumption occurred with loss of $CD4^+$, $CD8^+$ and IgA^+ from the intestinal lamina propria and Peyerls patches (6). Similarly, a recent report (7) showed poor production

Table 1. Effects of prior ethanol treatment and retrovirus infection on fecal oocysts after *Cryptosporidium* challenge.[1]

Treatment		Days Post *Cryptosporidium* Infection		
Retrovirus Infection	Dietary Alcohol	10	20	27
		oocysts/mg feces		
-	-	O	O	O
-	+	O	O	O
+	-	3.07+2.96*	1.88+0.42*	1.87+1.22*
+	+	12.00+11.37*	4.14+3.72*	1.36 + 0.10*

*Significantly different from controls (p < .05 student's t-test).
Values are mean ± S.D.
[1]Measured 20 wks post-retrovirus infection. Animals were fed 5% (v/v) ethanol in Lieber-DeCarli liquid diet for 4 wks after 16 wks post retrovirus infection. The alcohol containing diets were stopped the day before parasite inoculation. All animals were inoculated with *C. parvum*.

Table 2. Effects of prior ethanol treatment and retrovirus infection on *Cryptosporidium* colonization of intestinal villae[1]

Treatment		Days Post *Cryptosporidium* Infection		
Retrovirus Infection	Dietary Alcohol	10	20	27
		oocysts/villus section		
-	-	3.0+1.4	0	0
-	+	5.7+2.1	0	0
+	-	25.0+15.7*	41.0+25.5*	44.5+13.7*
+	+	25.5+21.9*	36.5+3.5*	36.7+13.3*

*Significantly different from controls (p < .05 student's t-test). Value are mean + S.D.
[1]Animals were fed 5% (v/v) ethanol in Lieber-DeCarli liquid diet for 4 wks after 16 wks post retrovirus infection. The alcohol containing diets were stopped the day before parasite inoculation. All animals were infected with *C. parvum*.

of IL-4 by Peyer's patches cells during *Giardia muris* infection in mice with murine AIDS as well as secretory anti-Giardia antibodies in the intestine. IL-4 is critical to both retention of B cells in the intestines and their maturation to produce IgA which is important in gut protective immunity to parasitic invasion. Therefore, failure to efficiently regulate cytokine and antibody production after retrovirus infection helps explain the progressive immunodeficiency which predisposed mice to opportunistic infections including loss of resistance to *Cryptosporidium*. *C. parvum* persistently parasitized the intestinal epithelium particularly the distal ilium of all retrovirus infected mice but not untreated or alcohol fed non-retrovirus infected mice. Oocysts were also heavily shedded in the feces of mice with AIDS throughout the duration of the study and this was exacerbated by ethanol ingestion. Hence, immune alterations that accompanied retrovirus infection and concommitant chronic alcohol ingestion resulted in severe immunodeficiency and reduced resistance to *Cryptosporidium* infection. Consequently these immune changes enhanced the development of persistent cryptosporidiosis and accelerated death observed even though severe diarrhea was not exhibited frequently (data not shown) as is often seen in AIDS patients. Lack of frequent diarrhea in murine-AIDS may be due to facilitated fluid resorption by the cecum (11). Even so, the murine model of AIDS described in this study could be useful in evaluating various immunotherapeutic agents for the prophylaxis of cryptosporidiosis.

Acknowledgement

Supported by grants AA08037, 5G12RR03059-04NIH/RCMI and 3-G12RR03059-0451NIH/RCMI.

REFERENCES

1. H. Darban, J. Enriquez, D. R. Sterling, M. C. Lopez, g. Chen, M. Abbaszadegan, and R. R. Watson, Cryptosporidiosis facilitated by murine retroviral infection with LP-BM5, *J. Infect. Dis.* 164:741 (1991).
2. P. Kazlow, G., K. Shah, K. J. Benkov, R. Dische, and N. S. Leiko, Esophageal Cryptosporidiosis in a child with the acquired immune deficiency syndrome, *Gastroenterol.* 91:1301 (1986).
3. G. M. Connolly, M. S. Dryden, D. C. Shanson, and B. G. Gazzard. Cryptosporidial diarrhea in AIDS and its treatment. *Gut.* 29:573 (1988).
4. J . R. Mead, M. J. Arrowood, R. W. Sidwell, and M. C. Healey, Chronic *Cryptosporidium parvum* infections in congenitally immunodeficient SCID and nude mice, *J. Infect. Dis.* 163:1297 (1991).
5. J . R. Mead, M. J. Arrowood, and C. R. Sterling, Antigens of *Cryptosporidium sporozoites* recognized by immune sera of infected animals and humans, *J. Parasitol.* 74:135-143 (1988).
6. M. Lopez, L. L. Colombo, D. S. Huang, and R. R. Watson, Impairment of mucosal immunity by LP-BM5 murine leukemia virus infection producing murine AIDS, *Regional Immunol*, 4:162 (1992).
7. T. Petro, M., R. R. Watson, D. E. Feely, and H. Carban, Suppression of resistance to *Giardia muris* and cytokine production in a murine model of acquired immune deficiency syndrome, *Regional Immunol.*, accepted, (1992).
8. S. A. Kocoshis, M. L. Cibull, T. E. Davis, J. T. Hinton, M. Seip, and J. G. Banwell, Intestinal and pulmonary Cryptosporidiosis in an infant with severe combined immune deficiency. J. Pediatric *Gastroenterol. and Nutr.* 149 (1984).
9. H. C. Morse III, , R. A. Yetter, C. S. Via, R. R. Hardy, A. Cerny, K. Hayakawa, A. W. Hugin, M. W. Miller, K. L. Holmes, and G. M. Shearer, Functional and phenotypic alteration in T-cell subsets during the course of MAIDS, a murine retrovirus-induced immunodeficiency syndrome, *J. Immunol.* 143:844 (1989).
10. D. E.Mosier, R. A. Yetter, and H. C. Morse III, Retroviral induction of acute lymphoproliferative disease and profound immunosuppression in adult C57BL/6 mice, *J. Exp. Med.* 161:766 (1985).
11. C. E. Chrisp, W. C. Reid, H. G. Rush, M. A. Suckow, A. Bush, and M. J. Thomann, Cryptosporidiosis in guinea pigs: an animal model, *Infect. Immun.* 58:674 (1990).

ENHANCEMENT OF HIV-1 REPLICATION BY OPIATES AND COCAINE: THE CYTOKINE CONNECTION

Phillip K. Peterson, Genya Gekker, Ronald Schut, Shuxian Hu, Henry H. Balfour, Jr., and Chun C. Chao

Department of Medicine, Hennepin County Medical Center; Department of Laboratory Medicine and Pathology, University of Minnesota Health Sciences Center, University of Minnesota Medical School, Minneapolis, MN

INTRODUCTION

In recent years, drug abuse has been identified as the most important factor in the spread of the AIDS epidemic (1). In the injection drug use (IDU) population, the sharing of contaminated injection equipment is a major means of transmitting HIV-1 (2, 3), the primary etiologic agent of AIDS. Several reports suggest that the course of HIV-1 infection is accelerated and that the mortality is increased in IDU patients (4-7), although results of some studies are contradictory (8, 9). As in other AIDS risk groups, multiple co-factors have been considered as possible contributors to the development of AIDS in HIV-1-infected drug abusers (10). A special cofactor postulated to be important in this patient group has been drug-induced immunologic disturbances (11, 12). This "co-factor hypothesis" is supported by a large body of evidence from clinical studies, animal models, and *in vitro* investigations (reviewed in 13-19).

Over the past several years, our laboratory has investigated the hypothesis that opiates and cocaine suppress functional activities of human peripheral blood mononuclear cells (PBMC) that are known to play a role in host defense against intracellular opportunistic pathogens observed in AIDS. Since the major target cells of HIV-1, CD4 lymphocytes and monocytes, are contained within PBMC cultures, we have also tested the hypothesis that morphine and cocaine amplify HIV-1 replication in PBMC. During the course of these studies, we have found that both of these drugs affect the function and susceptibility to HIV- 1 infection of PBMC via altering the production of cytokines, mediators that are now recognized to play a central role in HIV-1 pathogenesis (20-22).

In this chapter, we will review studies carried out in our laboratory which demonstrate that morphine and cocaine amplify HIV-1 replication in co-cultures of human PBMC. Other investigators have described similar results with heroin (23) and with morphine using human Kupffer cells (24) and neuroblastoma cells (25). Also, we report the results of recent studies indicating that morphine potentiates the release of

Drugs of Abuse, Immunity, and AIDS, Edited by
H. Friedman *et al.*, Plenum Press, New York, 1993

cytokines from microglial cells and astrocytes (the brain's immune cells) and discuss the implications of these findings for the neuroimmunopathogenesis of AIDS.

MORPHINE, COCAINE, AND LECTIN-ACTIVATED PBMC

In our initial studies of the effects of morphine on HIV-1 replication, we used a standard clinical virology laboratory assay in which PBMC from HIV-1-infected patients are co-cultured with PBMC obtained from normal donors. In this assay, HIV-1 p24 antigen levels in co-culture supernatants are quantified by an enzyme-linked immunoassay as an index of viral replication. Since it had been established early on that an activating signal was required for optimal stimulation of HIV-1 growth in cell culture, the normal donor PBMC were first activated with the plant lectin phytohemagglutinin (PHA) for 3 days prior to constitution of the co-cultures with HIV-1-infected patient PBMC. Significant potentiation of HIV-1 replication by morphine was demonstrated in these studies; however, considerable variability of morphine's stimulatory effect was found which appeared to be related primarily to the use of different patient donors of HIV-1-infected PBMC (26).

To allow us to study the mechanism of morphine's stimulatory effect on HIV-1 replication, we eliminated the variability of the PBMC standard co-culture assay by using the same HIV-1 isolate and the same pool of acutely infected PBMC for all experiments (27). With this modified co-culture assay, a highly reproducible, marked augmentation of viral replication was observed. We demonstrated: (1) the stimulatory activity of morphine was dose-dependent (a bell-shaped dose-response relationship existed with maximal enhancement occuring at $1O^{-12}$M morphine), (ii) an interaction of morphine with the PHA-activated donor PBMC was required, and (iii) morphine acted via an opiate receptor mechanism (27).

In our initial studies demonstrating an amplifying effect of morphine on viral replication, we used acutely HIV-1-infected PBMC as a cell culture model of HIV-1 infection. Since chronically ("latently") HIV-1-infected cell lines have been more commonly used as an *in vitro* model to explore potential co-factors that upregulate HIV-1 expression, we next investigated the effects of morphine on the induction of HIV-1 replication in two such cell lines: U1 cells (a promonocytic cell line) and the ACH-2 clone (a CD4 lymphocyte line). When morphine was added directly to these cell lines, low levels of HIV-1 p24 antigen were detected in culture supernatants, but no evidence of a stimulatory effect of morphine was found (28). Likewise, morphine had no effect on the upregulation of HIV-1 expression in U1 or ACH-2 cells when viral induction was triggered by recombinant tumor necrosis factor (TNF)-α When the U1 and ACH-2 clones were co-cultured with PBMC that had been activated with PHA in the presence of morphine, however, an opiate induced enhancement of HIV-1 expression was observed (28).

Parallel studies of cocaine in the modified PHA-activated PBMC co-culture assay demonstrated that this drug shared the potentiating effect on HIV-1 replication of morphine (29). Because we recently had determined that cocaine alters the respiratory burst activity of monocytes within PBMC cultures via a mechanism involving transforming growth factor (TGF)-β, we immediately investigated the contribution of this cytokine to cocaine's effect on HIV-1 replication. The observations that TGF-β potentiated HIV-1 replication in a manner similar to cocaine and that antibodies to TGF-β, blocked the potentiating effects of both TGF-β, and cocaine suggested that this multifunctional cytokine played a mediator role in cocaine-induced amplification of HIV-1 replication (29).

To test whether morphine treatment of PBMC would modify the production of TGF-β in response to PHA, we cultured PBMC from normal donors in varying concentrations of morphine during 72 hr activation with this lectin. Using a highly sensitive and specific bioassay for TGF-β, we found that supernatants from cultures containing morphine, in concentrations as low as 10^{-12} M, had significantly elevated levels of TGF-β when compared to control cultures lacking morphine (30). Thus we postulated that the mechanism whereby morphine and cocaine amplify HIV-1 replication in PBMC co-cultures containing PHA-activated PBMC involves enhanced production of TGF-β by drug-exposed cells. The cell type(s) and site(s) of action of morphine and cocaine underlying this phenomenon, however, remain to be determined.

MORPHINE, COCAINE, AND CYTOMEGALOVIRUS (CMV)-ACTIVATED PBMC

To extend our studies to a cell-activating signal of greater clinical relevance, we replaced PHA with CMV in the PBMC co-culture assay. This virus is not only an important cause of opportunistic infection in AIDS patients (31), but CMV also has been proposed to act as a co-factor in accelerating the progression of HIV-1 infection (32, 33). Prior to investigating the effects of morphine and cocaine, we first characterized the features required for HIV-1 replication in acutely infected PBMC when co-cultures contained CMV-activated PBMC. In this study, we found: (i) CMV could trigger HIV-1 replication, provided that the PBMC were obtained from CMV-seropositive donors, and (ii) the upregulation of HIV-1 expression by CMV-stimulated PBMC involved TNF-α (34).

The hypothesis that substances of abuse potentiate HIV-1 replication in PBMC co-cultures containing CMV-activated cells recently has been tested with morphine and cocaine. For these studies, PBMC were obtained from CMV-seropositive donors, and a suboptimal concentration of CMV was used to activate these PBMC. As shown in Fig. 1, when PBMC that had been activated with CMV in the presence of morphine were incorporated in the co-culture assay, significant amplification of HIV-1 replication was observed by day 6 of co-culture. As had been described for PHA (27), the dose-response relationship of morphine in co-cultures containing CMV-activated PBMC is bell-shaped; however, the optimal amplifying dose of morphine is extraordinarily low (10^{-15} M) when CMV is used as an activating signal (Fig. 1). In studies with cocaine, a similar bell-shaped dose-response relationship also was found with optimal enhancement of HIV-1 replication observed at 10^{-12} M cocaine (35). Based upon the results of our earlier studies with PHA (29) and the findings with CMV as an activating signal (34), we examined the role of TGF-β and TNF-α in cocaine's amplifying effect. Using specific antibodies to block the activity of these cytokines, evidence was provided that both TGF-β and TNF-α are involved in the mechanism of cocaine-induced enhancement of HIV-1 replication (35).

The relevance of these *in vitro* studies to HIV-1 infection in opiate or cocaine addicts is unknown. If our findings are clinically pertinent, however, it appears that neither opiates nor cocaine fosters HIV-1 infection independently of an activating signal, e.g., CMV. Thus epidemiologic studies of substances of abuse as potential co-factors in the acceleration of HIV-1 infection may need to examine the interaction of multiple co-factors to delineate an effect. Given the complexity of such studies in the IDU population, testing of the "substance of abuse co-factor hypothesis" in HIV-1 infection, may have to await development of an appropriate animal model.

MORPHINE AND THE BRAIN'S IMMUNE CELLS

In the past decade, the traditional view of the brain as an "immunologically privileged" site has been dramatically changed by the results of a large series of studies.

The central nervous system (CNS) has been found to be populated by two groups of glial cells - microglia and astrocytes - that share many of the functions of macrophages and lymphocytes in the periphery, including the production of cytokines (36-39).

HIV-induced encephalopathy, or AIDS dementia complex (ADC), affects up to 70% of patients prior to death. Although the pathogenesis of ADC is incompletely understood, several distinctive features have been delineated (40-43). HIV is of etiologic importance, and an interaction among monocytes/microglial cells, astrocytes, and cytokines appears to play a central role in the pathogenesis of ADC (44-46).

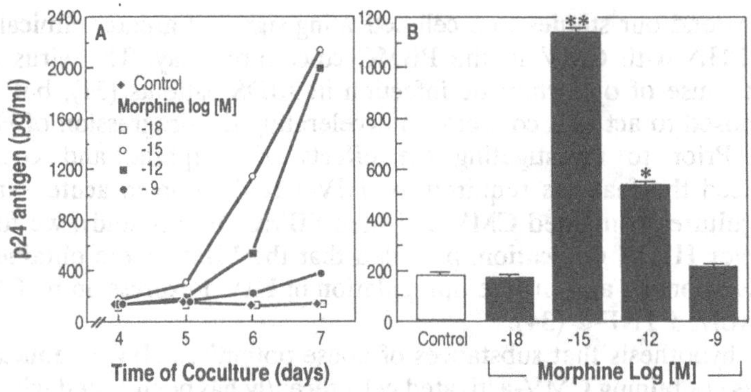

Fig. 1. Effect of morphine on HIV-1 replication in PBMC co-cultures containing CMV-activated PBMC. Previously described methods (2, 35) were adapted for this experiment. Prior to constitution of co-cultures with acutely HIV-1-infected PBMC, PBMC from healthy CMV seropositive donors were first incubated with CMV and then cultured for 3 days in the presence or absence (control) of morphine, at indicated concentrations. Co-cultures were then established, and supernatants were sampled for HIV- 1 p24 antigen levels on indicated days (Panel A) or on day 6 (Panel B). Results in Panel A are representative of three separate experiments. Values in Panel B are mean ± SE of experiments using PBMC from three donors (*P <0.05; ** P<0.01) compared to control value.

Since the brain is a principal target organ not only for drugs of abuse but also for HIV-1, we recently have initiated in *vitro* studies of the effects of morphine on cytokine production by microglial cells and astrocytes. Initially, we demonstrated that primary neonatal murine microglial cells produce abundant amounts of TNF when stimulated with lipopolysaccharide (LPS) (47). Using these cell cultures, preliminary studies in our laboratory suggest that exposure of microglial cells to morphine markedly potentiates the release of TNF from LPS-stimulated cells (Fig. 2). When primary neonatal murine astrocyte cultures are stimulated with LPS, we have found that morphine treatment results in significant enhancement of TGF-β release (Fig. 3).

Since both TNF-α and TGF-β are known to affect HIV-1 replication, our preliminary findings of the interaction of morphine with microglial cells and astrocytes could have implications for understanding the neuroimmunopathogenesis of ADC. Future studies in our laboratory will address this possibility and also will explore the potential effect of endogenous opioid peptides, the natural ligands of the opiate receptors, on cytokine ("immunotransmitter") production by immune cells of the brain.

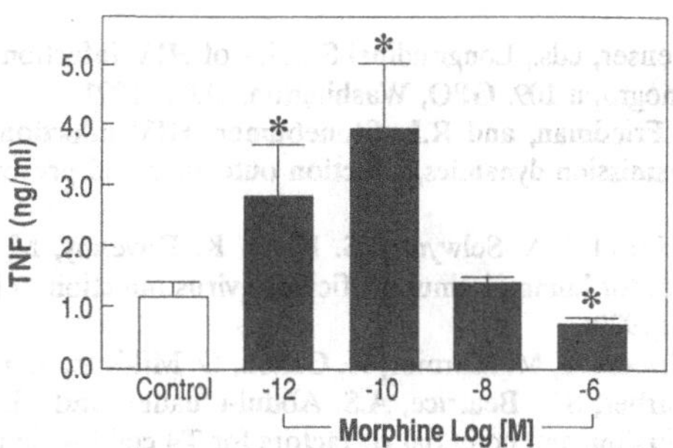

Fig. 2. Effect of morphine on microglial cell TNF production. Murine microglial cell cultures were prepared as previously described (47). Following 24 hr incubation with morphine, at indicated concentrations, or medium (control), microglial cell cultures (5 x 10^4 cells/well) were stimulated with 10 ng/ml LPS for 6 hr. Supernatants were then harvested for TNF bioassay. Data are mean ± SE of triplicate values and are representative of three separate experiments. *P<0.05, compared to control values.

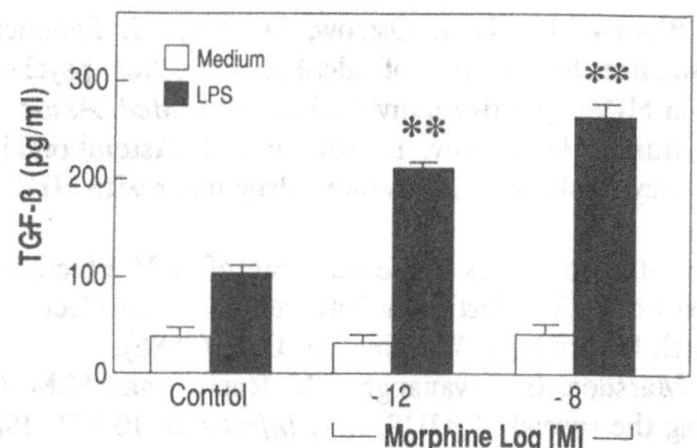

Fig. 3. Effect of morphine on astrocyte production of TGF-β. Murine astrocyte cultures (5 x 104 cells/well) were treated with morphine for 24 hr followed by incubation in medium alone or medium containing LPS (1 μg/ml) for 24 hr. Supernatants were then harvested for TGF-β bioassay. The methods used in this experiment were modified from those previously described for isolation of murine astrocytes (48) and for the measurement of TGF-β (49). Data are mean ± SE of triplicate values and are representative of three separate experiments. **P<0.01, compared to control values.

Acknowledgements

This work was supported in part by National Institute on Drug Abuse grant DA04381. The authors are grateful to Jacqueline Ostroum for secretarial assistance.

REFERENCES

1. P. Hartsock and S.G. Genser, eds., Longitudinal Studies of HIV Infection in Intravenous Drug Users. NIDA Research Monograph 109. GPO, Washington, D.C. (1991).
2. D. C. Des Jarlais, S.R. Friedman, and R.L. Stonebumer, HIV infection and intravenous drug use: Critical issues in transmission dynamics, infection outcomes and prevention, *Rev Infect Dis.* 10:151 (1988).
3. E. E. Schoenbaum, D Hartel, P.A. Selwyn, R.S. Klein, K. Davenny, M. Rogers, C. Feiner, and G. Friedland. Risk factors for human immunodeficiency virus infection in intravenous drug users, *New Engl. J Med.* 321:874 (1989).
4. D. C. Des Jarlais, S.R. Friedman, M. Marmor, H. Cohen, D. Mildvan, S. Yancovitz, U. Mathur, W. El-Sadr, T.J Spira, J. Garber, S.T. Beatrice, A.S. Abdul-Quader, and J.L. Sotheran, Development of AIDS, HIV seroconversion, and potential co-factors for T4 cell loss in a cohort of intravenous drug users, *AIDS* 1:105 (1987).
5. R. L. Stoneburner, D.C. Des Jarlais, D. Benezra, L. GoreLlcin, J.L. Sotheran, S.R. Friedman, S. Schultz, M. Marmor, D. Mildvan, and R. Maslansky, A larger spectrum of severe HIV-1-related disease in intravenous drug users in New York City, *Science* 242:916 (1988).
6. A. Munoz, V. Carey, A.J. Saah, J.P. Phair, L.A. Kingsley, J.L. Fahey, H.M. Ginzburg, and F.B. Polk, Predictors of decline in CD4 lymphocytes in a cohort of homosexual men infected with human immunodeficiency virus, *J. Acquir. Immune Defic. Syndr.* 1:396 (1988).
7. J. D. Sobel, Acquired immunodeficiency syndrome in intravenous drug abusers, *in*: "Infections in Intravenous Drug Abusers," D.P. Levine and J.D. Sobel, eds, Oxford University Press, New York (1991).
8. R. A. Kaslow, W.C. Blackwelder, D.G. Ostrow, D. Yerg, J. Palenicek, A.H. Coulson, and R.O. Valdiserri, No evidence for a role of alcohol or other psychoactive drugs in accelerating immunodeficiency in HIV-1-positive individuals, *J. Am. Med. Assoc.* 261:3424 (1989).
9. J. B. Margolick, A. Munoz, D. Vlahov, L. Solomon, J. Astemborski, S. Cohn, and K.E. Nelson, Changes in T-lymphocyte subsets in intravenous drug users with HIV-1 infection, *J. Am. Med. Assoc.* 267:1631 (1992).
10. D. C. Des Jarlais, "Potential co-factors in the outcome of HIV infection in intravenous drug users. *in*: "Longitudinal Studies of HIV Infection in Intravenous Drug Users," P. Hastsock and S.G Genser, eds., NIDA Research Monograph, Washington, D.C. (1986).
11. R. L. Hubbard, M.E. Marsden, E. Cavanaugh, J.V. Rachal, and H.M. Ginzburg, Role of drug-abuse treatment in limiting the spread of AIDS, *Rev. Infect Dis.* 10:377 (1988).
12. R. M. Donahoe and A. Falek, Neuroimmunomodulation by opiates and other drugs of abuse: Relationship to HIV infection and AIDS. *in:* "Psychological, Neuropsychiatric, and Substance Abuse Aspects of AIDS". T.P. Bridge, et al., eds. Raven Press, New York (1988).
13. R. M. Donahoe, Drug abuse and AIDS: Causes for the connection, *in:* "Drugs of Abuse: Chemistry, Pharmacology, Immunology, and AIDS". P.T.K Pham, and K. Rice, eds. NIDA Research Monograph 96 GPO. Washington, D.C. (1990).
14. M. J. Kreek, Immune function in heroin addicts and former heroin addicts in treatment: Pre-and post-AIDS epidemic. *in*: "Drugs of Abuse: Chemistry, Pharmacology, Immunology, and AIDS". P.T.K. Pham and K. Rick, eds. NIDA Research Monograph 96. GPO, Washington, D.C. (1990).
15. H. U. Bryant, E.W. Bemton, and J.W. Holaday, Immunomodulatory effects of chronic morphine treatment: Pharmacologic and mechanistic studies, *in*: "Drugs of Abuse: Chemistry, Pharmacology, Immunology, and AIDS", P.T.K. Pham and K. Rick, eds. NIDA Research Monograph 96. GPO, Washington, D.C. (1990).
16. P. K. Peterson, T.W. Molitor, C.C. Chao, and B. Sharp, "Opiates and cell-mediated immunity. *in*: "Drugs of Abuse and Immune Function," R.R. Watson, ed. CRC Press, Boca Raton (1990).
17. B. M. Bayer and C.M. Flores, Effects of morphine on lymphocyte function: Possible mechanisms of interaction. *in:* "Drugs of Abuse and Immune Function," R.R. Watson, ed. CRC Press, Boca Raton (1990).

18. J. J. Madden and R.M. Donahoe, Opiate binding to cells of the immune system, *in:* "Drugs of Abuse and Immune Function," R.R. Watson, ed. CRC Press, Boca Raton (1990).
19. R. Pillai, B.S. Nair and R.R. Watson, AIDS, drugs of abuse and the immune system: A complex immunotoxicological network, *Arch Toxicol.* 65:609 (1991).
20. Z. F. Rosenberg and A.S. Fauci, Immunopathogenic mechanisms of HIV infection: Cytokine induction of HIV expression. *in:* "HIV and the Immune System," R.B. Gallagher, ed. Elsevier Trends Journals, Cambridge (1991).
21. W. L. Farrar, M. Komer and K.A. Clouse, Cytokine regulation of human immunodeficiency virus expression, *Cytokine*, 3:531 (1991).
22. T. Matsuyama, N. Kobayashi and N. Yamamoto. Cytokines and HIV infection: Is AIDS a tumor necrosis factor disease? *AIDS* 5:1405 (1991).
23. E. Henderson, T. Eisenstein, J. Jr. Meissler, J. Yang et al, Increased proliferation of HIV by heroin *in vitro.* Problems of Drug Dependence 1991: Proceedings of the 53rd Annual Scientific Meeting, The Committee on Problems of Drug Dependence, Inc., NIDA Research Monograph, in press.
24. C. Schweitzer, F. Keller, M.P. Schmitt, D. Jaeck, M. Adloff, C. Schmitt, C. Royer, A. Kirn and A.M. Aubertin, Morphine stimulates HIV replication in primary cultures of human Kupffer cells, *Res. Virol.* 142:189 (1991).
25. S. P. Squinto, D. Mondal, A.L. Block and O.M. Prakash, Morphine-induced transactivation of HIV-1 LTR in human neuroblastoma cells, *AIDS Res. Human Retrovir.* 6:1163 (1990).
26. P. K. Peterson, B.M. Sharp, G. Gekker, B. Jackson and H. H. Balfour, Jr. Opiates, human peripheral blood mononuclear cells, and HIV, *Adv. Exper. Med. Biol.* 288:171 (1991).
27. P. K. Peterson, B.M. Sharp, G. Gekker, P.S. Portoghese, K. Sannerud and H.H. Jr. Balfour, Morphine promotes the growth of HIV-1 in human peripheral blood mononuclear cell co-cultures, *AIDS* 4:869 (1990) .
28. P. K. Peterson, G. Gekker, C.C. Chao, J. Verhoef and H.H. Jr. Balfour, Effects of morphine on human immunodeficiency virus-1 expression in the chronically infected cell lines, U1 and ACH-2, *Immunol. Infect. Dis.* 1:313 (1991).
29. P. K. Peterson, G. Gekker, C.C. Chao, R. Schut, T.W. Molitor and H.H. Jr. Balfour, Cocaine potentiates HIV-1 replication in human peripheral blood mononuclear cell co-cultures: Involvement of transforming growth factor-ß. *J. Immunol.* 146:81 (1991).
30. C. C. Chao, S. Hu, T.W. Molitor, Y. Zhou, M.P. Murtaugh, M. Tsang and P.K. Peterson, Morphine potentiates transforming growth factor-β release from human peripheral blood mononuclear cell cultures, *J. Pharmacol. Exp Ther.*, in press (1992).
31. R. Schooley, Cytomegalovirus in the setting of infection with human immunodeficiency virus, *Rev. Infect Dis.* 12 (Suppl.):8 (1990).
32. A. Webster, Cytomegalovirus as a possible cofactor in HIV disease progression, *J. Acquired Immune Defic. Syndr.* 4 (Suppl.):47 (1991).
33. J. Laurence, Molecular interactions among herpesviruses and human immunodeficiency viruses, *J. Infect. Dis.* 162:338 (1990).
34. P. K. Peterson, G. Gekker, C.C. Chao, S. Hu, C. Edelman, H.H. Jr. Balfour and J. Verhoef, Human cytomegalovirus-stimulated peripheral blood mononuclear cells induce HIV-1 replication via a tumor necrosis factor-α-mediated mechanism, *J. Clin. Invest.* 89:574 (1992).
35. P. K. Peterson, G. Gekker, C.C. Chao, R. Schut, J. Verhoef, C.K. Edelman, A. Erice and H. H. Balfour, Jr., Cocaine amplifies HIV-1 replication in CMV-stimulated PBMC co-cultures, *J. Immunol.*, in press(l992).
36. W. L. Farrar, Evidence for the common expression of neuroendocrine hormones and cytokines in the immune and central nervous systems, *Brain Behav Immun.* 2:322 (1988).
37. K. Frei and A. Fontana, Immune regulatory functions of astrocytes and microglial cells within the central nervous system. *in:* "Physiology and Diseases. Neuroimmune Networks", Alan R. Liss, Inc. (1989).
38. S. L. Hauser and T. Hayashi, Major histocompatibility complex antigens and the nervous system. *in:* "Physiology and Diseases. Neuroimmune Networks", Alan R. Liss, Inc. (1989).
39. J. E. Merrill, Lymphokines and glial cells: Implications for disease. *in:* "Peripheral Signaling of the Brain". R.C.A. Frederickson, J.L. McGaugh, and D.L. Felten, eds. Hofgrefe & Huber Publishers, Toronto (1991).
40. R. W. Price, B. Brew, J. Sidtis, M. Rosenblum, A.C. Scheck and P. Cleary, The brain in AIDS: Central nervous system HIV-1 infection and AIDS dementia complex, *Science* 239:586 (1988) .
41. D. D. Ho, D.E. Bredesen, H.V. Vinters and E.S. Daar, The acquired immunodeficiency syndrome (AIDS) dementia complex, *Ann. Intern Med.* 111:400 (1989).
42. D. H. Gabuzda and R.T. Johnson, Nervous system infection with human immunodeficiency virus: Biology and pathogenesis, *Curr. Asp. Neurosci.* 1:285 (1990).

43. R. T. Johnson, J.C. McArthur and O. Narayan, The neurobiology of human immunodeficiency virus infections. *FASEB J.* 2:2970 (1988).
44. D. W. Dickson, L.A. Mattiace, K. Kure, K. Hutchins, W.D. Lyman and C.F. Brosnan, Microglia in human disease, with an emphasis on acquired immune deficiency syndrome, *Lab. Invest.* 64:135 (1991).
45. J. E. Merrill and I.S.Y. Chen, HIV-1, macrophages, glial cells and cytokines in AIDS nervous system disease, *FASEB J.* 5:2391 (1991).
46. C. Cheng-Mayer, J.T. Rutka, M.L. Rosenblum, T. McHugh, D.P. Stites and J.A. Levy, Human immunodeficiency virus can productively infect cultured human glial cells, *Proc. Natl. Acad. Sci.* 84:3526 (1987).
47. C. C. Chao, S. Hu, K. Close, C.S. Choi, T.W. Molitor, W.J. Novick and P.K. Peterson, Cytokine release from microglia: Differential inhibition by pentoxifylline and dexamethasone, *J. Infect. Dis.* in press (1992).
48. I. Y. Chung and E.N. Benveniste, Tumor necrosis factor-α production by astrocytes: Induction by lipopolysaccharide, IFN-γ, and IL-1β, *J. Immunol.* 144:2999 (1990).
49. P. K. Peterson, C.C. Chao, S. Hu and E.G. Shaskan, Glioblastoma, transforming growth and Candida meningitis: A potential link, *Am. J. Med.* 92:262 (1992).

SMALL ANIMAL MODEL OF AIDS

AND THE FELINE IMMUNODEFICIENCY VIRUS

M. Bendinelli[1], M. Pistello[1], D. Matteucci[1], S. Lombardi[1], F. Baldinotti[1], P. Bandecchi[2], R. Ghilarducci[1], L. Ceccherini-Nelli[1], C. Garzelli[1], A. Poli[2], F. Esposito[3], G. Malvaldi[1], and F. Tozzini[2]

[1]Dipartimento di Biomedicina e [2]Dipartimento di Patologia Animale
Università di Pisa e [3]Dipartimento di Biologia Cellulare e Molecolare
Università di Camerino, Italy

INTRODUCTION

Many aspects of the virology, epidemiology and prevention of AIDS are fairly well known, but the mechanisms whereby HIV produces the characteristic severe immune deficiency remain essentially obscure. Even more importantly, the armamentarium for controlling HIV infection is still extremely limited. For these reasons it is generally believed that AIDS research might profit greatly from the study of animal models.

HIV infects and replicates in chimpanzees and rabbits where, however, it does not induce overt disease. As no other species has been found consistently susceptible to HIV, attention has necessarily been directed on several retroviruses of animals that are markedly immunodepressive in their natural host species or in heterologous hosts. Of special interest are the immunosuppressive retroviruses that infect small animals as they are particularly practical to work with. The small animal models of AIDS that have been proposed are listed in Table 1. The list begins with the Friend leukemia complex and other murine oncoviruses, that should be considered "preexisting models" as their immunosuppressive properties were the subject of intensive investigation by Friedman, Salaman and others long before AIDS was recognized (1). The murine oncovirus LP-BM5 has few features in common with the AIDS virus apart the name that has cunningly been given to the disease it induces (murine AIDS or MAIDS). Other murine models have not stood up to their promises or are still under evaluation or confirmation, as discussed in a number of recent reviews and books (2,3). In this article we focus on feline immunodeficiency virus (FIV).

FIV was added to the list of models of AIDS in 1987 when Pedersen, et al., reported the isolation of a lentivirus from the peripheral blood mononuclear cells (PBMC) of cats with immunodeficiency disorders similar to human AIDS (4). As it is

Drugs of Abuse, Immunity, and AIDS, Edited by
H. Friedman *et al.*, Plenum Press, New York, 1993

Table 1. Small animal models of AIDS in the chronological order they have been proposed (for reviews, see ref. 1-3, 30).

VIRUS	HOST	PROPONENTS
Friend leukemia and other immunosuppressive oncoviruses	mouse	Friedman, *et al.*, 1966; Salaman *et al.*, 1966; Bendinelli *et al.*,1966
LP-BM5 oncovirus	mouse	Mosier *et al.*, 1985
FIV	cat	Pedersen *et al.*, 1987
HIV-1	hu-hemato lymphoid SCID mouse	McCune *et al.*,1988; Namikawa *et al.*, 1988
HIV-1	rabbit	Filice *et al.*, 1988
HIV-1	*tat* transgenic mouse	Vogel *et al.*, 1988
HIV-1	provirus transgenic mouse	Leonard *et al.*, 1988
HIV-1	LTR transgenic mouse	Leonard *et al.*, 1989
HIV-1	hu-PBL-SCID mouse	Mosier *et al.*, 1991
HIV-1	mouse	Locardi *et al.*, 1992

the known lentivirus which affects the smallest animal species (Table 2) and induces profound immunosuppressive changes, it was immediately proposed as an ideal system for investigating aspects of AIDS that cannot be easily approached in humans. The areas of research in which FIV investigation is thought to be most useful are the understanding of AIDS pathogenesis, the evaluation of new antilentiviral drugs, the development of strategies for the production of effective anti-HIV vaccines and, last but not least, the improvement of cat health. We will discuss the latter aspect first, for its inherent importance and because it allows a discussion of the immunological and clinical changes caused by FIV.

IMPROVEMENT OF CAT HEALTH

FIV is a substantial health problem for its natural host species. It is spread worldwide with a prevalence ranging between 1 and 30% among apparently healthy

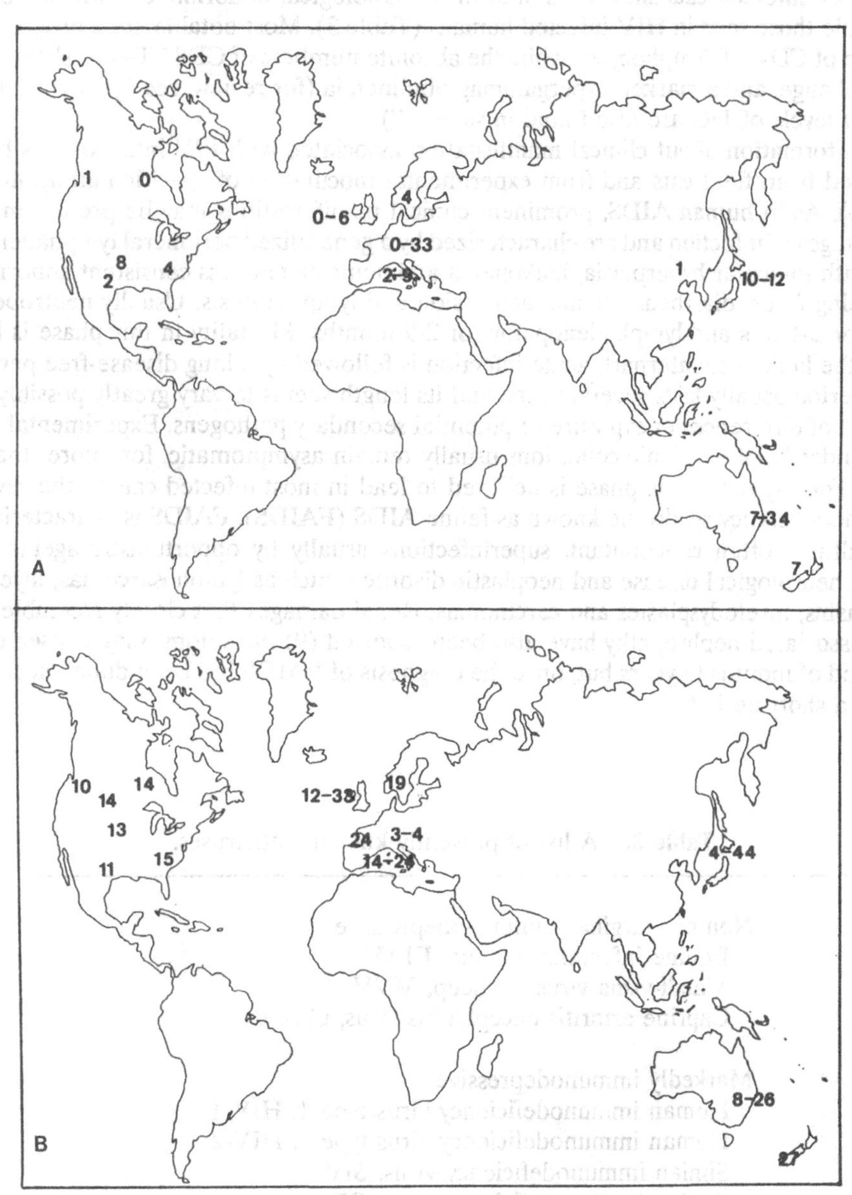

Fig. 1. **Prevalence of FIV infection in apparently healthy (A) and chronically sick domestic cats (B), as judged from serological studies performed in various countries.**

domestic cats and between 3 and 44% among cats seen by vets for long-lasting clinical ailments (Fig. 1). The large variations of prevalence in different countries may reflect differences in the lifestyle of cats. The high prevalence in adult male free-roaming cats and other evidence suggest that biting is a major means of FIV transmission (5,6), although others are also known.

FIV-infected cats show a number of immunological abnormalities which closely resemble those seen in HIV-infected humans (Table 3). Most notable are a progressive decline of $CD4^+$ T-lymphocytes, while the absolute numbers of $CD8^+$ T-cells show little or no change, and a marked hypergammaglobulinemia (for review, see 6). Higher than normal levels of IgG are also found in saliva (7).

Information about clinical manifestation associated with FIV infection has been obtained from field cats and from experimental inoculation of specific pathogen-free cats (6). As in human AIDS, prominent clinical manifestations may be present in the early stages of infection and are characterized by a generalized peripheral lymphadenopathy with follicular hyperplasia, leukopenia and neutropenia, less consistent abnormali ties being fever, diarrhea, anemia, depression and lymphocytosis. Usually neutropenia lasts for 2-4 wks and lymphadenopathy for 2-9 months. Mortality in this phase is low. As in the human counterpart, acute infection is followed by a long disease-free period. This period usually lasts several years, and its length seems to vary greatly possibly as a result of differences in exposure to potential secondary pathogens. Experimental cats kept under highly hygienic conditions usually remain asymptomatic for more than 5 years. The asymptomatic phase is believed to lead in most infected cats to the severe immunodeficiency syndrome known as feline AIDS (FAIDS). FAIDS is characterized by multiple, often concomitant, superinfections usually by opportunistic agents (8), severe neurological disease and neoplastic disorders such as lymphosarcomas, myeloid neoplasms, myelodysplasies and carcinomas. Renal damages that closely resemble the HIV-associated nephropathy have also been reported (9). Symptoms may worsen over a period of months to years but, once the diagnosis of FAIDS has been done, most cats die in a short period.

Table 2. A list of presently known lentiviruses.

Non or marginally immunodepressive
Equine infectious anemia, EIAV
Maedi-visna virus of sheep, MVV
Caprine arthritis-encephalitis virus, CAEV
Markedly immunodepressive
Human immunodeficiency virus type 1, HIV-1
Human immunodeficiency virus type 2, HIV-2
Simian immunodeficiency virus, SIV
Bovine immunodeficiency virus, BIV
Feline immunodeficiency virus, FIV
Others under characterization (dog, chimpanzee, etc.)

It is clear from this brief discussion that developing vaccines and other measures for prevention and treatment of FIV infection would be very important for the health of feline populations.

FIV AS A MODEL FOR HIV PATHOGENESIS

The cell types which have been shown to be susceptible to FIV are listed in Table 4. Although there is considerable similarity with HIV, two major differences should be noted. Firstly, $CD8^+$ T-lymphocytes appear to be capable of replicating FIV at least *in vitro* (10). Second, certain isolates of FIV can be grown on Crandell feline kidney (CrFK) fibroblasts, a continuous cell line routinely used as a convenient source of virus. Under appropriate culture conditions these adherent cells develop easily countable syncytia in response to FIV (Fig. 2). As the number of syncytia formed is linear over a wide range of virus inocula (Figure 3), this system has proved extremely useful for titrating FIV infectivity and FIV neutralizing antibodies (11).

Studies with CrFK cells indicate that the virus absorbs rapidly to cells (11), however the receptor(s) involved is still unknown. The ability to infect $CD8^+$ cells and other cell types that do not appear to express the $CD4^+$ molecule (12) suggests that such molecule is not the receptor or is not the only receptor for FIV. Indeed this might represent an important difference with HIV, whose relevance for pathogenesis remains to be evaluated.

Table 3. Immunologic abnormalities associated with FIV infection.

In vivo

- Hyperplasia, depletion, and dysplasia of lymphoid tissues
- Lymphopenia and neutropenia
- Progressive decline in circulating CD4+ T lymphocytes
- Gradual inversion of CD4+/CD8+ ratio
- Decreased lymphoproliferative responsiveness to mitogens
- Decreased IL 2 production in response to mitogens
- Decreased lymphoproliferative responsiveness to IL 2
- Hypergammaglobulinemia
- Reduced antibody responsiveness to T-dependent antigens
- Inhibition in the switch from IgM to IgG synthesis
- Increased susceptibility to superinfections
- Reduced protection conferred by vaccines

In vitro

- Transient down-regulation of CD4 expression
- Transient down-regulation of class II MHC expression

Table 4. Cell types that have been shown to be susceptible to FIV.

In vivo	*In vitro*
T lymphocytes	Activated T lymphocytes
Macrophages (peritoneum, brain)	Virus transformed T cell lines
Astrocytes	IL 2 dependent lymphoid cell lines
Megakariocytes	IL 2 independent lymphoid cell lines
	Crandell feline kidney fibroblast line

In experimentally infected cats the virus spreads rapidly. It has been isolated from all lymphoid tissues after one week from infection and from most nonlymphoid organs from the third week onwards. PCR and RT-PCR analysis shows that most tissues do not only contain the viral RNA but also the provirus indicating that at least some viral replication takes place in a variety of tissues and organs (13). The cell types which support viral replication in such organs have not yet been identified with certainty. Limited *in situ* hybridization and immunohistochemical studies suggest that the virus is present in macrophages and lymphocytes and, within the bone marrow, also in megakariocytes (6). The virus is easily isolated from PBMC at any stage of infection. Isolation is less frequent from plasma or saliva, although these fluids almost regularly contain FIV genomes detectable by PCR (14).

Table 5. Comparison between FIV and the ideal animal model of AIDS as envisioned by the World Health Organization (WHO).

WHO RECOMMENDATIONS	FIV
- should make use of HIV itself	-
- should be a small animal	+
- host's genetics, immunology and metabolism should be well known	±
- target cells should be CD4+ lymphocytes and macrophages	+
- target organs should include blood, lymphoid tissues and brain	+
- transmission should mimic that of HIV, including perinatal transmission	±
- infection should be possible with both virus-infected cells and free virus	+
- induced disease should have a short incubation period	-
- induced disease should resemble AIDS	+

Studies are in progress in many laboratories for understanding the mechanisms whereby the immunological and clinical effects of FIV are brought about. As manipulations are possible in this model that would be unethical in man, these studies are expected also to shed light on many unresolved problems that still hamper a full understanding of HIV-induced pathogenesis.

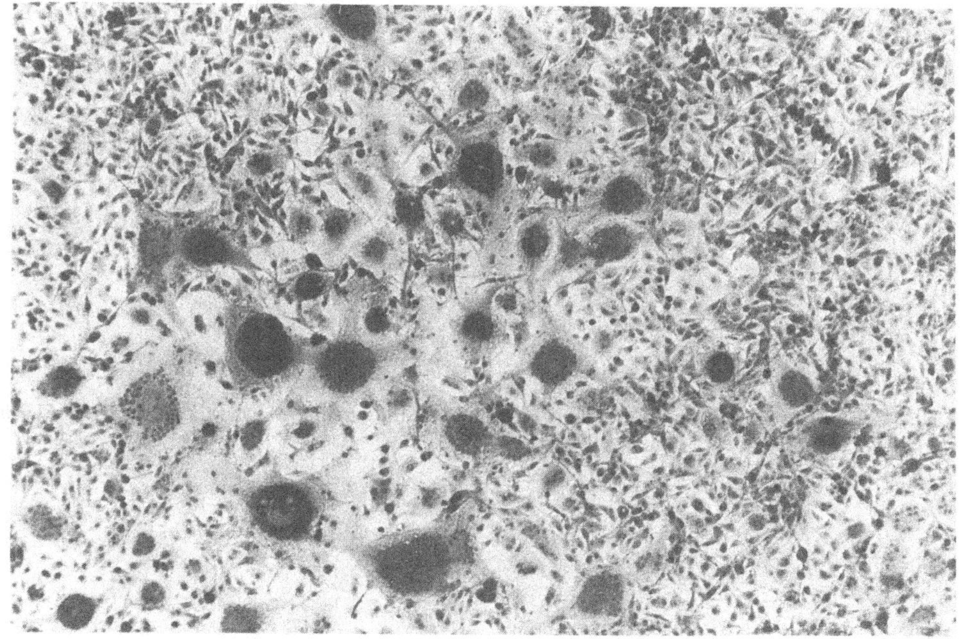

Fig. 2. Syncytia produced by FIV in CrFK cells. Cultures stained with crystal violet six days after infection, magnification ca. x 80.

FIV AS A MODEL FOR UNDERSTANDING THE ROLE OF CO-FACTORS

Table 5 compares FIV to requirements for an ideal animal model for AIDS studies as envisioned by the World Health Organization (3). The two major drawbacks of FIV as a model are that it does not make use of HIV itself and the long disease-free period. The first drawback is also an advantage because the laboratory does not need the restraint measures needed for working with HIV (FIV does not appear to infect humans). The second has its bright side too, because the long clinical latency provides opportunities to investigate whether co-factors can accelerate the decline of immune functions and/or the onset of FAIDS. Available information indicates that the feline leukemia virus can greatly precipitate the development of overt disease in FIV infected cats (15), thus reproducing what is known for humans doubly infected with HIV and HTLV-1 (16). Other viruses which might influence the outcome of FIV infection are listed in Table 6. Co-infection with the protozoa *Toxoplasma gondii* has also been shown to negatively influence the course of FIV infection (17).

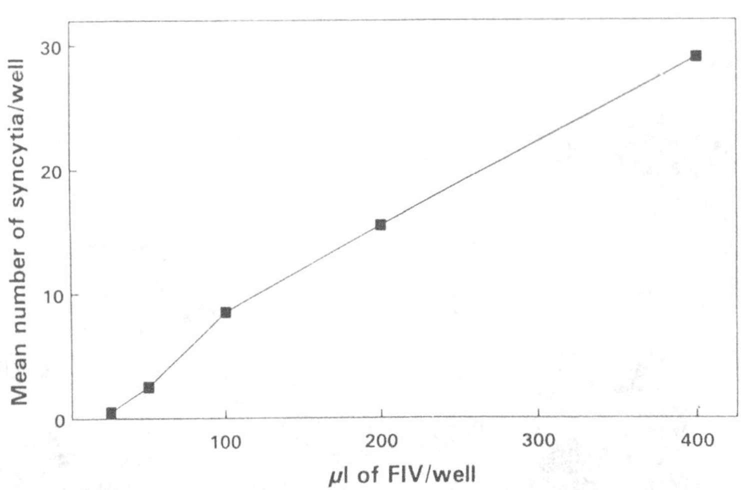

Fig. 3. **Effect of varying the dose of virus inoculated on the number of syncytia produced by FIV in CrFK cells.**

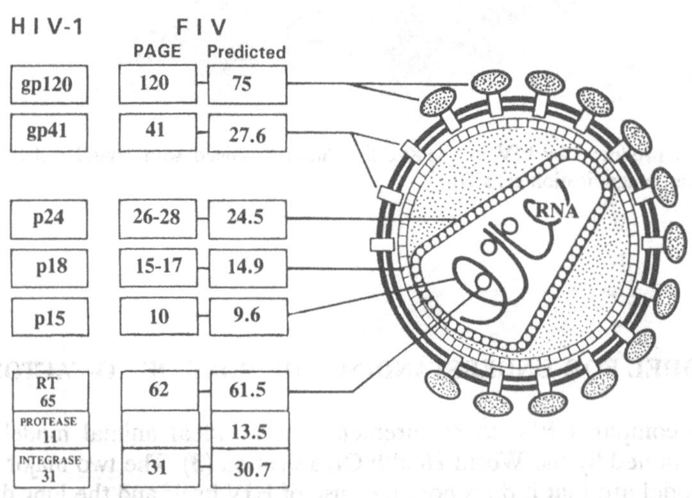

Fig. 4. **Comparative molecular anatomy of FIV and HIV-1.**

FIV AS A MODEL FOR HIV CHEMOTHERAPY

Shape and size of the FIV virion (Fig. 4) and the general organization of its genome (Fig. 5) are those characteristic of other lentiviruses. All the structural molecules of the FIV particle that have been characterized have mol. wt. and immunogenic properties (18) similar to the corresponding molecules of HIV. They also seem to share similar functional properties. For example, the reverse transcriptase activity of FIV and HIV have been shown to possess superimposible sensitivities to a number of inhibitors (19) and the same may be true for RNase activity (20). The emergence of drug-resistant strains following AZT treatment has also been described (21). It is therefore not surprising that currently FIV is extensively used for preclinical evaluation of anti-HIV drugs.

FIV AS A MODEL FOR DEVELOPING ANTI-HIV VACCINES

Cats experimentally infected with FIV develop a prompt antibody response detectable by ELISA, Western blot and indirect immunofluorescence. The presence of such antibodies can be considered indicative of an ongoing infection, as the virus can be isolated from 90% or more of seropositive animals (14). Antibody is present also in saliva, which can facilitate diagnosis (7). Infected cats also develop high titer neutralizing antibodies (Figure 6) that however fail to eradicate the infection. We have recently shown that sera obtained from different geographical areas effectively neutralize a given FIV isolate and that different geographical FIV isolates are neutralized to a similar extent by positive sera. These results indicate that, alike HIV, FIV possesses broadly reactive neutralization inducing epitopes (22). Whether cross-reacting antibodies are protective *in vivo* is still unknown.

Attempts to vaccinate cats have initially given contradictory results, but in more recent studies the administration of chemically inactivated whole virus or virus-infected cells has yielded promising results (Table 7). It should be noted however that in these studies vaccinated cats were challenged with the same viral isolate used to prepare the vaccines and grown on the same cells.

The number of isolates that have been cloned is still low (23-25), but the results clearly indicate that, as in HIV, a considerable degree of genetic diversity exists and may be significant even among isolates with the same geographical provenance. Such diversity is especially evident in the *env* gene, the predicted amino acid diversity in the *env* product being around 15% (26,27). It is noteworthy that in the surface *env* products of FIV and HIV-1 the variable regions have similar locations (Figure 7) indicating that, despite the scarce homology between these two viruses (around 50%), the overall structure of this important component of the virion might be conserved. Based on such observation and on the presence of important neutralization epitopes in the V3 region of HIV-1 (28), we have focused on the analogous region of FIV in the attempt to identify the epitopes responsible for neutralization. Synthetic peptide analysis has identified one or possibly two continuous B-cell epitopes in the carboxy-terminal portion of V3 recognized by most if not all the sera of the infected animals tested. Such results has been confirmed by PEPSCAN analysis, which has also lead to the identification of a sequence of 8 amino acids which reacted with all the sera examined (29). We are presently evaluating whether such epitope(s) is involved in cross-neutralization. Preliminary results also suggest that the V3 region contains continuous T-cell epitopes, indicating that such region might be of great interest for the engineering of better vaccines than those tested so far.

Table 6. Viruses that have been shown to accelerate or are potentially capable of accelerating FIV pathogenesis.

VIRUS[1]	FREQUENCY OF CO-INFECTION	FORMATION OF PSEUDOTYPES	CO-PATHO-GENESIS	Ref.
FeLV	relatively high	?	+++	15
FeSFV	high	?	?	5
RD114	constant	+	?	31
FeHV-1	presumably high	?	LTR activation	32

[1] FeLV: feline leukemia virus; FeSFV: feline syncytium forming virus; FeHV-1: feline herpesvirus type 1.

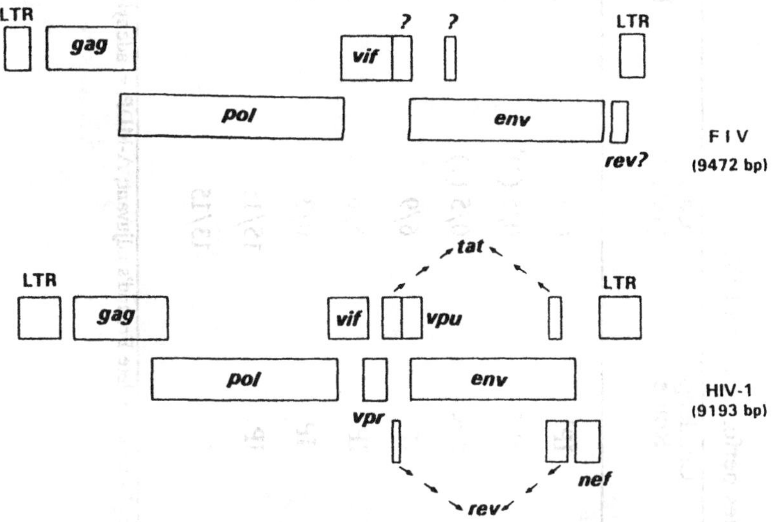

Fig. 5. Genomic organization of FIV and HIV-1. A notable difference is the shorter LTR of FIV (355-362 bp vs 637 bp). The regulatory sequences of FIV are still poorly known.

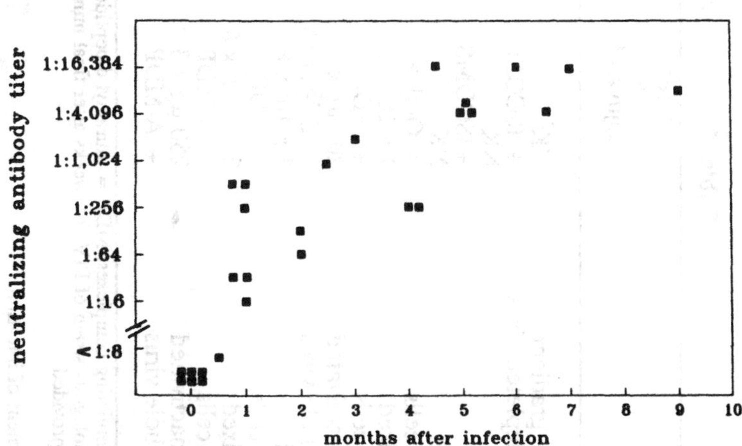

Fig. 6. The development of neutralizing antibodies following infection of cats with FIV. Specific pathogen free cats were infected with the Pisa-M2 isolate while neutralizing antibodies were assayed against the Petaluma isolate as described in Ref. 11.

Table 7. Vaccination studies performed with FIV.

Vaccine	Doses + Adjuvant[1]	Dose (ID50)	Challenge[2] Route	Cats protected	Ref.
Detergent disrupted, gradient purified envelope depleted virus	NK[3] + ISCOMS	20	IP[4]	0/4	33
Recombinant p24	NK +ISCOMS	NK	NK	0/5 (↑)[5]	33
Glutaraldehyde-fixed allogeneic infected cells	NK + Quil A	NK	NK	0/5 (↑)	33
Paraformaldehyde-fixed allogeneic infected cells	1 x 10^7 x 6 + MDP	10	IP	6/9	34, 35
Paraformaldehyde inactivated cell-free pelleted whole virus	200 μg x 4 + CFA/IFA	10	IP	5/6	34, 35
Glutaradehyde-fixed allogeneic infected cells	1 x 10^7 x 8 + MDP	5 x 10^4	IP	0/3	35
Paraformaldehyde-fixed allogeneic infected cells	2.5 x 10^7 x 6 + A-MDP	10	IP	15/15	31, 14
Paraformaldehyde-inactivated cell-free pelleted whole virus	250 μg x 3 + A-MDP	10	IP	13/15	31, 14

[1]ISCOMS = immune stimulating complexes; MDP = muramyl dipeptide; CFA/IFA = complete/incomplete Freund's adjuvant; A-MDP = adenyl-muramyl dipeptide.
[2]Challenge with the homologous strain of FIV, 2-6 weeks after final immunization.
[3]NK = information not provided.
[4]IP = intraperitoneal
[5](↑) = possible enhancement of infection.

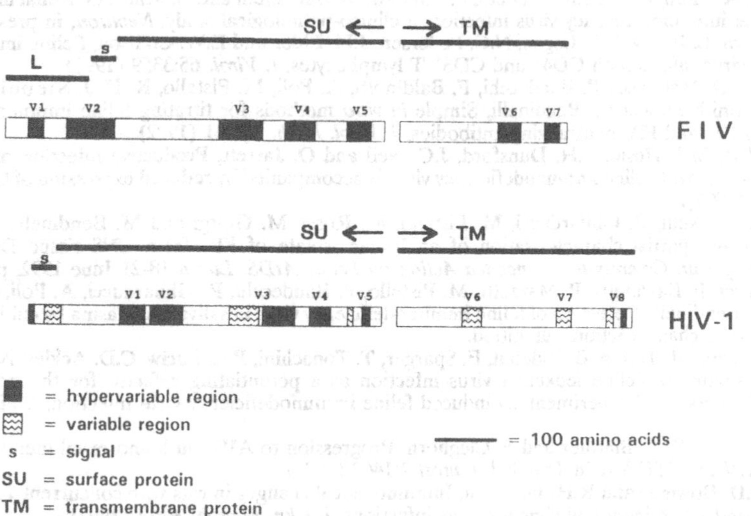

Fig. 7. **Variable regions in the predicted *env* gene products of FIV and HIV-1.**

CONCLUSIONS

We have reviewed the potential value of FIV as a animal model of AIDS. There is no doubt that, together with SIV, it is the best model presently available. At a difference with SIV, FIV induces an AIDS-like disease in its natural host. Thus, the large numbers of domestic cats that are naturally infected with FIV may be extremely valuable for many studies. Of particular interest in the context of this book is that FIV, better than any other model, lends itself to the investigation of co-factors that are currently believed to play a potentiating role in lentiviral pathogenesis such as the drugs of abuse.

Acknowledgements

The personal work discussed in this review was supported by grants from Ministero della Sanità - Istituto Superiore di Sanità "Progetto Allestimento Modelli Animali per l'AIDS", and Ministero Università e Ricerca Scientifica, Rome, Italy.

REFERENCES

1. M. Bendinelli, D. Matteucci and H. Friedman, Retrovirus induced acquired immunodeficiencies, *Adv. Cancer Res.* 45:125 (1985).
2. M. B. Gardner and P.A. Luciw, Animal models of AIDS, *FASEB J.* 3:2593 (1989).
3. H. Schellekens and M.C. Horzinek, "Animal models in AIDS," Elsevier, Amsterdam (1990).
4. N. C. Pedersen, E.W. Ho, M.L. Brown and J.H. Yamamoto, Isolation of a T lymphotropic virus from domestic cats with an immunodeficiency-like syndrome, *Science* 235:790 (1987).
5. P. Bandecchi, D. Matteucci, F. Baldinotti, G. Guidi, F. Abramo, F. Tozzini F. and M. Bendinelli, Prevalence of feline immunodeficiency virus and other retroviral infections in Italy, *Vet. Immunol. Immunopathol.* 31:337 (1992).
6. N. C. Pedersen, Feline immunodeficiency virus infection, *in*: "The Retroviruses" vol. 2, in press, J.A. Levy, ed., Plenum Press, New York (1992).
7. A. Poli, C. Giannelli, M. Pistello, L. Zaccaro, D. Pieracci, M. Bendinelli and G. Malvaldi, Detection of salivary antibodies in cats infected with feline immunodeficiency virus, *J. Clin. Microb.* 30:2038 (1992).
8. F. Mancianti, C. Giannelli, M. Bendinelli M. and A. Poli, Mycological findings in feline immunodeficiency virus-infected cats, *Med. Vet. Mycol.*, 30:257 (1992).

9. A. Poli, F. Abramo, E. Taccini, G. Guidi, P. Barsotti, M. Bendinelli and G. Malvaldi, Renal involvement in feline immunodeficiency virus infection: a clinico-pathological study, *Nephron*, in press.
10. W. C. Brown, L. Bissey, K.S. Logan, N.C. Pedersen, J.H. Elder and E.W. Collison, Feline immunodeficiency virus infects both $CD4^+$ and $CD8^+$ T lymphocytes, *J. Virol.* 65:3359 (1991).
11. F. Tozzini, D. Matteucci, P. Bandecchi, F. Baldinotti, A. Poli, M. Pistello, K. H. J. Siebelink, L. Ceccherini-Nelli and M. Bendinelli, Simple *in vitro* methods for titrating feline immunodeficiency virus (FIV) and FIV neutralizing antibodies, *J. Virol. Meth.* 37:241 (1992).
12. B. J. Willett, M.J. Hosie, T.H. Dunsford, J.C. Neil and O. Jarrett, Productive infection of T helper lymphocytes with feline immunodeficiency virus is accompanied by reduced expression of CD4, *AIDS* 5:1469 (1991).
13. L. Ceccherini-Nelli, R. Ghilarducci, M. Pistello, M. Rossi, M. Giorgi and M. Bendinelli, Molecular cloning and partial characterization of an Italian isolate of FIV from CNS tissue DNA, *Proc. Workshop Eur. Commission Concerted Action on Feline AIDS, Lucca* 18-21 June 1992, p. 11.
14. D. Matteucci, F. Baldinotti, P. Mazzetti, M. Pistello, P. Bandecchi, R. Ghilarducci, A. Poli, F. Tozzini and M. Bendinelli, Detection of feline immunodeficiency virus in saliva and plasma by cultivation and polymerase chain reaction, submitted.
15. N. C. Pedersen, M. Torten, B. Rideout, E. Sparger, T. Tonachini, P.A. Luciw, C.D. Ackley, N. Levy and J.H. Yamamoto, Feline leukemia virus infection as a potentiating cofactor for the primary and secondary stages of experimentally induced feline immunodeficiency virus infection, *J. Virol.* 64:598 (1990).
16. C. Bartolomew, W.A. Blattner and F. Cleghorn, Progression to AIDS in homosexual men co-infected with HIV and HTLV-1 in Trinidad, *Lancet* 2:1469 (1987).
17. D. Lin, D.D. Bowman and R.H. Jacobson, Immunological changes in cats with concurrent *Toxoplasma gondii* and feline immunodeficiency virus infections, *J. Clin. Microb.* 30:17 (1992).
18. S. Lombardi, M. Bendinelli and C. Garzelli, Detection of B epitopes on the p24 *gag* protein of feline immunodeficiency virus by monoclonal antibodies, Submitted.
19. T. W. North, R.C. Cronn, K.M. Remington and R.T. Tandberg, Direct comparison of inhibitor sensitivities of reverse transcriptases from feline and human immunodeficiency viruses, *Antimicrob. Agents Chemother.* 34:1505 (1990).
20. R. C. Cronn, J.D. Whitmer and T.W. North, RNase H activity associated with reverse transcriptase from feline immunodeficiency virus, *J. Virol.* 66:1215 (1992).
21. K. M. Remington, B. Chesebro, K. Wehrly, N.C. Pedersen and T.W. North, Mutants of feline immunodeficiency virus resistant to 3'-azido-3'-deoxythymidine, *J. Virol.* 65:308 (1991).
22. F. Tozzini, D. Matteucci, P. Bandecchi, F. Baldinotti, K.H.J. Siebelink, A. Osterhaus and M. Bendinelli, Neutralizing antibodies in feline immunodeficiency virus infected cats, submitted.
23. T. Miyazawa, M. Fukasawa, A. Hasegawa, N. Maki, K. Ikuta, E. Takahashi, M. Hayami and T. Mikami, Molecular cloning of a novel isolate of feline immunodeficiency virus biologically and genetically different from the original U.S. isolate, *J. Virol.* 65:1572 (1991).
24. K. H. J. Siebelink, I. Chu, G.F. Rimmelzwaan, K. Weijer, A.D.M.E. Osterhaus and M. L. Bosch, Isolation and partial characterization of infectious molecular clones of feline immunodeficiency virus obtained directly from bone marrow DNA of a naturally infected cat, *J. Virol.* 66:1091 (1992).
25. T. R. Phillips, R.L. Talbott, C. Lamont, S. Muir, K. Lovelace and J.H. Elder, Comparison of two host cell range variants of feline immunodeficiency virus, *J. Virol.* 64:4605 (1990).
26. S. Morikawa, H. Lutz, A. Aubert and D.H.L. Bishop, Identification of conserved and variable regions in the envelope glycoprotein sequences of two feline immunodeficiency viruses isolated in Zurich, Switzerland, *Virus Res.* 21:53 (1991).
27. M. Rigby, N. Macckay, J. Neil, E. Holmes, M. Pistello and M. Bosch, Sequence variation in FIV *env*: Evidence of distinct geographical clusters of isolates and of selection for change at variable regions, *Proc. Workshop Eur. Commission Concerted Action on Feline AIDS, Lucca* 18-21 June 1992, p. 9.
28. P. Nara, R.R. Garrity and J. Gousmit, Neutralization of HIV-1: A paradox of humoral proportions, *FASEB. J.* 5:2437 (1991).
29. F. Esposito, C. La Rosa, A. Habluetzel, S. Lombardi, C. Garzelli, D. Matteucci, and M. Bendinelli, Mapping of linear B epitopes on the V3 region of feline immunodeficiency virus surface glycoprotein, *Proc. Workshop Eur. Commission Concerted Action on Feline AIDS, Lucca* 18-21 June 1992, p. 14.
30. C. Locardi, P. Puddu, M. Ferrantini, E. Parlanti, P. Sestili, F. Varano and F. Belardelli, Persistent infection of normal mice with human immunodeficiency virus, *J. Virol.* 66:1649 (1992).
31. H. F. Egberink and M.C Horzinek, Phenotypic mixing leads to broadening of cell spectrum of feline immunodeficiency virus, *Proc. 1st Inter. Conf. FIV Res.*, Davis 4-7 September, 1991, p. 20.
32. Y. Kawaguchi, T. Miyazawa, T. Horimoto, S.-I. Itagaki, M. Fukasawa, E. Takahashi and T. Mikami, Activation of feline immunodeficiency virus long terminal repeat by feline herpesvirus type 1, *Virol.* 184:449 (1991).
33. M. J. Hosie, G. Reid, J.C. Neil and O. Jarrett, Enhancement of FIV infection after vaccination, *Proc. 1st Inter. Conf. FIV Res.*, Davis 4-7 September, 1991, p. 64.
34. J. K. Yamamoto, T. Okuda, C.D. Ackley, H. Zochlinski, E. Penbroke, and M.B. Gardner, Experimental vaccine protection against FIV, *Proc. 1st Inter. Conf. FIV Res.*, Davis 4-7 September, 1991, p. 63.
35. J. K. Yamamoto, T. Okuda, C.D. Ackley, H. Louie, E. Penbroke, H. Zochlinski, R.J. Munn and M.B. Gardner, Experimental vaccine protection against feline immunodeficiency virus, *AIDS Res. Hum. Retrov.* 7:911 (1991).

CURRENT STATUS AND FUTURE PROSPECTS IN THE IMMUNOTHERAPY OF HUMAN IMMUNODEFICIENCY VIRUS (HIV) INFECTION

John W. Hadden

Division of Immunopharmacology, University of South Florida Medical College, Tampa, FL 33612

INTRODUCTION

I reviewed recently the status of immunotherapy of HIV infection in Trends in Pharmacology (1). To recount briefly, a large number of trials involving acquired immunodeficiency syndrome (AIDS) and pre-AIDS patients have been performed with relatively meager results. Intravenous gamma globulin (IVIG) therapy is thought to be of benefit for children with AIDS and a large scale study has been initiated to document this impression. Similar studies have been proposed for adults with or without azidothymidine (AZT) (2). Recombinant alpha interferon, particularly with AZT, has proven successful for managing Kaposi's sarcoma in AIDS and is now licensed by the FDA for this use. Similarly, recombinant granulocyte-macrophage colony stimulating factor (GM-CSF) has proven useful and is licensed for leukopenia due to AZT in AIDS. Interleukin II (IL-2) by continuous infusion has been shown to induce T lymphocytosis and combined trials with AZT are in progress. Diethyl dithiocarbamate (DTC; Imuthiol) was reported to reduce the incidence of infection in AIDS patients in one study (3). The other immunotherapeutic agents have proven of no value in AIDS.

In studies with asymptomatic HIV individuals and pre-AIDS patients, the picture seemed a little brighter. Four agents, two thymomimetic drugs, imuthiol and isoprinosine and two thymomimetic peptides, thymopentin and IMREG-1, have been reported to be of some benefit. Imuthiol was reported to reduce infection in pre-AIDS patients in association with stabilization of CD4 T cell levels. Isoprinosine was reported to reduce infections in a study of 866 HIV patients (4). Preliminary smaller studies supported similar effects for thymopentin and IMREG-1 (5,6).

Collectively, these and related studies emphasized several important features about the immunotherapy of HIV infection. Attempts to restore T lymphocyte numbers have not been successful. Only IL-2 seems to affect T lymphocyte levels and the origin of these T lymphocytes and their HIV status are unclear. Attempts to preserve T lymphocyte levels have been more meaningful; however, only when the initial CD4 counts were greater than 250 mm^3 did these treatments appear to have some meaning in terms of reduction of opportunistic infections. Improvement of function of existing uninfected T lymphocytes has not been well documented in any of these studies.

Drugs of Abuse, Immunity, and AIDS, Edited by
H. Friedman *et al.*, Plenum Press, New York, 1993

Much information has evolved about the immune responses elicited by components of HIV and a strong prejudice has developed that HIV progression is favored by both immunosuppressive viruses (CMV, HSV, EBV) and factors like poor nutrition, recreational drugs, intrarectal sperm, and mycoplasma. A body of information has been developed (see 7) which describes how HIV itself contributes to immunosuppression through the generation of immunosuppressive constituents (gpl60, gpl20, gp41) and induced factors (prostaglandins, interferons).

Finally, initial attempts have begun using vaccinations to manage the infection (8) by enhancing resistance mechanisms. Despite the evolving understandings about the importance of resistance mechanisms and attempts to enhance them in HIV infection, reliance on antiviral drugs (AZT, DDI, DDC) has dominated the therapeutic approach to HIV infection, including now pre-AIDS. As a result, the immmunotherapeutic agents have been thrust into use in combination with AZT. Despite increasing information about the toxicity of AZT and the other antiviral drugs, their ability to be used compatibly with immunorestorative agents remain obscured by the immunosuppressive impact of the virus itself. Nevertheless, increasing numbers of combined trials are being planned or are in progress.

UPDATE ON IMMUNOTHERAPY

Since the review in 1991 (1), a number of significant events have occurred. Imuthiol, which looked so encouraging in its effects on infection in both pre-AIDS and AIDS patients (3) failed to show effects in 1,600 and HIV asymptomatic individuals and was abandoned for development by Merieux (9). Isoprinosine, which also looked encouraging, went off patent and is no longer being developed by Newport Pharmaceuticals. Thymopentin and IMREG-1 studies were revamped into combined AZT protocols currently in progress or in the planning stages, respectively (9; personal communication, A. Gottlieb). Interleukin II has been combined with AZT and studies are ongoing. The modification of IL-2 with polyethylene glycol (PEG IL-2) to inhibit the clearance and catabolism of IL-2 has provided the basis of one combined protocol at Stanford University. Merrigan reported at the 2nd International Conference on Combined Therapies (Catania, Italy, May 1992, in press) that PEG-IL-2 has been employed with AZT in a study of 20 HIV patients to induce sustained increases in CD4 T lymphocytes. He indicated evidence of new T lymphocyte production, presumably from the thymus. This is important since replenishment of virus free T cells is an important goal for treatment of HIV infection.

Another recent development concerns thymic humoral factor (THF). This octapeptide, derived from the thymus by Nathan Trainin and coworkers, is being employed in multicenter trials in pre-AIDS patients with and without AZT. THF was reported earlier to modulate T lymphocyte number and responses in 7 patients with asymptomatic HIV infection. Federico Spreafico presented work in progress on THF at the 2nd International Conference on Combined Therapies (in press).

It is difficult at this time to envision where immunotherapy will place itself relevant to vaccine development and its use to prevent progression of disease. The initial efforts with the gpl60 vaccine with alum as adjuvant showed that these AIDS patients are remarkably poor responders to the vaccine (8). It is clear that further adjuvant approaches must be undertaken to increase the efficacy of the vaccine. It also seems appropriate to consider contrasuppression, that is, effects to overcome virus-induced immunosuppression, as part of that approach. In terms of present understandings, the best we can offer for the management of HIV infection resides in a combined approach using antiviral therapy (to minimize toxicity and emergence of mutant HIV), immunotherapy (directed at T cell restoration and improved T cell function) and continued immunization (to promote relevant resistance mechanisms). The general issues underlying this discussion of combined approach were recently detailed (11).

NEW APPROACHES TO IMMUNOTHERAPY

For the remainder of this presentation, I would like to describe two new approaches to the immunotherapy of HIV infection with which we have been involved. Isoprinosine provided an impetus for drug development which is interesting to us. Although no longer in development, this drug has a respectable literature on its immunopharmacology involving more than 100 publications which describe immunomodulatory effects on T and B lymphocytes, macrophages, and granulocytes including natural killer cells. On the basis of an analysis of its immunopharmacology, particularly those actions which relate to T lymphocytes, we classified this drug as a thymomimetic drug of the purine type (12). In 1976, we launched a synthetic program to improve on isoprinosine. Compounds like NPT 15392 and NPT 16416 followed. Here I will discuss the most recent compound from this program, methyl ester 5' inosine monophosphate (MIMP). This compound was first presented at the 5th International Conference on Immunopharmacology (13-18) and a summary of its immunopharmacology has been published (19). The data papers are in press (20, 21, 22).

Methyl Inosine Monophosphate to Promote T Lymphocyte Function

MIMP is also to be classified as a thymomimetic drug. It promotes T lymphocyte differentiation as measured by the induction of markers (CD3, CD25)in human bone marrow prothymocytes *in vitro* and promotes T lymphocyte proliferation induced by mitogens like phytohemagglutinin (PHA) and concanavalin A (Con A).

Additionally, MIMP has small effects on lymphocyte proliferation induced by endotoxin (LPS, murine) or pokeweed (PKW, human) which presumably relates to B lymphocytes. Macrophages are also targets of its action. The effect of MIMP *in vitro* is observed between 0.1 - 100 μg/ml depending on the assay and requires in most assays the concomitant presence of mitogen or antigen. Effects plateau or decline above 100 μg/ml.

MIMP has been tested *in vitro* on PHA responses of normal lymphocytes depressed by a variety of stimuli including hydrocortisone (stress), prostaglandin PGE2 (inflammation), interferon (infection) and a gp41 analog (HIV infection). In each case, MIMP reversed the depressed PHA response when the depression was mild to moderate ($<50\%$) but not when it was severe ($>50\%$). With a defective IL-2-dependent CTLL line in which response to IL2 had been lost, MIMP stimulated thymidine incorporation and restored IL-2 responsiveness. With lymphocytes from aged individuals (mean age 84) whose PHA responses were mildly impaired, MIMP restored the responses to normal adult levels. With lymphocytes from ARC patients, MIMP restored the depressed PHA responses to the normal range and was additive with the restorative effects of both IL-2 or indomethacin. With lymphocytes from AIDS patients, MIMP had little effect to improve the markedly impaired responses.

In vivo experiments with mice show MIMP to be non-toxic (LD50 p.o. > 5000 mg/kg) and both orally and parenterally active. Single or multiple treatments with MIMP (1-100 mg/kg) augmented spleen responses to T cell mitogens (PHA and Con A), plaque forming cells (PFC) responses to sheep erythrocytes (SRBC), and delayed hypersensitivity to SRBC. In mice infected with Friend leukemia virus (FLV) or inoculated with Meth A tumor and endotoxin (LPS), MIMP prolonged life significantly. Preliminary experiments (T. Semenenko, personal communication) indicate that MIMP prolongs survival of mice following challenge with Listeria and Salmonella and enhances immune response to hepatitis B vaccine. In summary, MIMP is a safe, orally active thymomimetic drug which should be an interesting candidate to replace the other orally active thymomimetic drugs employed in HIV infection if toxicology studies in animals and man warrant.

Strategies to Promote T Lymphocyte Development

Another approach to immunorestoration in HIV infection relates to attempts to generate new T cells through enhanced thymic processing. Previously it was thought that the thymus once involuted could no longer process new T lymphocytes; however, it is now clear that when the T cell system is depressed due to intense radiation or chemotherapy with or without bone marrow transplantation, the thymus can rejuvenate and repopulate the system. Additionally, in experiments with aged animals having involuted thymuses, treatment with pituitary hormone secreting cells (23) or with zinc (24) will restore youthful thymic morphology and function. In AIDS, the thymus undergoes a profound involution and it is unclear whether the stromal and epithelial cells are also targets of virus infection and destruction. In any case, under these circumstances T cell depletion is not followed by restoration of normal levels. What the defective signals and mechanisms are remains unknown and when, in the course of HIV infection, this process becomes irreversible is not known. While appealing, the idea of promoting new virus-free T lymphocytes in HIV infection is frought with unknowns. IL-2 has been implicated by us and others (Cf25) to be an important regulator of intrathymic T lymphocyte development and, as indicated, clinical efforts with AZT and IL-2 are in progress. These are destined to be limited because IL-2 is only one of the possible mediators.

***In vitro* Studies**

The thymus is known to produce and to respond to a large variety of hormonal and peptide signals. Central to T cell development are both interleukin peptides and so-called "thymic hormone" peptides. These two types of peptides have recently been cast in complementary roles in which thymic hormones provide the endocrine "umbrella" under which T cell commitment and development proceed and interleukins regulate the stepwise development on a demand basis. Central to this hypothesis is that thymic hormones program the T cells to express the patterned response to IL-1 to yield high affinity IL-2 receptors, to produce IL-2 and to respond to the combination with clonal proliferation. In this scenario, it would seem logical that treatment of animals with a mixture of peptides of both types would be necessary to achieve immune restoration.

Other recent insights into methods for promoting T lymphocyte development and thymic restoration derive from the studies on the importance of zinc in thymus function. It has been noted for some time that zinc deficiency leads to thymic involution. Bach and coworkers found a thymic peptide from thymic epithelial cells called thymulin which binds and requires zinc for its thymic hormone action (26). N. Fabris and co-workers (24) observed that age-dependent thymic involution is associated with zinc deficiency and treatment with zinc restores thymus morphology and the production of zinc-thymulin complex. Others found that interleukin 1 promotes zinc uptake by thymus at the expense of other tissues (27). We have recently observed that IL-1 induces zinc uptake into thymic epithelial cells and promotes the secretion of zinc-thymulin complex (28). Further, we observed that zinc-thymulin complex potentiates the effect of IL-1 to promote proliferation of high affinity IL-2 receptor positive T lymphocytes in the presence of low doses of PHA and the absence of serum. This effect is paralleled by a similar synergistic effects on protein kinase C of isolated lymphocyte nuclei. These studies point to a central role of IL-1 and zinc-thymulin to deliver zinc to T lymphocytes at pg/ml levels and to facilitate T lymphocyte expansion.

In Vivo Studies

We recently embarked on a series of studies in which we performed a chemical thymectomy in aged retired breeder mice using hydrocortisone (28). As expected, these middle aged female mice, in whom partial thymic involution had occurred, showed a profound loss of thymic weight and depletion of cortical thymocytes on day 2 followed by a slow return to pre-treatment weight and cellularity by day 8. Similar but less dramatic reduction of spleen was observed followed by recovery. We asked the question: Will interleukin and thymic peptide treatment hasten thymic recovery in a way in which new thymocytes would derive from precursors and perhaps new T lymphocytes would derive from thymocytes? The second part of this question is more difficult to approach since expansion of existing T lymphocytes would create the same result. We treated the mice from day 3-7 with daily injections of:

1) mixed natural interleukins (50 units IL-2 equivalence)
2) rIL-l - 4 ng
3) rIL-2 - 50 units
4) combination of 2 and 3
5) thymosin fraction V (a mixture of thymic peptides, 100 μg)
6) combination of 1 and 5

We measured spleen and thymic weight, cellularity, and T cell number and subsets (Thy 1.2, CD4 and CD8) and assessed cellular responses *in vitro* to rIL-1, rIL-2, mixed natural interleukins, or the T mitogens Con A or PHA. We observed that only treatment 1 and 6, which included the natural interleukin mixture, promoted the return of thymus and spleen weight and cellularity (including T cell number) to above the pretreatment levels. These treatments also promoted splenic and thymic T lymphocyte responses *in vitro* to interleukins and Con A. Thymic peptides as thymosin fraction V and interleukins as IL-1, IL-2 or their combination were not by themselves significantly active. Importantly, thymosin fraction V greatly potentiated the effect of treatments with the mixed natural interleukins.

These results are revealing in a number of aspects. First, they show that interleukins injected peripherally (i.p. here) act like hormones to influence lymphoid organ weight and function. They sensitize the cells to show enhanced responsiveness to interleukin signals. They promote an increase in the numbers of immature and mature T lymphocytes, presumably through effects to promote their development. The potentiative effect of thymosin peptides is consistent with the foregoing hypothesis that they provide the "endocrine umbrella" which promote these pre-programmed responses.

The implication of the foregoing is that perhaps humans with thymic involution would respond in a similar manner. In order to test this premise, three patients with secondary immunodeficiency due to head and neck cancer were treated with a 10 day course of regional administration of mixed natural interleukins (200 IL-2 units/dose) and oral zinc. The treatment also included pretreatment by a single low dose of cyclophosphamide followed by oral indomethacin. The tumor responses have been reported elsewhere (29). Notable here is the impact of the treatment on T lymphocyte counts in blood (Fig. 1).

We observed a marked increase in total T lymphocyte levels including both CD4 and CD8 subsets. It is not clear whether these T cells were derived from thymus. We

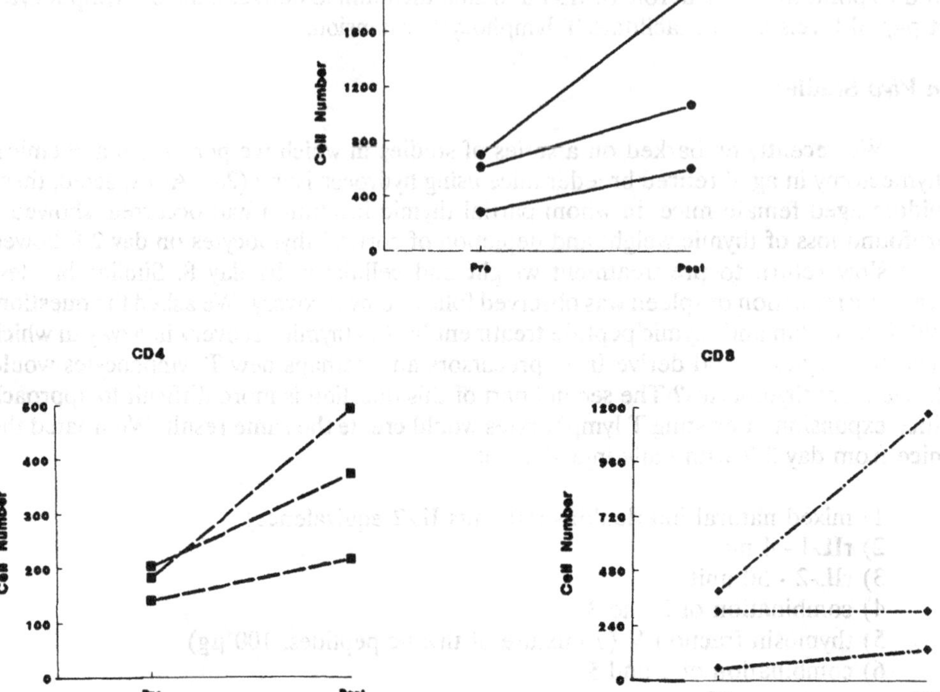

Fig. 1. T lymphocyte counts in patients with head and neck cancer. Three patients were treated with mixed natural interleukins (x 10) and total T, CD^4, CD^8 lymphocytes were assessed in blood before and after treatment. Data are expressed as cells/mm^3.

plan to extend these studies with the natural interleukin to the treatment of pre-AIDS patients (CD4 counts > 250) with AZT and zinc.

These studies are admittedly preliminary but they offer important encouragement to the notion that if we can understand better the molecular communications which regulate T lymphocyte development we can use this information to devise treatments to promote their development, in diseases like HIV infection.

REFERENCES

1. J. W. Hadden, Immunotherapy of human immunodeficiency virus (HIV), *Trends in Pharmacol.* 12:107 (1991).
2. C. DeSimone, S. Antonaci, M. Chirigos, S. Delia, S. Difabio, R.A. Good, J.W. Hadden, E. Jirillo, R. Lockey, F. Milazzo, G. Scalise, M. Tinelli, Report of the symposium on the use of intravenous gamma globulin (IVIG) in adults infected with HIV, *J. Clin. Lab. Analysis* 4:313 (1990).
3. E. M. Hersh, G. Brewton, D. Adams, J. Galpin, J. Bartlett, P. Gill, R. Gorter, M. Gottlieb, J. Jonikas, S. Landesman, A. Levine, A. Marcel, E.A. Peterson, M. Whiteside, J. Zahradnik, C. Negron, F. Boutitie, J. Caraux, J.M. Dupuy and L.R. Salmi, Ditiocarb sodium (diethyldithiocarbamate) therapy in patients with symptomatic HIV infection and AIDS. A randomized, double blind, placebo-controlled, multicenter study, *JAMA* 265(12):1538 (1991).
4. C. Pederson, E. Sandstrom, C.S. Peterson, G. Norkrans, J. Gersteft, A. Karlsonn, K.C. Christianson, C. Hadansson, P. Pehrson, J.O. Nielson, H.J. Jurgensen and the Scandinavian Isoprinosine Study Group, The efficacy of inosine pranobex in preventing the acquired immunodeficiency virus infection, *New Eng. J. Med.* 322:1757 (1990).

5. S. E. Thompson et al., Effects of thymopentin on disease progression and surrogate markers in HIV infection, *VI Int. Conf. AIDS*, San Francisco 3:207 (1990).
6. M. S. Gottlieb, R.A. Zackin, M. Fiala, D.H. Henry, A.J. Marcel, K.L. Combs, J. Vieria, H.A. Leibman, L.A. Cone, K.S. Hillman, A.A. Gottlieb, Response to treatment with the leukocyte derived immunomodulator IMREG-1 in immunocompromised patients with AIDS-related complex, *Ann. Int. Med.* 115:84 (1991).
7. R. A. Good, S. Haraguchi, E. Lorenz and N.K. Day, *In vitro* immunomodulation and in vivo immunotherapy of retrovirus induced immunosuppression, *Int. J. Immunopharmacol.* 13(S1):1 (1991).
8. D. L. Birx and R.R. Redfield, HIV vaccine therapy, *Int. J. Immunopharmacol.* 13(S1):129 (1991).
9. D. Abrams, D. Cotton, K. Mayer, eds., "AIDS/HIV Treatment Directory", AmFAR, New York, Vol. 5(3), (1992).
10. Z. T. Handzel, Y. Berner, O. Segal, Y. Burstein, V. Buchner, M. Pecht, S. Levin, R. Burstein, R. Milchan, Z. Bentwich, Z. Ben-shai and N. Trainin, Immunoconstruction of T cell impairments in asymptomatic male homosexuals by thymic humoral factor (THF), *Int. J. Immunopharmacol.* 9(2):165 (1987).
11. J. Hadden and M. Nonoyama, Guest eds. *Internatl. J. Immunopharmacol.*, Vol. 6, Pergamon Press, Oxford, (1991).
12. J. W. Hadden, Thymomimetic drugs, *in*: "Serono Symposium on Immunopharmacology", P.A. Miescher, L. Bolis, and M. Ghione, eds., Vol. 23, Raven Press, New York, p. 183 (1985).
13. J. W. Hadden, E.M. Hadden, Y. Wang, M. Sosa, R. Coffey and A. Giner-Sorolla: Methyl Inosine Monophosphate (MIMP), a new purine immunomodulator, *Int'l. J. Immunopharmacol.* 13:761 (abstract) (1991).
14. M. Sosa, Y. Wang, A. Saha, T. Wadsworth and J.W. Hadden, Methyl inosine monophosphate (MIMP) promotes immune responses in mice, *Int. J. Immunopharmacol.* 13:761 (abstract) (1991).
15J-L. Touraine, K. Sanhadji, O. deBouteiller and J.W. Hadden, *In vitro* effects of inosine monophosphate methyl (Me-Imp) on human prothymocyte differentiation, *Int. J. Immunopharmacol.* 13:761 (abstract) (1991).
16. M. Sosa, Y. Noso and J.W. Hadden, Methyl inosine monophosphate (MIMP) stimulates macrophage related functions *in vitro* and *in vivo*, *Int'l. J. Immunopharmacol.* 13:762 (abstract) (1991).
17. E. M. Hadden, M. Sosa, M. Strand, R.G. Coffey and J.W. Hadden, Methyl inosine monophosphate (MIMP) restores depressed lymphoproliferative response of normal human and murine T lymphocytes, *Int. J. Immunopharmacol.* 13:762 (abstract) (1991).
18. J. W. Hadden, J. Ongradi, S. Specter, R. Nelson, E.M. Hadden, M. Sosa, C. Monell and M. Strand, Methyl inosine monophosphate (MIMP) restores HIV-associated suppression of the proliferative responses of human lymphocytes *in vitro*, *Int. J. Immunopharmacol.* 13:762 (abstract) (1991).
19. J. W. Hadden, A. Giner-Sorolla and E.M. Hadden, Methyl inosine monophosphate (MIMP), a new purine immunomodulator for HIV infection, *Int. J. Immunopharmacol.* 13(S1):49 (1991).
20. J. W. Hadden, J. Ongradi, S. Specter, R. Nelson, M. Sosa, C. Monell, M. Strand, A. Giner-Sorolla and E.M. Hadden, Methyl inosine monophosphate: a potential immunotherapeutic for early human immunodeficiency virus (HIV) infection, *Int. J. Immunopharmacol.* 14(4):555-563 (1992).
21. M. Sosa, A.R. Saha, Y. Wang, T. Wadsworth, J. Coto, A. GinerSorolla, E.M. Hadden and J.W. Hadden, Potentiation of immune responses in mice by a new inosine derivative - methyl inosine monophosphate (MIMP), *Int. J. Immunopharmacol.* (in press, 1992).
22. E. M. Hadden, P.M. Malec, M. Sosa, and J.W. Hadden, Mixed interleukins and thymosin fraction V synergistically induce T lymphocyte development in hydrocortisone-treated aged mice, *Cell. Immunol.* 144:228 (1992).
23. K. W. Kelley, S. Brief, H.J. Westly, J. Novakofsky, P.J. Bechtal, J. Simon and E.R. Walker, Hormonal regulation of the age-associated decline in immune function, *in*: "Neuroimmune interaction: Proc. 2nd Internatl. Workshop on Neuroimmune Modulation", B.D. Jankovic, B.M. Markovic and N.H. Specter, eds, New York Academy of Science, New York, (1987).
24. E. Mocchegiani and N. Fabris, *In vivo* and *in vitro* effects of zinc on thymic efficacy in old age, *in*: *Abstracts of the 6th Int. Congress of Int. Assoc. Biol. Gerontol.*, Ancona, Italy, abstract #197, p. 279 (1991).
25. J. W. Hadden, Thymic endocrinology, *Int. J. Immunopharmacol.* 14(3):345 (1992).
26. M. Dardenne, W. Savino, L. Gastel and J-F. Bach, Thymulin new biochemical aspects, *in*: Thymic Hormones and Lymphokines, A.L. Goldstein, ed., Plenum Press, New York, (1984).
27. R. J. Cousins and A.S. Leinart, Tissue-specific regulation of zinc metabolism and methallothionein genes by interleukin 1, *FASEB J.* 2:2884 (1988).

28. J. A. Coto, E.M. Hadden, M. Sauro, N. Zorn and J.W. Hadden, Interleukin 1 regulates secretion of zinc-thymulin by thymic epithelial cells and its action on T lymphocyte proliferation and nuclear protein kinase C, *Proc. Natl. Acad. Sci.*, 89:7752 (1992).
29. J. W. Hadden, P.H. Malec, M. Sosa and E.M. Hadden, The case for synergy of thymic hormones and interleukins in immune reconstitution, *in*: "Combination Therapies", A.L. Goldstein and E. Garaci, eds., Plenum Press, New York, p. 177-184, (1992).
30. J. W. Hadden, E.M. Hadden, P. Baekey, P. Skipper and J.N. Endicott, Adjuvant nonrecombinant interleukins and contrasuppressive agents induces immune regression in head and neck cancer, 3rd *Int. Conf. Head & Neck Cancer*, San Francisco, and *Arch. Otolaryngol.* (in press, 1993).

PERINATAL AIDS: DRUGS OF ABUSE AND TRANSPLACENTAL INFECTION

William D. Lyman

Department of Pathology, Albert Einstein College of Medicine
Bronx, NY 10461 (U.S.A.)

INTRODUCTION

Type-1 human immunodeficiency virus (HIV-1) infection of children has been recognized since 1983 (1,2). The description of both the general signs and the specific infections which define AIDS in children has been well-outlined (3). The number of HIV-1 infected children has increased in recent years in parallel with the increase in HIV-1 infected women of child-bearing age (4,5). Although children have been infected by the inadvertent use of HIV-1 contaminated blood or blood products, in the United States, the overwhelming majority of childhood HIV-1 infection is believed to be transmitted pre- or perinatally from infected women (6-8). These observations are also consistent with data obtained from European patient cohorts although the frequency of transplacental HIV-1 infection in Europe appears to be different from that in the United States (8,9). This discrepancy may be the result of differences including that of the drugs of abuse that are associated with HIV-1 infection. In Europe, the major drug of abuse amongst pregnant women is heroine (10) while in the United States the drug that is predominant is "crack" cocaine (11).

MECHANISMS OF PATHOGENESIS

There are a number of reasons that drugs of abuse are an important co-factor in HIV infection and can impact directly on the frequency and morbidity of pediatric AIDS. The first set of reasons is related to the effect of psychoactive drugs on noninfected and HIV-infected females and their male sex-partners. It is well-documented that the use of a number of different illicit drugs is related closely with sexual behavior including promiscuity, prostitution and bisexualism (12,13). Each of these, in turn, correlates positively with HIV infection. However, because of the inability to document, in many cases, the nature of illicit drug abuse (eg. frequency, type of drugs used, amount of drugs used) it is often difficult to separate, in a female population, the incidence of HIV infection which is purely the result of heterosexual transmission from that which is the product of intravenous drug use.

Drugs of Abuse, Immunity, and AIDS, Edited by
H. Friedman *et al.*, Plenum Press, New York, 1993

In the HIV-positive female, illicit drugs can have a direct effect on fetal or neonatal infection. For example, because some drugs of abuse, (eg. cocaine) are associated with vasculitis (14); this drug can directly impact on the maternal-fetal interface. Either a placentitis or, more specifically, the documented association between cocaine and chorioamnionitis (15) could permit an accumulation of potentially HIV-infected inflammatory cells at the maternal-fetal interface and an increased maternal blood leakage into the fetal circulation. In addition, some drugs have been associated with an alteration in maternal immunocompetency (16) which may have an indirect effect on the progression of HIV infection either in the pregnant female or in the fetus. Such drugs may also facilitate the development of opportunistic infections. An example of this might be cytomegalovirus (CMV) infection and as a result CMV-placentitis (17). As in the case of chorioamnionitis, this condition might also lead to the accumulation of potentially HIV-infected cells in the placenta and increased leakage of maternal cells into the fetal circulation. Additionally, CMV placentitis may increase the possibility of herpetic infection of the fetus or antigenic stimulation of some fetal cells. This, in turn, may facilitate HIV infection of fetal lymphocytes and monocytes. Such a scenario could lead to an ablation of some lymphocyte populations and therefore contribute to alterations in immunoregulation or immunosuppression in the fetus.

Lastly, drugs of abuse can have direct effects on the fetus rendering it more susceptible to HIV infection. Clearly, all of the aforementioned effects within the female can potentially occur in the fetus. Either immunosuppression of the developing fetal immune system, or activation of certain components of it creating a reservoir of increased numbers of susceptible cells are clearly possible. Additionally, vasculitis may be a factor in the developing fetus exposed to drugs of abuse (18). This could have direct effect on the developing fetal blood-brain barrier and infection of the fetal central nervous system.

TIMING OF INFECTION

Although the incidence of pediatric AIDS is increasing and its relationship to intravenous drug abuse seems compelling, there are still questions related to the time of infection of the fetus, neonate or infant (19-23). For example, it has been documented that, at least in the African population, HIV can be transmitted from lactating females to their infants. Although this mechanism seems unquestionable, nevertheless, in the European and American communities it is probably less of a cause of pediatric AIDS than transmission of the virus directly from the mother to the fetus either during gestation or at the time of parturition (22). For example, in a study conducted under the aegis of the European Collaborative Study (9), it was determined that a significant number of fetuses are infected during pregnancy and that the frequency of infection was approximately 15%. It is interesting to note that in the North American population, and in areas of Africa, the transmission rate is believed to be higher and approximately 30% (20). In fact, in a series of studies, it was concluded that transmission of HIV to the fetus can occur as early as the 13th week of gestation (24) and that by the end of the second trimester approximately 30% of fetuses examined in one study from the Bronx found fetuses are infected (25).

Although the evidence for fetal infection appears quite strong, nonetheless it is still not apparent what the mechanism of infection is. That is, is the virus transmitted from the infected female via infected maternal cells across the placenta and into the fetal circulation or via cell-free virus. An additional component of this mechanism that has not been adequately resolved is in fact the events that occur within the placenta that may either inhibit or facilitate fetal infection. For example, nonspecific inflammation of the placenta possibly due to the use of intravenous drugs could contribute towards fetal infection. Either a villitus secondary to an altered maternal immune system or direct action of drugs of abuse could allow for a concentration of inflammatory cells at the maternal fetal interface and thereby increase the potential for fetal infection. Some information exists in the literature that tropoblasts and Hofbauer cells are infected by HIV (26). However, conclusive evidence is still lacking.

EFFECT OF DRUGS OF ABUSE ON THE FETUS

It has been well-documented that drugs of abuse can move across the placenta from the pregnant female to the fetus (27). The effect of these drugs are varied and are believed cause a spectrum of manifestations in the fetus ranging from an embryopathy to more subtle cognitive disorders (28,29). With respect to the major drug of abuse in the New York female drug abusing population, "crack" cocaine, some evidence exists that this may be a contributing factor towards the pathophysiology of pediatric AIDS. For instance, the craniofacial anomaly called "AIDS embryopathy" is a striking feature in some of the children who are born to HIV seropositive drug abusing females (28). This embryopathy is reminiscent of alcohol fetal syndrome and consistent with other observations made of drug induced embryopathy. Additional evidence that transplacental cocaine may induce significant pathology in the fetus is provided in the number of studies that described in children with HIV disease a calcific vasculopathy as an important finding (30). For instance, in one study, aneurysmal dilatations of a number of subarachnoid vessels including the Circle of Willis have been noted (31). Upon examination of these lesions, it was clearly shown that there was pronounced intimal thickening which could be a response to the vasoactive (vasospasmotic) action of "crack" cocaine. However, other major findings in children infected by HIV also comprise marked leukoencephalopathy and microcephaly (32). While each of these components of the neuropathology of pediatric AIDS may be attributable directly to HIV, nevertheless, one cannot exclude the possibility that in fact they are in part contributed to by cofactors such as cocaine or heroine.

MODEL SYSTEMS

In order to investigate the direct effects of HIV and drugs of abuse either alone or in consort, we have developed a model system which employs human fetal central nervous system tissue that is explanted into organotypic culture (33,34). Over time, the cells in this explant model differentiate and are comprised of all of the major neural cell types. For instance, there is differentiation of neurons that is hallmarked by their expression of nerve growth factor receptor, neurofilament proteins and formation of synapses. Astrocytes are also observed in these cultures and represent both classes (protoplasmic and fibrous cells) that are strongly positive for glial fibrillary acidic protein. Cultures obtained from the spinal cord of human fetuses contain significant numbers of oligodendrocytes and myelin (35). Over time in culture, although there is some degradation of the myelin from the initial explantation, nevertheless, strong evidence also exists that there is de novo myelin synthesis. In fact, myelin in these cultures can be observed to be organized into functional internodes with morphologically appropriate terminal loops. Endothelial cells are also found in these cultures and are in the form of microvessels that are captured in the initial explantation process. These endothelial cells maintain their morphological characteristics and vessel integrity for extended periods of time. Lastly, microglia are also observed. These cells are both of the amoeboid and ramified types and stain with the appropriate markers that identify microglia in tissue sections obtained during *in vivo* studies from both man and other animals (36,37). In order to provide an adequate model for development and differentiation of the CNS when exposed either to drugs of abuse or to viruses, numerous mitoses can also be observed which allow for alterations in cell development and as a substrate for viral replication.

RESULTS OF PRELIMINARY STUDIES

These cultures have been exposed to a number of different HIV isolates including both lymphocytotropic and monocytotropic strains (38). Demonstration of viral infection can be achieved by many methods including nucleic acid hybridization. It was found that upon exposure to lymphocytotropic isolates, both microglia and astrocytes identified by double stains for either cell type specific markers and the gp-41 transmembrane protein of HIV could be observed. However, when the monocytotropic variants of HIV were used, only microglia could be demonstrated to be infected. It was interesting to note that some cells which stained positive for GFAP and for HIV proteins also were multinucleated as determined by propidium iodine staining.

Although these cultures are exposed to HIV and viral and nucleic acids can be identified in specific cell types, nevertheless the results of reverse transcriptase, p24 antigen and syncytium forming assays do not indicate that there is a florid infection. These observations are consistent with those obtained *in vivo* wherein the central nervous system of fetuses infected during gestation appear not to support a productive viral infection. This implies that a productive infection coincides with the release from the immunosuppression of pregnancy and only appears after delivery.

This model system is yet to be exploited in terms of the direct effects of drugs of abuse on CNS neurodevelopment and as a co-factor in HIV infection. These studies are currently being planned and initiated in our laboratories.

OTHER MODELS

In addition to the organotypic culture model, our laboratories have also developed a model of the human blood brain barrier which utilizes autologous endothelial cells and astrocytes (39). The endothelial cells are isolated from the umbilical vein of second trimester fetuses, maintained in culture and characterized through the expression of factor VIII. Concurrently, astrocytes are isolated from the central nervous system of the same fetus, maintained in culture and characterized for the expression of GFAP. Subsequently, the endothelial cells and astrocytes are seeded onto the opposite sides of a permeable membrane and permitted to adhere and interact through the porous membrane. Using this model system, endothelial cells have been demonstrated to express a number of CNS endothelial cell-type specific markers, namely: the glucose-1 transporter and gamma glutamyl transpeptidase. Additionally, junctional complexes are observed in ultrastructural studies between the individual endothelial cells. This model is currently being exploited to investigate the ability of cytokines to induce adhesion molecules and the interaction of this model system with both infected and noninfected lymphocytes and monocytes obtained from the same fetus. The use of this model in conjunction with the organotypic model may provide a valuable resource for the ultimate dissection of the pathogenic mechanisms associated with the neuropathology of pediatric AIDS. In addition, this model will undoubtedly provide much new information about the effects of drugs of abuse on the developing human fetal central nervous system either by themselves or as cofactors during viral infection.

SUMMARY

The number of children infected by the human immunodeficiency virus type-1 (HIV-1) who develop the acquired immunodeficiency syndrome (AIDS) continues to increase. While some children become infected after birth and others at the time of parturition, a significant percentage are infected during gestation and there is a positive correlation between maternal illicit intravenous drug use and fetal HIV-1 infection. Drugs can contribute in, at least, four ways to vertical transmission of HIV-1. These four ways are divisible into 2 main catagories that are comprised of both direct and indirect mechanisms. For example, drugs of abuse can have a direct effect on the maternal-fetal interface. Cocaine is associated with vasculitis. If this occurs as a placentitis or chorioamnionitis, it can alter the permeability of these barriers to maternal blood and increase the number of potentially infected inflammatory cells in this tissue and as a result in the fetus. Another direct mechanism wherein drugs of abuse can increase the probability that a fetus will become infected is via an inflammatory reaction such as a vasculitis in the fetus rendering it more susceptible to viral infection. Drugs can also affect the course of HIV-1 infection via indirect mechanisms. An example of this may be by modulating the female immune system. This effect can exacerbate the woman's immunodeficiency and accelerate opportunistic infections. For example, cytomegalovirus infection resulting in placentitis might facilitate fetal HIV-1 infection. Lastly, a similar type of indirect mechanism can be postulated for the fetus wherein its developing immune system can be adversely effected. Although the precise mechanisms by which drugs of abuse contribute to vertical transmission of HIV-1 are undefined, nevertheless variations in the incidence of vertical transmission of HIV-1 between drug users and non-users tend to support the conclusion that illicit drug use impacts directly on this growing public health concern.

Many of these hypotheses can be adequately explored with current technologies. Most certainly, the effect of drugs of abuse on the female immune system can be conducted both *in vivo* with human patients as well as in animal models. These can then easily be correlated with *in vitro* systems. It is of critical significance to explore not only illicit drugs that are abused in our society but also therapeutic drugs such as methadone and other drugs which may be abused but may not be defined as illicit. With respect to the direct effects of drugs of abuse on the maternal-fetal interface, these hypotheses can be explored using human tissue obtained at the time of termination of pregnancy by either abortion or full-term delivery, in animal models and in *in vitro* systems. Exploration of the hypothesis that CMV placentitis may affect the progression of HIV disease in the fetus can be explored initially, at least, using epidemiological methods. The effect of abused drugs on the development of the fetus itself can also be explored using human systems as well as animal models and also *in vitro*.

With respect to methodology, current techniques allow for the exploration of many of these issues and should permit adequate answers to be obtained. Additionally, one could easily prioritize all of these issues into a coherent strategy that would permit the optimal utilization of limited research resources.

Acknowledgments

We thank Agnes Geoghan and Barbara Shea for their excellent secretarial assistance. We also want to acknowledge cooperation from New York City Health and Hospitals Corporation and the Bronx Municipal Hospital Center with its excellent nursing staffs at Van Etten and Jacobi Hospitals. This work was supported by United States Public Health Service grants MH 46815 and MH 47667.

REFERENCES

1. A. Rubinstein, M. Sicklick, A. Gupta, et a., Acquired immunodeficiency with reversed T4/T8 ratio in infants born to promiscuous and drug-addicted mothers, *JAMA* 249:2350 (1983).
2. J. Oleske, A. Minnefor, R. Cooper, et al., Immune deficiency syndrome in children, *JAMA* 249:2345 (1983).
3. Centers for Disease Control. Classification system for human immunodeficiency virus (HIV) infection in children under 13 years of age, *MMWR* 36:1 (1987).
4. New York State Department of Health. AIDS among New York State children, *Epidemiol. Notes* 10:1 (1988).
5. L. F. Novick, D. Berns, R. Strickoff, R. Stevens, HIV seroprevalence in newborn infants in New York State, *in*: "4th Internatl. Conf. on AIDS", 7221 (abstract) (1988).
6. J. Falloon, J. Eddy, L. Wiener, P. Pizzo, Human immunodeficiency virus in children, *J. Pediatr.* 46:154 (1989).
7. A. Wiznia, and A. Rubinstein, Acquired immunodeficiency syndrome in infants and children, *Ann. Nestle* 46:154 (1988).
8. A. Rubinstein, Pediatric AIDS, *in*: "Current Problems in Pediatrics", 6:361 (1986).
9. European Collaborative Study, Children born to women with HIV-1 infection: natural history and risk of transmission, *Lancet* 37:253 (1991)
10. Review of drug abuse and measure to reduce the illicit demand for drugs by region. Division of Narcotic Drugs of the United Nations Secretariat, *Bull. Narc.* 9:3 (1987).
11. J. Feldman, H. L. Minkoff, S. McCalla, and M. Salwan, A cohort study of the impact of perinatal drug use on prematurity in an inner-city population, *Am. J. Public Health.* 82:726 (1992).
12. J. A. Gayle, R. M. Selik, and S. Y. Chu, Surveillance for AIDS and HIV infection among black and hispanic children and women of child bearing age, *MMWR CDC Surveillance Summaries* 39:23 (1990).
13. A. I. Trachtenber, J. A. Gaudino, and C. V. Hanson, Human kkKT-cell lymphotropic virus in California's injection drug users, *J. Psychoactive Drugs* 23:225 (1991).
14. D. A. Krendel, S. M. Ditter, M. R. Frankel, and W. K. Ross, Biopsy-proven cerebral vasculitis associated with cocaine abuse, *Neurology* 40:1092 (1990).
15. W. M. Gilbert, C. M. Lafferty, K. Benirschke, and R. Resnik, Lack of specific placental abnormality associated with cocaine use, *Am. J. Obstet. Gynecol.* 163:998 (1990).
16. M. W. Kline, and W. T. Shearer, Impact of human immunodeficiency virus infection on women and infants, *Infect. Dis. Clin. North Am.* 6:1 (1992).
17. Y. Mehraein, H. Rehder, and H. G. Draeger, Froster-Iskenius, U.G. Diagnosis of fetal virus infections by *in situ* hybridization, Geburtshilfe-Frauenheildk, 51:984 (1991).
18. H. el-Bizri, I. Guest, and D. R. Varma, Effects of cocaine on rat embryo development in vivo and in cultures, *Pediatr. Res.* 29:187 (1991).
19. N. A. Halsey, R. Boulos, E. Holt, et al., Transmission of HIV-1 infections from mothers to infants in Haiti, *JAMA* 264:2088 (1990).
20. R. W.Ryder, W. Nsa, S. E. Hassig, et al., Perinatal transmission of the human immunodeficiency virus type 1 to infants of seropositive women in Zaire, *N. Engl. J. Med.* 320:1637 (1989).
21. S. Blanche, C. Rouzioux, M-LG. Moscato, et al., A prospective study of infants born to women seropositive for human immunodeficiency virus type 1, *N. Engl. J. Med.* 320:1643 (1989).
22. J. J. Goedert,J. E. Drummond, H. L. Minkoff, et al., Mother-to-infant transmission of human immunodeficiency virus type 1: Association with prematurity or low anti-gp 120, *Lancet* ii:1351 (1989).
23. G. G. Scott, C. Hutto, R. W. Makuch, et al., Survival in children with perinatally acquired human immunodeficiency virus type 1 infection, *N. Engl. J. Med.* 321:1791 (1989).
24. W. D. Lyman, Y. Kress, K. Jure, W. K. Rashbaum, A. Rubinstein, and R. Soeiro, Detection of HIV in fetal central nervous system tissue, (Short communication) *AIDS* 4:917 (1990).
25. R. Soeiro, A. Rubinstein, W. K. Rashbaum, and W.D. Lyman, Maternofetal transmission of AIDS: frequency of HIV-1 nucleic acid sequences in human fetal tissue DNA, *J. Inf. Dis.* (in press) (1992).
26. W. Page Faulk, and C. A. Labarrere, HIV proteins in normal human placentae, *Am. J. Reproduct. Immunol.* 25:99 (1991).
27. A. G. Fantel, R. E. Person, C. J. Burroughs-Gleim, and B. Mackler, Direct embryotoxicity of cocaine in rats: effects on mitochondrial activity, cardiac function, and growth and development in vitro, *Teratology* 42:35 (1990).
28. A. Wiznia, and A. Rubinstein, Acquired immunodeficiency syndrome in infants and children, *Ann. Nestle* 46:154 (1988).
29. A. Rubinstein, Pediatric AIDS, *in*: "Current Problems in Pediatrics", 16:361 (1986).

30. W. D. Lyman, R. Soeiro, and W. K. Rashbaum, HIV-1 infection of human fetal central nervous system tissue, *in*: "Brain in Pediatric AIDS," Kozlowski, P.B., Snider, D.A., Vietze, P.M. and H.M. Wisniewski, eds. pp 183-196, (1990).
31. D. W. Dickson, A. L. Belman, Y. D. Park, C. Wiley, D. S. Horoupian, J. Llena, K. Kure, W. D. Lyman, R. Morecki, S. Sitsudo and S. Cho, Central nervous system pathology in pediatric AIDS: An autopsy study, *Acta Pathologica, Microbiologica et Immunologica Scandinavica* 8:40 (1989).
32. K. Kure, Y. D. Park, T. S. Kim, W. D. Lyman, G. Lantos, S. Lee, S. Cho, A. L. Belman, K. M. Weidenheim, and D.W. Dickson, Immunohistochemical localization of an HIV epitope in cerebral aneurysmal arteriopathy in pediatric AIDS, *Pediatric Pathol.* 9:655 (1989).
33. W. D. Lyman, M. Tricoche, W. C. Hatch, Y. Kress, and W.K. Rashbaum, Human fetal central nervous system organotypic cultures, *Developmental Brain Res.* 60:155 (1991).
34. W. D. Lyman, W. C. Hatch, E. Pousada, G. Stepney, W. K. Rashbaum, and K. M. Weidenheim, Human fetal myelinated organotypic cultures, (submitted).
35. K. M. Weidenheim, Y. Kress, I. Epshteyn, W. K. Rashbaum, and W. D. Lyman, Early myelination in the human fetal spinal cord: Characterization by light and electron microscopy, *J. Neuropathol. and Experimental Neurol.* 51:142 (1992).
36. K. Hutchins, D. W. Dickson, W. K. Rashbaum, and W. D. Lyman, Localization of morphologically distinct populations of microglia in the human fetal brain, *Developmental Brain Res.* 55:95 (1990).
37. K. Hutchins, D. Dickson, W. K. Rashbaum, and W. D. Lyman, Localization of microglia in the human fetal cervical spinal cord, *Developmental Brain Res.* 66:270 (1992).
38. W. C. Hatch, E. Pousada, L. Losev, W. K. Rashbaum, and W. D. Lyman, L- and M-tropic isolates of HIV-1 infect human fetal neural cells, (submitted).
39. A. A. Hurwitz, J. W. Berman, Y. Kress, W. K. Rashbaum, and W. D. Lyman, Cocultivation of autologous human fetal endothelial cells and astrocytes: A model for the blood-brain barrier, (submitted).

SOLID TUMORS IN HIV-INFECTED PATIENTS OTHER THAN AIDS-DEFINING NEOPLASMS

Scot C. Remick[1], Ann Boguniewicz[2], and Barbara Wolf[2]

[1]Division of Medical Oncology and AIDS Program
[2]Department of Pathology and Laboratory Medicine
Albany Medical College, Albany, NY, USA, 12208

INTRODUCTION

The first reported cases of Kaposi's sarcoma (KS) in homosexual men appeared in 1981 and heralded the onset of the AIDS epidemic (1,2). A year later the first four cases of non-Hodgkin lymphoma (NHL) were reported (3). In 1983 the first cases of primary central nervous system lymphoma (PCL) were described (4). By 1985, NHL was added to KS and PCL as index AIDS-defining neoplasms (5). The incidence of PCL and NHL in particular is sharply on the rise (6,7). All three AIDS-defining neoplasms are characterized by higher grade lesions, more advanced stage, and shorter survival when compared to similar tumors in non-HIV infected patients. The epidemiology and clinical characteristics of these neoplasms is well described. (8-10). Today epidemic KS, PCL and NHL represent major causes of morbidity and mortality in AIDS patients.

As we enter the second decade of the HIV epidemic, it is apparent that other solid tumors are seen in these patients as well. This paper will briefly review the epidemiology and clinical characteristics of Hodgkin's disease (HD), cervical intraepithelial neoplasia (CIN) or squamous intraepithelial lesions (SIL), and other solid tumors. Discussion of the pathogenetic mechanisms and the molecular biology of HIV infection and associated neoplasia is beyond the scope of this report. The reader is referred to the references cited at the end of this paper for thoughtful reviews on this topic (12-14).

HODGKINS DISEASE

Epidemiologic studies in the United States have failed to report a clear rise in the incidence of HD in populations at risk for HIV infection (7). Several European studies have noted a greater frequency of HD, where there is a greater proportion of HIV infection associated with intravenous drug use (IVDU) (15-17). More large, population--based epidemiologic studies are needed to further define this relationship. It has been suggested that the risk of HIV-associated malignancies may vary among risk-behavior groups. HIV-related KS is seen predominantly among gay men and bisexuals. KS is

Drugs of Abuse, Immunity, and AIDS, Edited by
H. Friedman *et al.*, Plenum Press, New York, 1993

rarely seen in patients with IVDU or transfusion-associated AIDS. As the proportion of AIDS cases associated with IVDU increases in the United States, it will be important to determine if the frequency of HIV-associated HD increases as well.

It is clear that the natural history of HD in patients with underlying HIV-infection is different than that observed in HIV-uninfected patients. The clinical presentation and course of HD in patients with HIV infection is reminiscent of HD that develops in other immunosuppressive states. As in developing areas of the world where malnutrition and chronic infection, especially malaria may contribute to immunosuppression, HD that develops in this setting is characterized by poor prognostic histopathologic subtypes and constitutional disease or B symptoms (18). The majority of patients with HIV-associated HD will present with a constellation of unfavorable prognostic features (18-22). Approximately 80% of patients will have advanced stage disease, clinicopathological stage III or IV; the majority will have B symptoms at time of diagnosis; extranodal dissemination, especially bone marrow involvement is common; and mixed cellularity and lymphocyte depletion are the predominant histologies. Mediastinal involvement is much less frequent in HIV-infected HD patients.

As the majority of patients with HIV infection and HD have advanced stage of disease at diagnosis, systemic chemotherapy is recommended. MOPP and ABVD, alternating or hybrid combinations of these regimens are most commonly employed in treating HIV-associated HD. The complete response rate ranges between 25% and 55%, which is considerably less than that observed in HD patients without underlying HIV infection (11). Responses when seen are often shortlived and not durable. Median survival ranges between 14 and 36 months (11). Radiation therapy is reserved for the occasional HIV-infected patient with early stage disease (stage I and sometimes stage II). The majority of patients with HIV-associated HD will die as a result of subsequent opportunistic infection (21,22).

CERVICAL NEOPLASIA

It is now well established that human papillomavirus (HPV) infection is linked to the development of squamous cell carcinoma of the anogenital tract, and the cervix in particular (23). HPV-associated malignancy of the anogenital tract has been observed in increased frequency in immunosuppressed patients as a result of renal transplantation and in other immunocompromised settings as well (24). Not surprisingly, HIV-infected women have high rates of HPV infection, since patients at risk for HIV and HPV infection share common risk behaviors. Similarly, HIV-infected patients are at increased risk for the development of other forms of cancer, notably KS and lymphoma. Therefore, HIV-infected women are at increased risk for the development of cervical intraepithelial neoplasia (CIN) and potentially invasive carcinoma. It remains to be seen how serious a problem this represents but it is imperative that prospective large-scale population-based studies of HIV-infected women be undertaken to define the risk of CIN and development of invasive carcinoma.

The prevalence of CIN in HIV-infected women has been reported between 30%-40% (25-27). It is probably underestimated as this problem has only recently been recognized. The incidence is likely rapidly increasing. Common observations in various studies include the following: HIV-seropositive patients have higher grade cytological and histological lesions than HIV-seronegative patients or patients at risk for HIV infection; the frequency and severity of dysplasia increases with lower CD4 lymphocyte count; and HIV infection exacerbates HPV-mediated cervical cytological abnormalities (25-30). We have observed similar findings in HIV-infected women seen at our center (31).

Invasive cervical carcinoma is less well characterized in HIV-infected patients. In the limited number of cases reported it is fair to say that the clinical course is much more aggressive when compared to women without HIV infection (27,30,32,33). Surgery and radiation for the present remain the standard therapeutic modalities. Systemic chemotherapy data is very limited. In one series, the median survival of HIV-infected patients with cervical carcinoma was 10 months (30).

The natural history of CIN and what triggers the progression to invasive disease needs to be defined. It is paradoxical that this problem will likely increase as improvements in antiretroviral therapy prolong life. As patients survive longer, the period of underlying immunosuppression is extended resulting in the emergence of CIN and ultimately invasive carcinoma.

SOLID TUMORS

Preliminary reviews of tumor registry data from the United States and parts of western Europe have suggested that basal cell carcinoma of the skin, squamous cell carcinoma of the anus and other anorectal tumors, and condylomata accuminata are seen in increased frequency in HIV-infected patients (34-37). The majority of these tumors occurred in homosexual men. In a recent report of 49 patients with HIV infection and solid tumors, the majority of whom were IVDU's, only a single case of anorectal carcinoma and oral carcinoma were described (38). Squamous cell carcinoma of the head and neck has been described in homosexual men though not in increased incidence (34). These observations suggest that the pattern of solid tumors in HIV-infected patients may differ among risk-behavior groups as well in that gay men are more likely to develop head and neck or anorectal tumors than IVDU's. Further follow-up of these observations is needed.

Anal intraepithelial neoplasia (AIN) is a well recognized clinical entity in HIV-infected homosexual men (23,39,40). HPV infection appears implicated in the pathogenesis of AIN (23,39,40). In one series up to 40% of HIV-infected gay men with advanced AIDS had evidence of AIN (38). The model of concurrent and/or compounding HPV and HIV infection in CIN may also be applicable in the development of AIN, in which long term dysplasia with prolonged periods of immunosuppression precedes the onset of invasive disease (23,41). It is not surprising therefore that patients with HIV infection are at increased risk for developing anorectal malignancy.

A variety of other solid tumors have also been described in HIV-infected patients and these include melanoma, brain, breast, lung, colon, pancreas, and testicular cancers (38,42-47). Upon review of these cases it is clear that solid tumors in HIV-infected patients generally present at a younger age and have shorter survival when compared to similar tumors in patients without HIV infection. In many instances, patients present with advanced stage of disease but it remains to be seen if this is more commonly encountered in HIV-infected patients than in patients without underlying HIV infection.

Sridhar and colleagues have recently reported a series of 19 HIV-infected lung cancer patients and compared them to 1335 HIV-indeterminate lung cancer patients (45). This is the largest series of HIV-infected lung cancer patients reported to date. Their data support the following conclusions that HIV-infected lung cancer patients are male, have significant smoking histories, are younger, have similar stage and pathology of disease and shorter median survival (3 vs 10 months) when compared to non-HIV infected patients with lung cancer. It appears that many of these observations are generalizable to other solid tumors in HIV-infected patients upon review of previously published cases.

SUMMARY

As the HIV epidemic advances and patients live longer as a result of improvements in antiretroviral therapy, and recognition, management and prophylaxis of opportunistic infections we might anticipate seeing more solid tumors other than AIDS-defining neoplasms in our patients. Recent reports have suggested that patients on prolonged zidovudine therapy with progressive and severe underlying immunosuppression with CD4 lymphocyte counts less than 50/mm , may have an increased risk of developing lymphoma (48,49). It is likely that prolonged periods of immunosuppression contribute to the development of both CIN and AIN and ultimately invasive disease as well. The spectrum of solid tumors in HIV-infected patients is no doubt expanding (Table 1). For primary practitioners and general internists solid tumors are becoming an increasing cause of morbidity and mortality in HIV-infected patients. And for the clinical investigator and scientist, it will be important to track the epidemiology and biology of these solid tumors and the underlying HIV infection itself to further define the natural history and pathogenesis of these neoplasms.

Table 1. Spectrum of Solid Tumor Malignancy in HIV Infection

AIDS-defining neoplasms:

1. Kaposi sarcoma
2. Primary CNS lymphoma
3. Non-Hodgkin lymphoma

Neoplasms with increased incidence:

1. Basal cell carcinoma skin
2. Squamous cell carcinoma anus
3. Condylomata accuminata

Neoplasms that are well characterized (possible increased incidence):

1. Cervical carcinoma
2. Hodgkin's disease
3. Head and neck carcinoma
4. Melanoma
5. Lung carcinoma

Acknowledgement

(This project supported in part by AmFAR Project Grant Nos. 600027-9-CT and Operating Grant Nos. 400069-11-CGR. Dr. Remick is a recipient of an American Cancer Society Cancer Development Award.)

REFERENCES

1. Centers for Disease Control, Kaposi sarcoma and pneumonia among homosexual men-New York and California, *MMWR* 30:305 (1981).
2. K. B. Hymes, J. B. Greene, A. Marcus , et al., Kaposi's sarcoma in homosexual men-a report of eight cases, *Lancet* 2:598 (1981).
3. J. L. Ziegler, R. L. Miner, E. Rosenbaum, et al., Outbreak of Burkitt's-like lymphoma in homosexual men, *Lancet* 2:631 (1982).
4. W. D. Snider, D. M. Simpson, K. E. Aronyk, Primary lymphoma of the nervous system associated with acquired immune-deficiency syndrome, *N. Engl. J. Med.* 308:45, (1983). (Letter.)
5. Centers for Disease Control, Revision of the case definition of acquired immunodeficiency syndrome for national reporting, United States, *MMWR* 34:373 (1985).
6. M. H. Gail, J. M. Pluda, C. S. Rabkin, et al., Projections of the incidence of non-Hodgkin's lymphoma related to acquired immunodeficiency syndrome, *JNCI* 83:695 (1991).
7. R. J. Biggar, Cancer in acquired immunodeficiency syndrome: an epidemiological assessment, *Semin. Oncol.* 17:251 (199O).
8. B. Safir, J. J.Schwartz, Kaposi's sarcoma and the acquired immunodeficiency syndrome, *in*: "AIDS Etiology, Diagnosis, Treatment and Prevention", V. T. DeVita Jr., S. Hellman, and S. A. Rosenberg, eds. J.B. Lippincott Co., Philadelphia, 3rd ed, pp. 209-223, 1992.
9. S. C. Remick, C. Diamond, J. A. Migliozzi, et al., Primary central nervous system lymphoma in patients with and without the acquired immune deficiency syndrome, A retrospective analysis and review of the literature, *Medicine* 69:345 (1990).
10. J. L. Ziegler, J. A. Beckstead, P. A. Volberding, et al., Non-Hodgkin's lymphoma in 90 homosexual men: relation to generalized lymphadenopathy and acquired immunodeficiency syndrome, *N. Engl. J. Med.* 311:565 (1984).
11. S. C. Remick, H. Wagner, Jr., J. C. Ruckdeschel, Management of the patient with HIV-associated lymphomas and Hodgkin's disease, AIDS Reader
12. K. J. Cremer, S. B. Spring, J. Gruber, Role of human immunodeficiency virus type I and other viruses in malignancies associated with acquired immunodeficiency syndrome, *JNCI* 82:1016 (1990).
13. B. Ensoli, G. Barillari, R. C. Gallo, Pathogenesis of AIDS-associated Kaposi's sarcoma, *Hematology/-Oncology Clin. N. Amer.* 5:281 (1991).
14. B. Shiramizu, and M. S. McGrath, Molecular pathogenesis of AIDS-associated non-Hodgkin's lymphoma, *Hematology/Oncology Clin. N. Am.* 5:323 (1991).
15. S. Roithman, J. M. Tourani, J. M. Andriev, Hodgkin's disease in HIV-infected intravenous drug abusers, *N. Engl. J. Med.* 323:275 (1990). (Letter.)
16. E. Senaldi, M. H, Lee, I. Toth, et al., Hodgkin's disease after non-Hodgkin's malignant lymphoma in acquired immune deficiency syndrome, *Cancer* 66:960 (1990).
17. M. Serrano, C. Bellas, E. Campo, et al., Hodgkin's disease in patients with antibodies to human immunodeficiency virus: a study of 22 patients, *Cancer* 65:2248 (1990).
18. A. M. Levine, Lymphoma and other miscellaneous cancers, *in*: "AIDS Etiology, Diagnosis, Treatment and Prevention", V. T. DeVita Jr., S. Hellman, and S. A. Rosenberg, eds., JB Lippincott Co., Philadelphia, 3rd ed, pp. 209-223, (1992).
19. E. D. Ames, M. S. Conjalka, A. F. Goldberg, et al., Hodgkin's disease and AIDS. Twenty-three new cases and a review of the literature, *Hematology/Oncology Clin. N. Am.* 5:343 (1991).
20. J. E. Gold, D. Altarac, A. Khan, et al., HIV-associated Hodgkin disease: A clinical study of 18 cases and review of the literature, *Am. J. Hematol.* 36:93 (1991).
21. Italian Cooperative Group for AIDS-related tumors, Malignant lymphomas in patients with or at risk for AIDS in Italy, *JNCI* 80:855 (1988).
22. S. Monfardini, V. Tirelli, E. Vaccher, et al., Hodgkin's disease in 50 intravenous drug users with HIV infection, *Leuk Lymphoma* 24 3:375 (1991).
23. J. Palefsky, Human papillomavirus infection among HIV-infected individuals, *Hematology/Oncology Clin. N. Am.* 5:357 (1991).
24. I. Penn, Cancers of the anogenital region in renal transplant recipients: analysis of 65 cases, *Cancer* 58:611 (1986).
25. L. K. Schrager, G. H. Friedland, D. Maude, et al., Cervical and vaginal squamous cell abnormalities in women infected with human immunodeficiency virus, *J. AIDS* 2:570 (1989).
26. A. R. Feingold, S. H. Vermond, R. D. Burk, et al., Cervical cytologic abnormalities and papillomavirus in women infected with human immunodeficiency virus, *J. AIDS* 3:896 (1990).

27. A. Schafer, W. Friedmann, M. Mielke, et al., The increased frequency of cervical dysplasia-neoplasia in women infected with the human immunodeficiency virus is related to degree of immunosuppression, *Am. J. Obstet. Gynecol.* 164:593 (1991).
28. D. Provencher, B. Valme, H. E. Averette, et al., HIV status and positive Papanicolau screening: identification of a high-risk population, *Gynecol. Oncol.* 31:184 (1988).
29. S. H. Vermund, K. E. Kelley, R. S. Klein, et al., High risk of human papillomavirus infection and cervical squamous intraepithelial lesions among women with symptomatic human immunodeficiency virus infection, *Am. J. Obstet. Gynecol.* 165:392 (1991).
30. M. Maiman, N. Tarricone, J. Vieira, et al., Colposcopic evaluation of human immunodeficiency virus-seropositive women, *Obstet. Gynecol.* 8:84 (1991).
31. A. Boguniewicz, A. Mudgil, K. O'Neil, R. Weiss, S. Remick, and B. Wolf, Cytopathologic and epidemiologic findings in HIV seropositive women, United States and Canadian Academy of Pathology, Atlanta, GA, March 14-20, (1992).
32. M. A. Rellihan, D. P. Dooley, T. W. Burke, et al., Rapidly progressing cervical cancer in a patient with human immunodeficiency virus infection, *Gynecol. Oncol.* 36:435 (1990).
33. L. B. Schwartz, M. L. Carcangiu, L. Bradham, P. E. Schwartz, Rapidly progressive squamous cell carcinoma of the cervix coexisting with human immunodeficiency virus infection: clinical opinion, *Gynecol. Oncol.* 41:255 (1991).
34. D. M. Heyer, S. Desmond, P. Volberding, J. Kahn, Changing prevalence of ' malignancies in men at San Francisco General Hospital during the HIV epidemic, *Fifth Internatl. Conf. on AIDS*, Montreal, p.206, June 1989.
35. M. Rarick, D. Sharma, P. S. Gill, M. Berstein-Singer, A. M. Levine, et al., Miscellaneous carcinomas developing in patients with HIV infection, *Fifth Internatl Conf. on AIDS,* Montreal, June 1989, p.600.
36. C. S. Rabkin, R. J. Biggar, J. Horm, Cancer trends associated with increasing incidence of AIDS, *Sixth Internatl Conf. on AIDS*, San Francisco, June, 1:295, (1990).
37. I. Gilson, J. Barnett, J. Snow, Basal cell carcinoma in HIV disease, *Fifth Internatl Conf. on AIDS*, Montreal, p.252, June (1989).
38. S. Monfardini, E. Vaccher, G. Pizzocaro, et al., Unusual malignant tumors in 49 patients with HIV infection, *AIDS* 3:449 (1989).
39. J. M. Palefsky, J. Gonzales, R. M. Greenblatt, et al., Anal intraepithelial neoplasia and anal papillomavirus infection among homosexual males with group IV HIV disease, *JAMA* 263:2911 (1990).
40. J. Paavonen, and M. Lehtinen, Human papillomavirus and anogenital neoplasia, *AIDS Reader* 1:116 (1991).
41. J. H. Scholefield, I. C. Talbot, C. Whatrup, et al., Anal and cervical intraepithelial neoplasia possible parallel, *Lancet* 2:765 (1989).
42. B. Tindall, R. Finlayson, K. Mutimer, et al., Malignant melanoma associated with human immunodeficiency virus infection in three homosexual men, *J. Am. Acad. Dermatol.* 20:587, (1989).
43. S. Remick, G. R. Harper, M. A. Abdullah, J. J. McSharry, J. S. Ross, and J. C. Ruckdeschel, Metastatic breast cancer in a young HIV-seropositive patient, *JNCI* 83:447 (1991).
44. M. A. Braun, D. A. Killam, S. C. Remick, and J. C. Ruckdeschel, Lung cancer in HIV seropositive patients, *Radiol.* 175:341 (1990).
45. K. S. Sridhar, M. R. Flores, W. A. Raub, Jr, and M. Saldana, Lung cancer in patients with human immunodeficiency virus infection compared with historical controls, *Chest* 102:1704 (1992).
46. M. H. Kaplan, M. Susin, S. G. Pahwa, et al., Neoplastic complications of HTLV-III infection. Lymphomas and solid tumors, *Am. J. Med.* 82:389 (1987).
47. A. N. Tessler, and N. Catanese, AIDS and germ cell tumors of the testis, *Urol.* 3:203 (1987).
48. J. M. Pluda, R. Yarchoan, and E. S. Jaffe, Development of non-Hodgkin lymphoma in a cohort of patients with severe human immunodeficiency (HIV) infection on long-term antiretroviral therapy. *Ann. Intern. Med.* 13:276 (1990).
49. R. D. Moore, H. Kessler, D. D. Richman, C. Flexner, and R. E. Chaisson, Non-Hodgkin's lymphoma in patients with advanced HIV infection treated with zidovudine, *JAMA* 265:2208 (1991).

STRESS, ENDOCRINE RESPONSES, IMMUNITY AND HIV-1 SPECTRUM DISEASE

Neil Schneiderman, Michael H. Antoni, Mary Ann Fletcher, Gail Ironson, Nancy Klimas, Mahendra Kumar and Arthur LaPerriere

Departments of Psychology, Psychiatry and Medicine, University of Miami, Miami, FL

The immunodeficiency virus, type 1 (HIV-1), which is the cause of the acquired immunodeficiency syndrome (AIDS), is a retrovirus of the human T-cell leukemia/lymphoma line. Well-documented quantitative and qualitative decrements in immunologic functioning occur during the course of HIV-1 spectrum disease (1,2,3). Because the HIV-1 infected person typically goes through several stages of progressive quantitative and qualitative decrements in immunologic functioning that may be associated with disease progression over many years, the disease is increasingly being viewed as a chronic disorder. Subsequent to a brief, frequently unrecognized, acute phase lasting a few weeks, the HIV-1 infected individual enters a clinically latent period characterized by low viral expression. The usual period from onset of acute infection to seropositivity (seroconversion) is 4-12 wks (4,5). After seroconversion, the clinically latent phase of seropositivity begins and may last as long as 10-15 years (6). Then, as the disease progresses, a loss in overall immunocompetence leaves the HIV-1 infected individual susceptible to opportunistic infections. These infections commonly include *Pneumocystis carnii* pneumonia, cryptococcal meningitis and toxoplasmosis-related phenomena, including meningoencephalitis, candidal esophagitis, and herpes simplex encephalitis.

During the past six years our research program has been examining the influence of psychosocial stressors upon affective, endocrine and immune responses in asymptomatic HIV-1 seropositive gay men. The reason that we are examining these relationships is because the literature suggests that psychosocial factors may impact upon the immune system, and because the possibility exists that in HIV-1 infected individuals, who experience quantitative and qualitative decrements in immune functioning, psychosocial stressors could conceivably facilitate disease progression. The purpose of this chapter is to review briefly some of our recent findings within the context of the research literature in order to explore the possibility that affective, endocrine and immune responses are interactive in asymptomatic individuals suffering from HIV-1 spectrum disease.

Drugs of Abuse, Immunity, and AIDS, Edited by
H. Friedman *et al.*, Plenum Press, New York, 1993

STRESS HORMONES AND IMMUNE FUNCTION

The exact functional relations among behavior, immune function, and disease progression are unknown. This is especially true of the relationships among behavior, immune function, and HIV-1 progression. Relationships between various neurohormones and immune function, however, have been sufficiently established to permit the advancement of hypotheses relating psychological and behavioral variables on the one hand and immunomodulation on the other.

An individual's perception of a stressor or the availability or unavailability of a coping response to that stressor, or both, may trigger a series of physiological events leading to specific autonomic nervous system (ANS), neuroendocrine, and neuropeptide changes (7). A specific pattern of ANS activation, which occurs when coping responses are available and potentially adequate to meet stressful demands, is often associated with active coping. The sympathoadrenomedullary (SAM) system, activated during such active coping episodes, releases norepinephrine (NE) and epinephrine(E), and may promote increases in heart rate (HR), cardiac contractility and cardiac output. Another physiological pattern appears to be dominant when coping responses are unavailable, as in those stressful situations defined as unpredictable, uncontrollable, or *unrelenting*. This pattern, associated with hypervigilance and lack of adequate coping resources is characterized by behavioral inhibition, increases in NE and total peripheral resistance and activation of the hypothalamic-pituitary-adrenocortical system (HPAC). Activation of the HPAC system is associated with adrenocorticotropic hormone (ACTH) and cortisol release, the ACTH release following signaling by corticotropin releasing hormone (CRH). It should be noted, however, that many stimulus situations in humans elicit mixed patterns of response in which both the SAM and the HPAC system are activated (8). Individual difference variables also need to be considered (9).

Preliminary findings suggest that elevations in CRH, ACTH, cortisol, NE, and E may be accompanied by decrements in immune function. Corticotropin releasing hormone has been shown to inhibit human natural killer cell cytotoxicity (NKCC) and may do so by stimulating cyclic adenosine monophosphate (cAMP) in large granular lymphocytes (10). This finding is significant in that CRH release from the parvocellular subdivision of the paraventricular nucleus of the hypothalamus is the initiating step in HPAC activation (7). Downstream, HPAC products (i.e., ACTH, cortisol) appear to be important as well. Physiologic doses of ACTH have been shown to impair the responsiveness of T (thymus-derived) lymphocytes to antigenic (CD3 antibody) and mitogenic stimuli such as Concanavalin A (ConA), and may do so by interfering with intracellular levels of calcium, an important second messenger for T-cell activation (11).

Evidence has accumulated indicating that corticosteroids directly impair or modify several components of cellular immunity including T lymphocytes (12,13), macrophages (14,15,16), and NKCC (17,18). Corticosteroids are also known to inhibit both humoral and cellular responses to several antigens such as tetanus toxoid (19), and these suppressive effects include decreases in T-cell subpopulations (12); decreased production of macrophage mitogenic factor, chemotaxis factor, and macrophage migration inhibitory factor (20); and impaired production of interleukin-I (IL-l) and plasmogen activator by monocytes (12). Furthermore, corticosteroids appear to decrease leukocyte migration inhibitory factor production in response to the plant mitogen phytohemagglutinin (PHA) (21); impair NKCC and gamma interferon production (19); and diminish lymphotoxin release by lymphocytes (12). Cortisol as well as ACTH receptors have been established on lymphocytes, and the interaction of cortisol receptors with appropriate cortisol levels may inhibit cellular immune responses via changes in DNA and RNA synthesis and uptake (see 22 for review). Hence, the literature supports the notion that elevated levels of cortisol may be associated with altered immune system function and accompanying depression of lymphokine production.

Although the research literature shows some consistency, several caveats concerning corticosteroid-immune interactions deserve mention. First, milieu factors need to be taken into account in interpreting the data since some studies have used *in vivo* and others *in vitro* analyses. Second, dosage factors need to be considered since some studies have manipulated physiologic and others pharmacologic levels of hormonal independent variables. Third, species factors need to be evaluated since some species appear to be steroid-sensitive while others appear to be steroid-resistant and this can profoundly affect endocrine-immune relationships. Fourth, duration of corticosteroid activation needs to be taken into account since this can influence endocrine immune interactions.

Elevations in peripheral catecholamines have also been shown to depress immune functioning ostensibly via beta-adrenergic receptors on lymphocytes (13,23,24,25,26). Sympathetic noradrenergic fibers innervate the vasculature as well as the parenchymal regions of lymphocytes and associated cells in several lymphoid organs in which nerve terminals are generally directed into zones of T lymphocytes (13). The administration of beta-adrenergic agonists such as E has been associated with decreases in mouse and human NKCC and decreased T-lymphocyte proliferation; these effects appear to be mediated by increases in intracellular cAMP levels (26,27). In sum, evidence exists for immunomodulatory effects of catecholamines and corticosteroids on several aspects of cellular immunity including lymphocyte and NK cell functioning.

BEHAVIORAL STRESSORS AND IMMUNE FUNCTION

Several behavioral variables have been associated with both neuroendocrine changes and altered immune functioning. Animals subjected to uncontrollable stressors, for instance, have been noted to display elevated plasma corticosteroids and depleted brain NE levels (28,29) and increased peripheral catecholamine release (30) as well as immune system decrements such as thymic involution (31), suppressed lymphocyte proliferation (32), impaired plaque-forming cell response to sheep red blood cells (29) and decreased T-lymphocyte helper-inducer/suppressor-cytotoxic (CD4/CD8) ratios (33).

In research using naturally occurring uncontrollable stressors in human subjects, some parallels to the animal findings noted previously have been identified. The experience of chronic environmental stressors characterized by a loss of personal control (e.g., being a resident of Three-Mile Island during the nuclear reactor accident) among normal healthy subjects was accompanied by increased symptoms of psychological distress (e.g., anxiety, depression); elevations in urinary catecholamine levels; and decreases in total T-lymphocyte number (CD3), total macrophage number, and total CD4 number (34). In work with a geriatric population in which the effects of perceived controllable versus uncontrollable major events were evaluated for immunomodulatory effects, only uncontrollable events were associated with decrements in CD4/CD8 ratios and PHA mitogen responses (35).

Social stressors have been associated with elevations in stress hormone levels and altered immune functioning in both the animal and human research literature. Animal models of separation stress and social isolation in monkeys separated from their mothers show a behavioral response suggesting depression and helplessness, elevated cortisol level and compromised immune functioning (36,37). Separation associated with loss of a spouse (i.e., bereavement) in humans has also been associated with glucocorticoid elevation and cellular immunomodulation (38,39,40).

A series of studies conducted by Kiecolt-Glaser, Glaser and associates has documented impairments in lymphocyte response to mitogens, NK cell (CD56) counts, NKCC and percent of CD4 T-lymphocytes as well as elevated antibody titers to

Epstein-Barr virus (EBV), Herpes Simplex virus and cytomegalovirus (reflecting poorer immunological control of latent virus), and increased incidence of infectious disease among healthy students during the period preceding medical school examinations (see 41 for review). Other studies of examination stress support the above findings of impaired mitogen responsiveness (42,43).

Periods of adjustment *following* aversive events have also been associated with changes in endocrine and immune function. After the nuclear reactor accident at Three-Mile Island, for example, residents showed evidence of psychological distress, elevated urinary catecholamines and decreased total T-lymphocyte (CD3), total macrophage and CD4 cell number (34). Divorced individuals have shown decreased lymphocyte proliferative responses to PHA, decreased CD56 number, and higher EBV antibody titers compared to age-matched married control subjects (44). Other research has indicated that the death of a spouse is accompanied by up to a 10-fold decrease subsequently in lymphocyte response to mitogen stimulation (45,46,47). Caregivers of chronically ill Alzheimer's victims have shown a lower percent of CD3 and CD4 number as well as CD4/CD8 ratios, and higher antibody titers to EBV (48).

BEHAVIORAL STRESSORS, STRESS HORMONES, IMMUNE FUNCTION AND HIV-1

Immunologic Effects of Early HIV-1 Infection

We have examined immunologic function in a cohort of 71 gay men entered into a study in which they would learn their serostatus after several weeks and compared them with 25 matched laboratory control subjects not entered into the study (49). Of the study subjects, 25 turned out to be HIV-1 seropositive and 46 were seronegative. The HIV-1 seropositive men had a relatively high median CD4 count of 721/cmm at entry into the study. This is consistent with a similar value of 715 T4 cells/cmm observed in the Multicenter AIDS Cohort Study (MACS) within 6 mos. after seroconversion (50). MACS found a further drop after one year to 626/cmm; whereas, longer-term seropositive asymptomatic men in the MACS study had a CD4 count of 530/cmm. Thus, our seropositive men appear to have been in an early stage of infection.

The numbers of CD4 cells and their helper subset (CD4+CD29+) were significantly depressed in our HIV-1 seropositive men compared with the other two groups. There was a significant elevation in the percentages of CD8 and the subsets, CD8+12+ and CD8+12-, for both seropositive and seronegative study groups compared with the laboratory control group. The median ratio of CD4/CD8 cells was approximately 1.3 in the seronegative study group, which was significantly higher than in the seropositive study group but also significantly lower than the control group. Responses to the plant mitogens, PHA and PWM (pokeweed mitogen), in the HIV-1 seropositive group were lower than in the other two groups at the outset of the study. NKCC was lower in the two study groups than in the laboratory controls but was not related to HIV-1 serostatus. At baseline there were no differences in either seronegative group as compared to seropositives in total number of T cells (CD2), activated T cells (CD2+CDw26), T inducer cells (CD4+CD45RA), B cells (CD20) or NK Cells (CD56). In summary, early stage asymptomatic seropositive gay men showed a decrease in CD4 cells, in the helper subset CD4+CD29+, in CD4/CD8, and in response to PHA and PWM.

Psychosocial Stressor Effects

In the Klimas et al., (49) study we observed that seronegative gay men had decreased mitogen responses and NKCC, compared to age and sex matched laboratory controls. When we followed HIV-1 *seronegative* subjects until 5 weeks after serostatus notification we observed that NKCC and the responses to PHA and PWM returned to normal values (51). This suggested that the decision to enter the study in which HIV-1 antibody testing would occur was a potent acute stressor with immunologic effects.

Asymptomatic HIV-1 *seropositive* individuals had a dampened immune response at the baseline measurement as reflected in low NKCC and subnormal responses to PHA and PWM (51) as compared to controls. Despite significant changes in state anxiety and intrusive thoughts *following news of a positive test*, there was no change in lymphocyte response to mitogens. This lack of change in seropositives may reflect the observation that asymptomatic seropositives show significant decrements in enumerative indices (e.g., helper cell number) at baseline, which place an upper limit on any exogenously-induced (i.e., psychosocial stressors) changes in mitogen responsivity. Seropositives did show fluctuations in NKCC similar to those seen in seronegatives.

We next examined the relationship of psychological and neuroendocrine measures to functional immune changes in anticipation of HIV-1 serostatus notification in men who turned out to be seronegative (52). The results indicated that distress scores and cortisol levels were elevated at study entry and gradually decreased across the 10 wk study period. In contrast the mitogen response to PHA gradually increased over time and ultimately reached levels normally observed in nonstressed individuals. Analyses of individual differences showed that higher baseline cortisol and lower denial coping scores predicted lower PHA values at baseline. Persisting intrusive thoughts about risk of HIV-1 infectivity (after notification of seronegativity) were consistently associated with higher plasma cortisol levels and lower lymphocyte responses to PHA. Finally, beta-endorphin levels did not change significantly across the 10-wk observation period, were not associated with psychological variables, and were inconsistently associated with immune functioning.

Our next step was to assess concurrently, psychological distress, plasma cortisol concentrations and lymphocyte proliferative responses to PHA and PWM in the 5-week periods preceding and following serostatus notification among asymptomatic HIV-1 seropositive and seronegative gay men (53). Seropositives, as opposed to seronegatives, showed a disparity in predicted relationships among distress, cortisol, and immunologic measures across the notification period. That is, the seropositive men showed a marked increase in distress to serostatus notification, but a marked *decrease* in plasma cortisol that lasted for more than a week; response to PHA was low before and after serostatus notification. Individual difference analyses suggested that among seropositives, in contrast to seronegatives, plasma cortisol concentrations were negatively correlated with psychological distress and positively correlated with responses to PHA. This pattern in HIV-1 seropositives could not be explained by differences in perceived risk of infectivity prior to diagnosis, extraneous environmental stressors, or CD4 cell counts within the seropositive group.

In addition to the above published studies, we have assessed the lymphocyte proliferative responses to optimal concentrations of PHA (10 µg/ml) and PWM (diluted 1:40) while simultaneously pulsing the lymphocyte cultures with five successive concentrations of cortisol. The amounts of PHA and PWM used were the levels that give optimum proliferation in both HIV-1 seropositive and seronegative subjects (54). Compared to the laboratory controls, the lymphocytes of the seropositive men appeared to show a hypersensitivity to cortisol that was most pronounced at the 75 ng/ml concentration. These findings suggest the possibility of an upregulation in lymphocytes of individuals in the early stages of the HIV-1 infection process. At the least, they indicate that the paradoxical decrease in cortisol responses to notification of HIV-1 seropositivity is not related to the receptor properties of the lymphocytes.

Our finding that HIV-1 serostatus notification in seropositive gay men caused a paradoxical decrease in plasma cortisol and disrupted the significant negative correlation between plasma cortisol and PHA seen in noninfected individuals (53), prompted us to take a closer look in the behavioral laboratory at the relationship between stressors and plasma cortisol, and the relationship between plasma cortisol and lymphocyte proliferation to PHA that occurs when a psychological stressor is introduced. We therefore subjected eight HIV-1 seronegative and nine seropositive gay men to an evaluative speech stressor task (55). In response to the psychological stressor, significant increases occurred in HR, systolic blood pressure, diastolic blood pressure, ACTH and cortisol. Significant increases also occurred in CD8 and CD56 counts and in NKCC. In contrast, significant decreases occurred in CD4% counts as well as in lymphocyte mitosis to PHA. There were no significant differences in reactivity main effects between the HIV-1 seronegative and seropositive groups. (Using a larger sample and the cold pressor task in the laboratory, however, we have observed a larger response to ACTH but not in cortisol in HIV-1 seropositive as opposed to HIV-seronegative gay men[56,57]). In any event, significant increases in the cardiovascular measures and in CD8 and CD56 occurred as early as 4 min into the speech stressor task as did the decrease in CD4% and the mitogen response to PHA. These changes occurred well *before* plasma cortisol increased.

Based upon our laboratory reactivity findings it would appear that cortisol responses to stressors appear to be intact in HIV-1 seropositive individuals and that the decreased lymphocyte proliferation to PHA produced by psychological stressors in HIV-1 seronegative individuals can occur independent of changes in plasma cortisol. Moreover, the strong negative correlation (r= -.84) observed across multiple timepoints including baseline between cortisol and the mitogen response to PHA stimulation demonstrated by the seronegative subjects in the speech stressor experiment, does not imply that the lymphocyte proliferation response was inhibited by cortisol, since in direct response to the speech stressor the PHA response preceded the cortisol response. The rapidity of the PHA response (< 4 min) suggests that SNS activation may be a critical mediator.

We have begun to study the SNS reactivity responses of HIV-1 seronegative and seropositive gay men by examining their plasma catecholamine responses to the cold pressor test (56,57). Briefly, 76 HIV-1 seropositive and 19 seronegative gay men were each asked to immerse one of his hands in ice water for 2 min. The results indicated that the plasma NE response in HIV-1 seropositive men was blunted when compared to that of seronegative subjects.

DISCUSSION

The studies cited in this chapter indicate that important relationships exist among behavioral stressors, endocrine responses and immune functioning. In our research involving HIV-1 serostatus notification, for example, we have observed that high risk gay men who are awaiting serostatus diagnosis and turn out to be seronegative reveal <u>anticipatory</u> responses including elevated psychological distress and plasma cortisol levels accompanied by a decrease in lymphocyte proliferation to PHA (52,49). These responses are also associated with decreases in NKCC (51). Thus, the seronegative men demonstrated significant positive correlations between perceived distress and plasma cortisol and a significant negative correlation between each of these measures and functional immune measures.

Within the same serostatus notification paradigm, gay men who later turned out to be asymptomatic but HIV-1 seropositive showed significantly elevated distress (48) and an elevated level of plasma cortisol (53) prior to serostatus notification. Subsequent to diagnosis the seropositive men showed a further significant increase in distress accompanied by a reliable but paradoxical decrease in cortisol. Interestingly, there were no significant changes in any immune measure in response to diagnosis (49,51,53). The lack of change in functional immune measures appears to be related to our observation that asymptomatic seropositive individuals show significant decrements in enumerative indices upon entry into the study, and this may well place an upper limit upon any stressor induced change in functional measures.

Although our findings indicate that functional immune measures (i.e., NKCC, PHA, PWM) are lower in HIV-1 seropositive than in seronegative gay men before and after diagnosis and that no significant changes occur as a function of diagnosis (49), our data also suggest that the immune system of the seropositive men may not be totally unresponsive. Thus, for example, we found a significant positive correlation between plasma cortisol and PHA responses in the seropositive men at the outset of the study (r= 0.65) that was in contrast to the reliable negative correlation displayed by the seronegative men (r = -0.36). Postnotification, the correlation between cortisol and the mitogen response to PHA in the seropositive men was r = 0.56. Also, in the seropositive group cortisol and PWM were not associated at baseline, but were significantly positively correlated (r = 0.56) after diagnosis. The picture that emerges then among seronegative individuals, is of a strong relationship between increased distress scores and plasma cortisol on the one hand and decreased functional responses to a natural stressor on the other. In contrast, among HIV-1 seropositive gay men the picture is one of a "dampened" functional immune system and a paradoxical response to the stress of diagnosis. Thus, the seropositive men displayed increased distress that was associated with a decreased level of cortisol. Also, paradoxically, positive relationships were observed between cortisol and functional immune measures.

Our *in vitro* study examining the impact of cortisol on PHA indicated that lymphocyte proliferation of HIV-1 infected men was not impaired by cortisol simulation. The behavioral laboratory study using an evaluative speech stressor indicated that both seronegative and seropositive gay men responded appropriately in terms of ACTH and cortisol secretion. Our finding that major immune changes including CD8 and CD56 trafficking as well as the PHA response occurred before changes were observed in cortisol release, suggest that cortisol is not involved in these changes.

In our HIV-1 serostatus diagnosis study, however, we did observe a significant negative correlation between cortisol and immune functioning in seronegative gay men. In view of our behavioral laboratory and more naturalistic findings it would appear that in situations in which there is time for the adrenal cortical outflow to influence the adrenal medulla, the release of cortisol and catecholamines may be positively correlated (58), and the release of catecholamines may suppress lymphocyte proliferation (see 59 for details). This could account for the negative correlation we previously observed between cortisol and PHA (52). In contrast, in situations in which actions of the SNS become evident over a few minutes, as in our laboratory reactivity situation, the more direct linkage between SNS activation and the suppression of lymphocyte proliferation may be more obvious.

The findings that changes in CD8 and CD56 lymphocyte migration occur rapidly (< 4 min) and closely in time with increases in HR and blood pressure suggests that these changes in lymphocyte trafficking may occur as a function of sympathetic nervous system (SNS) activation. Previous research, of course, has demonstrated extensive SNS innervation of both primary and secondary lymphoid organs (13,25,60,61,62). Within 5 min after infusion of NE or isoproterenol, Ernstrom and Sandberg (63) found an increased splenic veno-arterial difference in lymphocyte numbers. The effects of NE were blocked by phentolamine and the effects of isoproterenol by propranolol. Thus, specific stimulation of alpha- or beta-adrenergic receptors causes considerable mobilization of lymphocytes from the spleen. Moreover, the finding in our study that SNS arousal was associated with the preferential increase in CD8 cell release into the systemic circulation may be due to specificity in SNS innervation and/or to T-suppressor cytotoxic cells simply having more beta-adrenergic receptors than other T cells (64).

In our study of HIV-1 serostatus notification we observed that the seropositive men responded to their diagnosis with a paradoxical decrease in cortisol. One conceivable explanation for this finding may be based upon disruption of the short-loop negative feedback system described by Axelrod and Reisine (58). According to these authors, the release of ACTH by the anterior pituitary results in the release of cortisol, which results in negative feedback to the pituitary, terminating the further release of ACTH. Concomitantly, the release of ACTH by the anterior pituitary when it results in the release of cortisol, in turn, facilitates the release of plasma catecholamines (primarily E) from the adrenal medulla. The release of catecholamines from the adrenal medulla, in turn, provides positive feedback to the system. In our behavioral study using the cold pressor test, we found that NE release to a stressor was impaired in asymptomatic HIV-1 gay men (57). To the extent that the release of plasma catecholamines is impaired in seropositive individuals, balanced negative and positive feedback to the anterior pituitary and hypothalamus could be disrupted and account for our paradoxical findings. Although this view at present remains speculative, the data do suggest the need for further investigation of endocrine-immune interactions in HIV-1 seropositive gay men with increased emphasis upon the SNS and biobehavioral responses to stressors.

REFERENCES

1. R. M. De Martini, R. R. Turner, S. C. Formenti, D. C. Boone, P. C. Bishop, A. M. Levine, and J. W. Parker, Peripheral blood mononuclear cell abnormalities and their relationship to clinical course in homosexual men with HIV infection, *Clin. Immunol. and Immunopathol.*, 46:258- (1988).
2. J. V. Giorgi and R. Detels, T-cell subset alterations in HIV infected homosexual men: NIAID Multicenter AIDS Cohort Study (MACS), *Clin. Immunol. Immunopathol.* 52:1018 (1989).
3. D. P. Stites, A. Moss, P. Bacchetti, D. Osmond, T. M. McHugh, Y. J. Wang, S. Hebert, and B. Colfer, Lymphocyte subset analysis to predict progression to AIDS in a cohort of homosexual men in San Francisco, *Clin. Immunol. Immunopathol.* 52:96 (1989).
4. M. Clerici, J. A. Berzofsky, G. M. Shearer, and C. O. Tacket, Exposure to human immunodeficiency virus type 1-specific T helper cell responses before detection of infection by polymerase chain reaction and serum antibodies, *J. Infect. Dis.* 164:178 (1991).
5. C. R. Horsburgh, C. Y. Ou, J. Jason, S. D. Holmberg, A. R. Lifson, and J. L. Moore, Concordance of polymerase chain reaction with human immunodeficiency virus antibody detection, *J. Infect. Dis.* 162:542 (1990).
6. A. Munoz, M. Wang, R. Good, H. Detels, L. Ginsberg, J. Kingsley, J. Phair, and B. F. Polk, Estimation of the AIDS-free times after HIV-1 seroconversion. Paper presented at the Fourth Annual Meeting of the International Conference on AIDS, Stockholm, Sweden.
7. M. McCabe and N. Schneiderman, Psychophysiologic responses to stress, *in*: "Behavioral Medicine: The Biopsychosocial Approach", N. Schneiderman, & J. T. Tapp, eds., Erlbaum, Hillsdale, NJ (1985).
8. N. Schneiderman, and P. M. McCabe, Psychophysiologic strategies in laboratory research, *in*: "Handbook and Research Methods in Cardiovascular Behavioral Medicine" N. Schneiderman, S. M. Weiss, & P. Kaufmann, eds., Plenum Press, New York (1989).
9. S. B. Manuck, A. L. Kasprowicz, S. M. Monroe, K. T. Larkin, and J. R. Kaplan, Psychophysiologic reactivity as a dimension of individual differences, *in*: "Handbook and Research Methods in Cardiovascular Behavioral Medicine", N. Schneiderman, S. M. Weiss, & P. Kaufmann, eds., Plenum Press, New York (1989).
10. M. Pawlikowski, P. Zelazowski, K. Dohler, and H. Stepien, Effects of two neuropeptides, somatoliberin (GRF) and corticoliberin (CRF), on human lymphocyte natural killer activity, *Br. Behav. Immun.* 2:50 (1988).

11. A. Kavelaars, R. E. Ballieux, and C. Heijnen, Modulation of the immune response by proopiomelanocortin derived peptides. II. Influence of adrenocorticotropic hormone on the rise in intracellular free calcium concentration after T cell activation, *Br. Behav. Immun.* 2:57 (1988).
12. T. Cupps and A. Fauci, Corticosterol-mediated immunoregulation in man, *Immunol. Rev.* 65:133 (1982).
13. D. Felten, S. Felten, S. Carlson, J. Olschawka, and S. Livnat, Noradrenergic and peptidergic innervation of lymphoid tissue, *J. Immunol.* 135 (Suppl 2):755s (1985).
14. N. Hall and A. Goldstein, Neurotransmitters and the immune system, *in*: "Psychoneuroimmunology" R. Ader, ed., Academic Press, New York (1981).
15. A. Monjan. Psychosocial factors, stress and immune processes, *in*: "Psychoneuroimmunology", R. Ader ed., Academic Press, New York (1981).
16. N. Pavlidis and M. Chirigos, Stress-induced impairment of macrophage tumoricidal function, *Psychosom. Med.* 4247 (1980).
17. R. Herberman and H. Holden, Natural cell-mediated immunity, *Adv. in Cancer Res.* 27:305 (1978).
18. S. Levy, R. Herberman, M. Lippman, and T. d'Angelo, Correlation of stress factors with sustained depression of natural killer cell activity and predicted prognosis in patients with breast cancer, *J. Clin. Oncol.* 5:348 (1987).
19. D. Stites, J. Stobo, H. Fudenberg, and J. Wells, *Basic Clin. Immunol.* (1982).
20. M. Duncan, J. Sadik, and J. Hadden, *Cellular Immunol.* (4th ed.) (1982).
21. T. Hahn, S. Levin, and Z. Handzel, Leukocyte migration inhibition factor (LIF) production by lymphocytes of normal children, newborns, and children with immune deficiency, *Clin. Exp. Immunol.* 24:448 (1976).
22. M. Antoni, Neuroendocrine influences in psychoimmunology and neoplasia: A review, *Psy. Hlth.* 1:3 (1987).
23. J. Hadden, Neuroendocrine modulation of the thymus-dependent immune system, Agonists and mechanisms, *Ann. NY Acad. Sci.* 496:39 (1987).
24. S. Hatfield, B. Petersen, and J. DiMicco, Beta adrenoceptor modulation of the generation of murine cytotoxic T lymphocytes *in vitro*, *J. Pharm. Exp. Therap.* 239:460 (1986).
25. S. Livnat, S. Felten, D. Carlson, D. L. Bellinger, and D. L. Felton, Involvement of peripheral and central catecholamine systems in neural-immune interactions, *Neuroimmunol.* 10:5 (1985).
26. M. Plaut, Lymphocyte hormone receptors, *Ann. Rev. Immunol.* 5:621 (1987).
27. P. Katz, A. Zeytoun, and A. Fauci, Mechanisms of human cell-mediated cytotoxicity. Modulation of natural killer cell activity by cyclic nucleotides, *J. Immunol.* 129:287 (1982).
28. J. M. Weiss, and P. G. Goodman, *in*: "Stress and Coping" (pp. 93-116), T. M. Field, P.M. McCabe, & N. Schneiderman, eds., Erlbaum, Hillsdale, NJ (1985).
29. D. Pericic, H. Manev, M. Boranic, M. Poljak-Blazi, and N. Lakic, Effect of diazepam on brain neurotransmitters, plasma corticosterone, and the immune system of stressed rats, *Ann. NY Acad. Sci.* 496:450 (1987).
30. J. Mason, A historical review of the stress field, *J. Human Stress*, 1:6 (1975).
31. H. Selye, *in*: "Stress in health and disease" Butterworths, Reading, MA (1976).
32. M. Laudenslager, S. Ryan, R. Drugan, R. Hyson, and S. Maier, Coping and immunosuppression: Inescapable but not escapable shock suppresses lymphocyte proliferation, *Science*, 221:568 (1983).
33. H. Teshima, H. Sogawa, S. Kihara, S. Nagata, Y. Ago, and T. Nakagawa, Changes in populations of T-cell subsets due to stress, *Ann. NY Acad. Sci.* 496:459 (1987).
34. A. Baum, Q. McKinnon, and C. Silvia, Paper presented at the Eighth Annual Scient. Mtg. of the Soc. of Behav. Med., Washington, DC (1987).
35. J. Rodin, Paper presented at the Ninth Annual Scientific Mtg. of the Soc. of Behav. Med. Boston (1988).
36. C. Coe and S. Levine, *in*: "Anxiety: New research and changing concepts" (pp. 155-177), D. Kline, & J. Rabkin, eds., Raven Press, New York (1981).
37. C. Coe, L. Rosenberg, and S. Levine, Prolonged effect of psychological disturbance on macrophage chemiluminescence in the squirrel monkey, *Brain. Behav Immun*, 2:151 (1988).
38. J. Calabrese, M. Kling, and P. Gold, Alterations in immunocompetence during stress, bereavement, and depression: focus on neuroendocrine regulation, *Am. J. Psych.* 144:1123 (1987).
39. M. Irwin, M. Daniels, and H. Weiner, Immune and neuroendocrine changes during bereavement, *Psych. Clin. North Am.* 10:449 (1987).
40. T. Kosten, S. Jacobs, and J. Mason, Psychosocial modulators of immune function, *J. Nerv Ment. Dis.* 172:359 (1984).
41. J. K. Kiecolt-Glaser, and R. Glaser, Psychosocial modulators of immune function, *Ann. Behav. Med.* 9:16 (1987).
42. B. Dorian and P. Garfinkel, Stress, immunity and illness--a review, *Psychol. Med.* 3:393 (1987).

43. R. Halvorsen and O. Vassend, Effects of examination stress on some cellular immunity functions, *J. Psychosom. Res.* 31:693 (1987).
44. J. K. Kiecolt-Glaser, L. Fisher, P. Ogrocki, J. C. Stout, C. E. Speicher, and R. Glaser, Marital quality, marital disruption, and immune function, *Psychosom. Med.* 49:13 (1987).
45. R. W. Bartrop, E. Luckhurst, L. Lazarus, L. G. Kiloh, and R. Penny, Depressed lymphocyte function after bereavement, *Lancet* 1:834 (1977).
46. S. J. Schleifer, S. E. Keller, M. Caminero, J. C. Thornton, and M. Stein, Suppression of lymphocyte stimulation following bereavement, *JAMA*, 15:374 (1983).
47. M. Stein, S. E. Keller, and S. J. Schliefer, Stress and immunomodulation: The role of depression and neuroendocrine function, *J. Immunol.* 135 (Suppl 2):827s (1985).
48. J. K. Kiecolt-Glaser, R. Glaser, E. C. Shuttleworth, C. S. Dyer, P. Ogrocki and C. E. Speicher, Chronic stress and immunity in family caregivers of Alzheimer's disease victims, *Psychosom. Med.*, 49:523 (1987).
49. N. Klimas, P. Caralis, A. LaPerriere, M. Antoni, G. Ironson, J. Simoneau, M. Ashman, N. Schneiderman and M. A. Fletcher, Immunologic function in a cohort of HIV-1 seropositive and negative healthy homosexual men, *J. Clin. Microbiol.* 29:1413 (1991).
50. J. Giorgi and R. Detels, T-cell subset alterations in HIV-infected homosexual men: NIAID multicenter AIDS cohort study, *Clin. Immunol. Immunopath.* (1989).
51. G. Ironson, A. LaPerriere, M. Antoni, P. O'Hearn, N. Schneiderman, N. Klimas and M. A. Fletcher, Changes in immune and psychological measures as a function of anticipation and reaction to news of HIV-1 antibody status, *Psychosom. Med.* 52:247 (1990).
52. M. H. Antoni, S. August, A. La Perriere, H. Baggett, N. Klimas, G. Ironson, N. Schneiderman and M. A. Fletcher, Psychological and neuroendocrine measures related to functional immune changes in anticipation of HIV-1 serostatus notification, *Psychosom. Med.* 52:496 (1990).
53. M. H. Antoni, N. Schneiderman, N. Klimas, A. LaPerriere, N. Klimas and M. A. Fletcher, Disparities in psychological, neuroendocrine, and immunologic patterns in HIV-1 infected gay men, *Bio. Psychiat.* 29:1023 (1991).
54. M. A. Fletcher, G. Baron, M. Ashman, M. A. Fischl and N. G. Klimas, Use of whole blood methods in assessment of immune parameters in immunodeficiency states, *Diagnostic Clin. Immunol.* 5:69 (1987).
55. N. Schneiderman, Psychoneuroendocrinology and HIV-1, Paper presented at the 23rd Congress of the *Internatl. Soc. of Psychoneuroendocrinol*, Madison, WI (1992).
56. M. Kumar, A. M. Kumar, R. Morgan, J. Szapocznik and C. Eisdorfer, Abnormal ACTH response in early HIV infection, *J. AIDS* (in press).
57. M. Kumar, R. Morgan, J. Szapocznik and C. Eisdorfer, Norepinephrine response in HIV+ subjects, *J. AIDS* 4.782 (1991).
58. J. Axelrod and T. Reisine, Stress hormones: Their interaction and regulation, *Science* 224:452 (1984).
59. T. L. Roszman and S. L. Carlson, Neurotransmitters and molecular signalling in the immune response, *in* "Psychoneuroimmunology" (2nd ed.) (pp. 311-335), R. Ader, D.L. Felten, & N. Cohen, eds., Academic Press, San Diego, CA (1991).
60. K. D. Ackerman, S. Y. Felten, D. L. Bellinger, S. Livnat and D. L. Felten, Noradrenergic sympathetic innervation of spleen and lymph nodes in relation to specific cellular compartments, *Prog. Immunol.* 6:588 (1987).
61. D. L. Bellinger, S. Y. Felten, D. Lorton and D. L. Felten, Origin of noradrenergic innervation of the spleen in rats, *Brain. Behav.Immunity*, 3:291 (1989).
62. D. L. Felten, K. D. Ackerman, S. J. Wiegand and S. Y. Felten, Noradrenergic sympathetic innervation of the spleen: Nerve fibers associate with lymphocytes and macrophages in specific compartments of the splenic white pulp, *J. Neurosci. Res.*, 18:28 (1987).
63. U. Ernstrom, and G. Sandberg, Venous output of 3-H-labelled lymphocytes from the spleen, *Scand. J. Hematol.* 11:275 (1973).
64. M. M. Khan, P. Sansoni, E. D. Silverman, E. G. Engleman and K. L. Melman, Beta adrenergic receptors on human supressor, helper, and cytolytic lymphocytes, *Biochem. Pharm.* 35:1137 (1986).

EPIDEMIOLOGY AND INFECTIOUS COMPLICATIONS OF HUMAN IMMUNODEFICIENCY VIRUS ANTIBODY POSITIVE PATIENTS

Bienvenido G. Yangco and Vicki S. Kenyon

St. Joseph's Hospital Infectious Disease Research Institute
Tampa, FL 33677-4227

ABSTRACT

From July 1, 1991 to March 31, 1992, 156 patients (pts) with positive antibody titers to the human immunodeficiency virus (HIV) were seen in our clinic. A retrospective review of the epidemiology and infectious complicaions of these patients is presented.

There were 129 males and 27 females (4.8:1, ratio). Only 10/156 (12.8%) were non-whites (13 blacks and 7 hispanics). The majority, 126 (80.7%), were 25 to 44 years old. The most common risk factor was homosexuality or bisexuality 100 (64.1%), followed by heterosexual acquisition 25 (16%), intravenous drug abuse 23 (13.7%), unknown 6 (3.8%) and transfusion-related 3 (1.9%).

Sixty-five pts had no infections. In the remaining 91 pts, the infections noted were: candidiasis (54 pts); *Pneumocystic carinii* pneumonia (25 pts); Herpes simplex (13 pts); cytomegalovirus (CMV) retinitis (11 pts) and CMV esophagitis (1 pt), central nervous system toxoplasmosis (8); *Herpes zoster* (6 pts); cryptococcal meningitis (5 pts); *Mycobacterium avium* complex bacteremia (4 pts); *Molluscum contagiosum*, hepatitis-B, staphylococcal infection, perirectal abscess and oral hairy leukoplakia (2 pts each); syphilis, cryptosporidiosis, nocardiosis, histoplasmosis and laryngeal papillomatosis (1 pt each). Infections were multiple in 57/91 (62%) pts and tend to occur more often when the helper cells are <200 47/57 (82%) pts. Appropriate antimicrobials for prophylaxis and maintenance therapy appeared to decrease the occurrence or relapse of infections such as pneumocystosis, candidiasis, cryptococcosis, tuberuclosis and toxoplasmosis.

INTRODUCTION

Infections are the most common the complications (HIV-infected individuals (1-4). These infections undoubtedly contribute to their morbidity and mortality (2-4). Infections may be newly-acquired, e.g., influenza, bacterial pneumonia, cryptococcal meningitis; or a reactivation of a pathogen suppressed by a previously intact immune system, e.g., cytomegalovirus, *Herpes zoster* and *Toxoplasma gondii*. While appropriate treatment and prophylaxis may satisfactorily control if not eradicate some infections,

Drugs of Abuse, Immunity, and AIDS, Edited by
H. Friedman *et al.*, Plenum Press, New York, 1993

persistence and/or relentless progression in spite of available antimicrobial therapy is the rule.

The main objectives of our study are to determine the epidemiology of HIV-positive patients in our institute; assess the type of infections affecting our HIV-infected patients determine the relationship between the CD_4 lymphocyte count and the occurrence of these infections; and further examine the impact of appropriate antimicrobials in the prophylaxis and treatment of these infections.

METHODS

A retrospective review of the clinic charts of patients referred to the St. Joseph's Hospital Infectious Disease Research Institute from July 1, 1991 to March 31, 1992 was conducted. Data collected included: epidemiologic profile, CD_4 lymphocyte count, type and number of specific infections per patient, and relapse of infections during antimicrobial therapy and/or prophylaxis.

RESULTS

The epidemiology of HIV-positive patients seen in our institution are shown on Table 1-3. The majority of patients (80.7%) were between 25 to 44 yrs old with a 4.8:1 male to female ratio (Table 1). Caucasians predominate in number (87.2%) over afro-americans and hispanics (Table 2). The most common risk factor was homosexuality or bisexuality in 100 (64.1%) patients followed by heterosexual acquisition in 25 (16%) patients, intravenous drug abuse in 23 (14.7%), unknown in 6 (3.8%) and transfusion-related in 3 (1.9%) (Table 3). Heterosexual acquisition was the most common risk factor among females.

Table 1. Epidemiology of HIV-positive patients at St. Joseph's Hospital Infectious Disease Research Institute: Gender and age distribution.

Age (Years)	Male	Female
<15	0	0
15 - 24	1	3
25 - 34	45	14
35 - 44	62	5
45 - 54	16	2
<55	5	3
Total	129	27

Table 2. Epidemiology of HIV-positive patients at St. Joseph's Hospital Infectious Disease Research Institute: race or ethnic origin

	No. pts
Caucasians	136
Afro-American	13
Hispanics	7

Table 3. Epidemiology of HIV-positive patients at St. Joseph's Hospital Infectious Disease Research Institute: Risk Factors.

	Males	Females
Homosexual	100	0
IV Drug abuse	18	5
Heterosexual	4	21
Transfusion	2	1
Unknown*		51

*Patients were unable to provide information.

Sixty-five patients had no associated infections. Of the remaining 91 patients, the infections noted are shown on Table 4. Infections were multiple in 57 (62%) patients and occurred with greater frequency when the CD4 lymphocyte count was <200 cells per cubic millimeter 47/57 (82%) patients (Fig. 1). Relapse of the opportunistic infection in spite of standard antimicrobial prophylaxis was noted in 19/54 (54%) patients with oropharyngeal and gastrointestinal candidiasis and 1/25 (8%) patients with pulmonary pneumocystosis, but not in patients with cryptococcal meningitis, toxoplasmosis or tuberculosis (Table 5).

Table 4. Infections of 91 HIV-positive patients at St. Joseph's Infectious Disease Research Institute

Infection	No. pts.	Infection	No. pts.
Candidiasis	54	*Mycobacterium tuberculosis*	2
Pneumocystosis	25	Hepatitis C	2
Herpes simplex	13	Staphylococcus	2
Cytomegalovirus retinitis	11	Perirectal abscess	2
CNS toxoplasmosis	8	Oral Hairy Leukoplakia	2
Herpes zoster	6	Syphilis	2
CNS crytococcosis	5	Cryptosporidiosis	2
Mycobacterium avium complex	4	Nocardiosis	2
Molluscum contagiosum	3	Histoplasmosis	2
Hepatitis B	3	Cytomegalovirus esophagitis	2
Bacterial pneumonia	3	Laryngeal papillomatosis	2

DISCUSSION AND CONCLUSION

Our retrospective study, to a certain extent, reflects the epidemiology of HIV-positive patients nationwide (5). Exceptions were: male-female ratio reflecting a slightly greater number of females compared to the nationwide ratio of 8.5:1, the relatively high heterosexual acquisition of 16% compared to 6% and the lower transfusion-related HIV infection 1.9% compared to 3-4% (5). One possible explanation for these differences is the selection of our patients who are likely to participate in clinical trials.

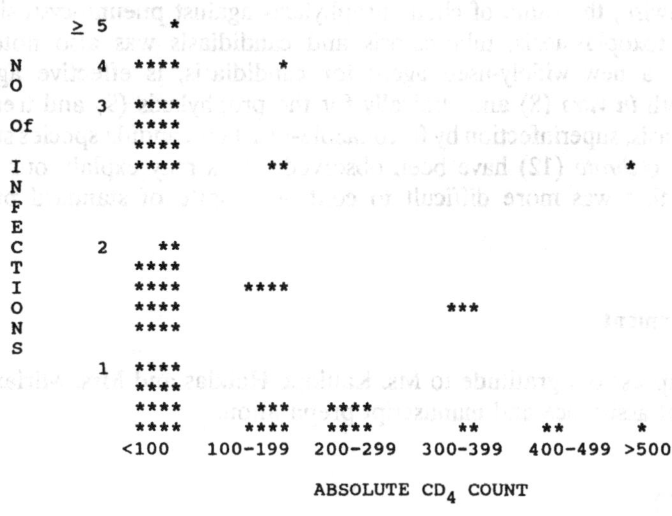

Fig. 1. **Relationship between absolute CD_4 counts and number of infections among HIV-positive patients at St. Joseph's Hospital Infectious Disease Research Institute**

Table 5. Relapse of opportunistic infection while on prophylaxis

Infection	Total no. pts	No. pts. with relapse	%
Candidiasis	54	29	54
Pneumocystosis	25	2	8
Cryptococcal meningitis	5	0	0
Toxoplasmosis	8	0	0
Tuberculosis	1	0	0

The occurrence of at least one infection in 58% of our patients underscores the importance of co-infections as a complication of HIV-positive patients. The inverse relationship of CD4 lymphocyte counts and the occurrence of multiple opportunistic infections has been noted previously (1,6,7) and was further underscored by our present study. Likewise, the value of chemoprophylaxis against pneumocystosis, cryptococcal meningitis, toxoplasmosis, tuberculosis and candidiasis was also noted. Although fluconazole, a new widely-used agent for candidiasis, is effective against *Candida albicans*, both *in vitro* (8) and clinically for the prophylaxis (9) and treatment (10) of oral candidiasis, superinfection by fluconazole-resistant candida species such as *C. krusei* (11) and *C. glabrata* (12) have been observed. This may explain our observation of candidiasis that was more difficult to control in spite of standard prophylaxis and therapy.

Acknowledgement

We express our gratitude to Ms. Kalliope Halkias and Mrs. Miriam Alojipan for the technical assistance and manuscript preparation.

REFERENCES

1. A. E. Glatt, K. Chirgwin, and S. H. Landesman, Treatment of infections associated with human immunodeficiency virus, *N. Engl. J. Med.* 318:1439 (1988).
2. R. Rothenberg, M. Woelfel, R. Stoneburner, J. Milberg, R. Parker, B. Truman, Survival with the acquired immunodeficiency syndrome, Experience with 5833 cases in New York City, *N. Engl. J. Med.* 317:1297 (1987).
3. P. Bacchetti, D. Osmond, R. E. Chaisson, S. Dritz, G. W. Rutherford, L. Swig, A. R. Moss, Survival patterns of the first 500 patients with AIDS in San Francisco, *J. Infect. Dis.* 157:1044 (1988).
4. L. Moskowitz, G. T. Hensley, J. C. chan, K. Adams, Immediate causes of death in acquired immunodeficiency syndrome, *Arch. Pathol. Lab. Med.* 109:735 (1985).
5. The HIV/AIDS Surveillance Report, Division of HIV/AIDS, National Center for Infectious Diseases, Centers for Disease Control, Atlanta, GA (Mar 1992).
6. H. C. Lane, H. Masur, E. P. Gellman, D. L. Longo, R. G. Steis, T. Chused, G. Whalen, L. C. Edgar, A. S. Fauci, Correlation between immunologic function and clinical subpopulations of patients with the acquired immunodeficiency syndrome, *Am. J. Med.* 78:417 (1985).
7. H. Masur, F. P. Ognibene, R. Yarchoan, J. H. Shelhamer, B. F. Baird, W. Travis, A. F. Suffredini, L. Deyton, J. A. Kovacs, J. Fallon, R. Davey, M. Polis, J. Metcalf, M. Baseler, R. Wesley, V. J. Gill, A Fauci, H. C. Lane, CD4 counts as predictors of opportunistic pneumonias in human immunodeficiency virus (HIV) infections, *Ann. Intern. Med.* 111:223 (1989).
8. M. Ruhnke, A. Eigler, B. Geiseler, Fluconazone resistance in *Candida albicans* isolates from patients with AIDS, *The VIII Internatl. Conf. on AIDS/III STD World Congress*, Amsterdam, the Netherlands, Abstract PoB 3246 (July 19-24, 1992).
9. A. Schmidt-Westhausen, T. Gruenewald, J. Sandfort, F. Bergman, B. Ruf, P. Reichart, Secondary prophylaxis of clinical symptomatic Candida infections using bi-weekly fluconazole in HIV-infected patients, *The VIII Internatl. Conf. on AIDS/III STD World Congress*, Amsterdam, the Netherlands, Abstract PoB 3251 (July 19-24, 1992).
10. S. DeWit, D. Weerts, H. Goosens, N. Clumeck, Comparison of fluconazole and ketoconazole for oropharyngeal candidiasis in AIDS, *Lancet*, 1:746 (1989).
11. J. R. Wingard, W. G. Merz, M. G. Rinaldi, T. R. Johnson, J. E. Karp, and R. Saral, Increase in Candida krusei infection among patients with bone marrow transplantation and enutropenia treated prophylactically with fluconazole, *N. Engl. J. Med.* 325:1274 (1991).
12. D. W. Warnack, J. Burke, N. J. Cope, E. M. Johnson, N. A. Fraunhofer, E. W. Williams, Fluconazole resistance in *Candida glabrata*, *Lancet* 2:1310 (1988).

IMMUNE FUNCTION AND DRUG TREATMENT IN ANTI-RETROVIRUS NEGATIVE INTRAVENOUS DRUG USERS

Mary Ann Fletcher[1,3], Nancy G. Klimas[1,3,4], and Robert O. Morgan[2,3]

[1]Departments of Medicine and [2]Psychiatry
[3]University of Miami School of Medicine
[4]Miami VA Medical Center, Miami, Florida 33101

INTRODUCTION

A recent cross-sectional study by Klimas, et al., (1) showed that a clinically significant degree of immune impairment exists in methadone treated intravenous drug users (IVDUs) in the absence of human T cell lymphotropic virus, subtypes I or II (HTLV) or human immunodeficiency virus (HIV-1) infection or use of street drugs. The methadone-treated group exhibited significant differences in lymphocyte phenotype with elevations in the numbers of CD4+CD29+ (T helper), CD8+ (T suppressor/cytotoxic), CD8+I2+ cells (activated T suppressor/cytotoxic), and CD2+CD29+ (activated total T) lymphocytes. Despite these increases in lymphocyte numbers, lymphocyte function was suppressed in the methadone group, with poor response to phytohemagglutinin (PHA) and pokeweed mitogen (PWM) in culture, except for the subset of subjects who were HTLV positive. Moreover, natural killer (NK) cell cytotoxicity was significantly reduced in the methadone group. These findings could not be ascribed to psychoimmunologic interactions, to concomitant use of street drug or alcohol (2). Other investigators have reported, in studies of peripheral blood mononuclear cells from patients on methadone, a significant impairment of the ability to generate superoxide anion (3). Morphine, and to a lesser extent, methadone reduced phagocytosis, intracellular killing and superoxide production in polymorphonuclear leukocytes and in monocytes (4). In heroin addicts, both before and after methadone treatment, skin test anergy to seven recall antigens was common (3). Other types of immunomodulation by methadone have been reported. Kreek (5) noted persistence of lymphocytosis in patients maintained on methadone for three or more years. However, in one study of 11 very long term methadone users who were 'successful', 'stable' former addicts who remained clear of other drugs and on methadone maintenance for more than a decade, Novick, et al., found no differences between these subjects and controls for certain lymphocyte subsets and in NK cell cytotoxicity (6). Because the published studies on the immunological effects of methadone have been largely cross-sectional, as well as contradictory, the present study was designed to determine changes in immune function over time. Observations were continued on the cohort of patients who were the subject of our prior cross-sectional study (1). No literature is available regarding the immunologic consequences of other treatment options for IVDUs, particularly detoxification. Another

Drugs of Abuse, Immunity, and AIDS, Edited by
H. Friedman *et al.*, Plenum Press, New York, 1993

objective of the present report was to evaluate the effects of 6 wks in an in-patient chemical dependence unit on immune function of HIV-1 seronegative IVDUs.

METHODS

A cohort of male anti-HIV-1, anti-HTLV seronegative patients (n = 19), on methadone maintenance were studied at six months intervals for 12 to 36 months. These were compared over the same time period to 5 age and sex matched seronegative, non-drug abusing controls. Anti-HIV-1, HTLV negative male IVDUs (n = 32) were studied in an in-patient Miami Veterans Administration Medical Center detoxification treatment unit. Samples were obtained within 1 week of entry into the unit and at weeks 2, 3 and at discharge (usually 6 wks).

Laboratory Studies

The *in vitro* assessment of T and B cells function was measured by proliferative response to plant mitogens, PHA and PWM in triplicate 72 hr cultures. A whole blood method was used and assessment of ^{3}H-thymidine incorporation during an additional 6 hr incubation was used to determine the degree of lymphocyte proliferation. Results were expressed as net counts per minute (cpm) per 10 mononuclear cells present in the sample of blood (8).

Cytotoxicity mediated by NK cells to tumor cell targets, K562 cells, was done using a whole blood, ^{57}Cr release assay (9,10). Four effector (defined as CD56+ cells) to target cells ratios were tested in triplicate. Results were expressed both as lytic index (LI), where LI = % cytotoxicity at an effector to target cell ratio of 1:1/number of effector cells and as kinetic lytic units (KLU) where KLU = the number of target cells killed per effector cell during the 4 hr assay period.

Serostatus to HIV-1 and HTLV was determined by repetitive enzyme-linked immunosorbent assays (Coulter) and confirmed by immunoblot. Lymphocyte subsets were determined by two color flow cytometry (7). Shown in Table 1 are the monoclonal antibodies used and subsets measured.

Analytical Strategy

Linear change coefficients were calculated separately for each individual and each immunologic measure. These change coefficients were defined as the linear slope parameters from separate within person regressions and utilized all available observations for each individual. The distributions of these coefficients were examined using Wilcoxon Sign Rank tests to determine if the methadone patients and inpatients, as groups, demonstrated significant change over the course of their observations. In addition, Wilcoxon Rank Sums analyses were used to test for statistically significant differences between the linear change coefficients estimated for the methadone and control subjects. Two-tailed tests of significance were used for all tests. Change estimates for the measure of cell functions (response to mitogens and NK cytotoxicity) were based on the log 1O transformed measures. The medium change coefficients and their 25 or 75th percentile cutoffs are used in Figures 1 through four.

RESULTS

The in-patient treatment group showed no change in the total number of white blood cells or lymphocytes over the period of observation. The results of flow cytometric analyses of lymphocyte subsets in the in-patient group are shown in Fig. 1. There was

Table 1. Functional Associations of Lymphocyte Markers

CD4	T cell subset with helper/inducer functions
CD4+CD29+	Subset which includes the inducers of help
CD4+CD45RA+	Subset which includes the naive (unprimed cells) and inducers of suppression
CD8	T suppressor/cytotoxic cells
CD8+DR+	Activated cells with class II marker
CD2+CD26+	Activated T cells
CD20	Mature B cells
CD21	Resting B cells
CD56	Active natural killer cell subset

no change noted in overall percentage of CD4 cells, but there were significant differences in beta coefficients (median change per day for marker) for CD4 cell subset distribution with a decrease in CD4+CD29+ and an increase in CD4+CD45RA+ cells. Although there were no changes in CD4 cells overall, total CD8 cells or in the CD4/CD8 ratios. There were increases in %CD56 (NK cells) and an increase in B cells. There were no changes in percent total T cells expressing an activation marker (CD2+CD26+), or in percent CD8 cells or activated CD8 cells (CD8+DR+).

Functional changes were observed (Fig. 2). There was a trend toward increase in several measures of NK cytotoxicity and the response to the T and B cell stimulant, PWM. The increase seen in PHA response was statistically significant. In the methadone treatment group, phenotypic change over the period of observation, as compared to baseline, was seen in B cells which decreased in number and in CD8 cells expressing DR, which also decreased. Comparison of beta coefficients for this group with the matched controls showed significant decreases for between the two groups for estimated change per month for B cell subsets, with $p<.007$ for %CD20+CD21+ and $p<.006$ for CD21+ cells (Fig. 3). Comparison of beta coefficients for the methadone treatment group with matched controls showed a very small and only marginally significant increase for cytotoxicity expressed as KLU ($p<.07$) and as LI ($p<.06$) in the treatment group (Figure 4). It should be noted, however, that the median NK cytotoxicity response of the methadone group was still depressed as compared to controls.

CONCLUSION

The aim of this study was further evaluate the effects of two standard methods of treatment of drug abuse on selected markers, both phenotypic and functional, of immune status. One facet of investigation was to make serial measures, over a six week period, of these markers on subjects following admission an inpatient chemical dependence unit. The results indicated that drug withdrawal in such a setting does not result in a major degree of immune enhancement or impairment. There was a redistribution of CD4 subsets with an increase in the naive subset, CD4+CD45RA+ cells. This change probably accounted for the increase over time in the PHA response. The decrease in %NK was not associated with a functional impairment in NK cytotoxicity. We have previously reported that methadone treated IV drug users as compared to controls had significant immunologic changes, including changes in subsets

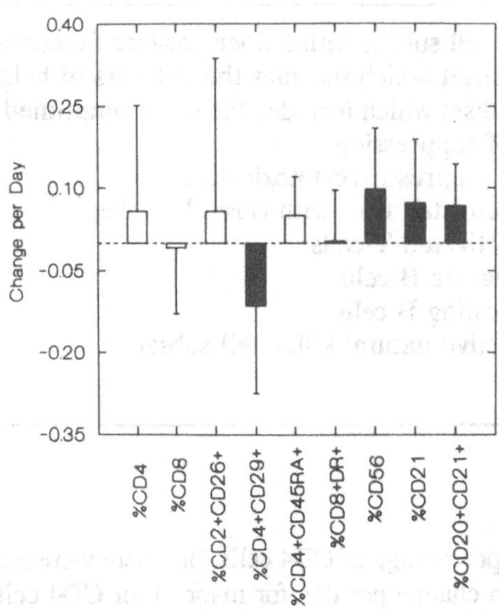

Fig. 1. **Change per day in beta coefficients (median ± 75th percentile) for measurements of lymphocyte surface markers for the in-patients undergoing detoxification. Filled bars represent significant change ($p<.05$).**

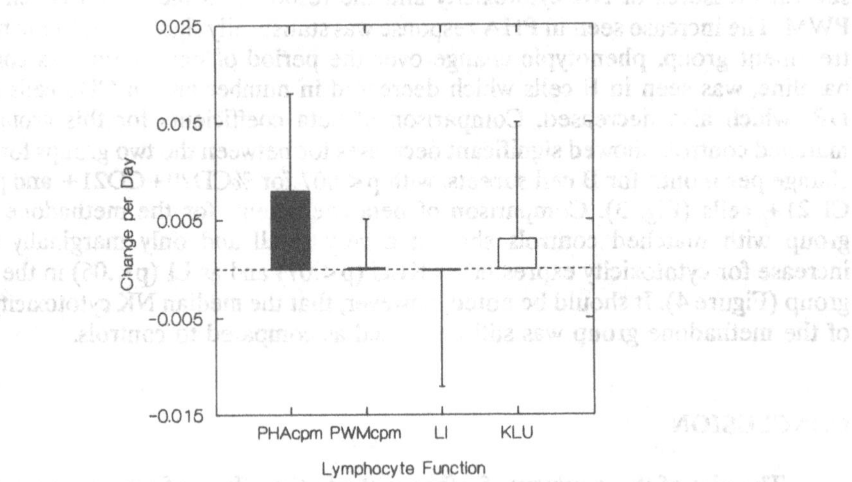

Fig. 2. **Change per day in beta coefficients (median ± 75th percentile) for measurements of lymphocyte function for the inpatients undergoing detoxification. Change in cell function was estimated on $\log_{10}$ transformed measures. Filled bars represent significant change ($p<.05$).**

of CD4, activation markers and suppressed elevations in CD4+CD29+, in CD8 and activated CD8, CD8+DR+ and activated total T lymphocytes, CD2+CD26+.

Lymphocyte function was suppressed in the methadone group, with poor response to PHA and PWM and low NK cytotoxicity (1). The results obtained on longitudinal follow-up showed a normalization in some aspects, namely CD8 subset and NK activity, in the methadone group. However, there was a loss of B cells, and no change in CD4 parameters nor in response to mitogens, suggesting continued immune impairment over the period of observation, which was a minimum of 12 months. The results of this study support concerns which have been raised regarding the possible consequences of methadone-mediated immunologic changes on HIV-1 susceptibility, in IVDUs, who are strongly at risk for retrovirus exposure. They suggest that inpatient detoxification is a more immunologically neutral approach to treatment of IVDU. The results of Novick, et al., (6) suggest that in patients maintained for very long term periods (over 10 on methadone, that complete immunologic normalization can occur. Obviously these are complex relationships. There is need for more methodologically controlled studies to assess the effect of the contributions of various co-factors to the interaction, or lack of interaction with immunologic status, of strategies for treatment of drug abusers.

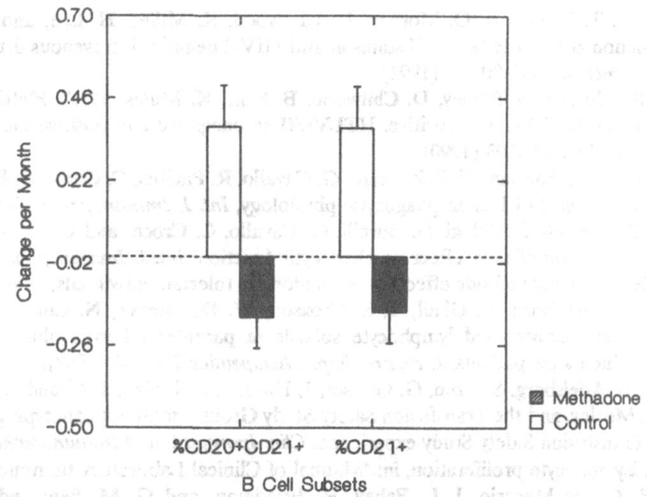

Fig. 3. **Change per month (median ± 75th percentile) in B cell subsets of IVDUs in methadone treatment as compared to controls.**

ACKNOWLEDGMENTS

This research was funded by the National Institute of Mental Health through a center award to the Center for the Biopsychosocial Study of AIDS (P50 MH42455).

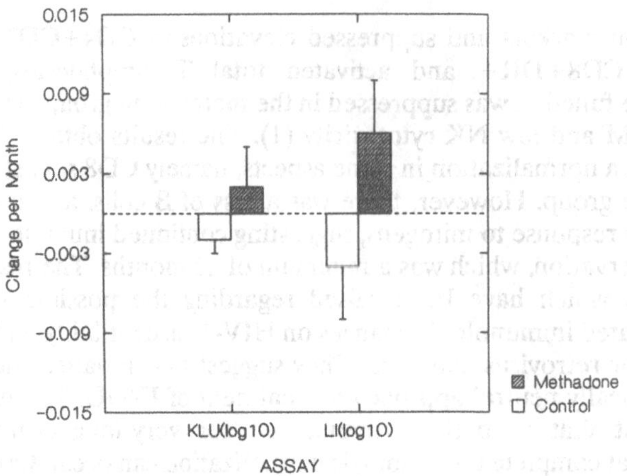

Fig. 4. Change per month (median ± 75th percentile) in NR cell cytotoxicity response of IVDUs in methadone treatment as compared to controls.

REFERENCES

1. N. G., Klimas, N. T. Blaney, R. O. Morgan, D. Chitwood, K. Milles, H. Lee, and M. A. Fletcher, Immune function and anti-HTLV-I/II status in anti-HIV-1 negative intravenous drug users receiving methadone, *Amer. J. Med.* 90:163 (1991).
2. N. G Klimas, R. Morgan, N. Blaney, D. Chitwood, B. Page, K. Milles, M. A. Fletcher, Alcohol and immune function in HIV-1 seropositive, HTLVI/II seronegative and positive men on methadone, *Prog. Clin. Biol. Res.* 325:103 (1990).
3. E. Tubaro, U. Avico, C. Santiangeli, P. Zuccaro, G. Cavallo, R. Pacifici, C. Croce, G. Borelli, Morphine and methadone impact of human phagocytic physiology, *Int. J. Immunopharm.* 7:865 (1985).
4. E. Tubaro, C. Santiangeli, L. Belogi, G. Borelli, G. Cavallo, C. Croce, and U. Avico, Methadone vs. morphine: comparison of their effect on phagocytic function, *Int. J. Immunopharm.* 9:79 (1987).
5. M. J. Kreek, Medical safety and side effects of methadone in tolerant individuals, *JAMA* 223:665 (1973).
6. D. M. Novick, M. Ochshorn, V. Ghall, T. S. Croxson, W. D. Mercer, N. Chiorazzi, M. J. Kreek, Natural killer cell activity and lymphocyte subsets in parenteral heroin abusers and long-term nethadone maintenance patients, *J. Pharm. Exp. Therapeutics* 250:606 (1989).
7. M. A. Fletcher, B. Adelsberg, S. Azen, G. Gjerset, J. Hassett, J. Kaplan, J. Niland, T. Odom-Maryon, J. Parker, J. Mosley, and the Transfusion Safety Study Group, Immunophenotyping in a multicenter study: The Transfusion Safety Study experience, *Clin. Immunol. and Immunopathol.* 52:38 (1989).
8. M. A Fletcher, Lymphocyte proliferation, *in*: "Manual of Clinical Laboratory Immunology", 4th ed., N. R. Rose, E. C. De Macario, J. L. Fahey, H. Friedman, and G. M. Penn, eds., *Am. Soc. for Microbiol.*, Wash. DC, pp. 213-219, 1992.
9. M. A. Fletcher, G. A. Baron, M. A. Ashman, N. G. Klimas, Use of whole blood methods in assessment of immune parameters in immunodeficiency syndromes, *Clin. Diag. Immunol.* 5:69 (1987).
10. G. A. Baron, N. G. Klimas, M. A. Fischel and M. A. Fletcher, Decreased natural cell-mediated cytotoxicity per effector cell in acquired immunodeficiency syndrome, *Diag. Immunol.* 3:197 (1985).

PSYCHOSOCIAL STRESS AND NK CELLS AMONG MEMBERS OF A COMMUNAL SETTLEMENT

M. Schlesinger[1,2], Y. Yodfat[3], R. Rabinowitz[1,2], S. Bronner[3] and J.D. Kark[4]

[1]The Hubert H. Humphrey Center for Experimental Medicine and Cancer Research, [2]The Paul Ehrlich Center for Study of WBC, [3]The Department of Family Medicine, and [4]The Department of Social Medicine, The Hebrew University-Hadassah Medical School and the Hadassah Medical Organization, Jerusalem, Israel

ABSTRACT

The aim of the present study was to assess the effect of daily psychosocial stress on the human immune system. We tested 38 couples living in a communal settlement (kibbutz) under similar economic and social conditions, sharing similar housing, nutrition and health care. They were tested repeatedly over a two year period for a number of psychosocial parameters including demoralization, social support, family cohesion, adaptational hardiness and hostility. In parallel, the natural killer "NK" cell system was analysed for distinctive markers and for cytotoxic activity. The proportion of CD16^{+} lymphocytes was found to correlate with cytotoxic NK activity in both men and women. In contrast, the proportion of CD57+ cells correlated with that of CD16+ cells only in women while in men only the CD57+CD8-lymphocyte subset correlated with CD16+ cells. For each individual tested, the values of NK activity and NK markers obtained in tests carried out more than a year apart showed a striking correlation. In males, NK cytotoxicity correlated with hostility but was negatively correlated with family cohesion, adaptability and hardiness. The level of CD16+ and CD57+ cells correlated positively with demoralization in males only. Changes in the level of NK activity and in the level of CD16+ cells occurring in husbands during the observation period correlated positively with changes in demoralization and negatively with changes in family cohesion and adaptability. The results indicate that daily psycholological stress and low family function may enhance the NK system, and that this response may differ between the sexes.

INTRODUCTION

The immune system is controlled by a complex network of regulatory mechanisms which include neurological and psychological factors (1-10). There is ample evidence that psychological stress affects the immune response (1-10) and increases the susceptibility to infection (11). The activity of natural killer cells was found to be impaired following examination (5), bereavement (6), or other stressful life events and hassles (8, 9).

Drugs of Abuse, Immunity, and AIDS, Edited by
H. Friedman *et al.*, Plenum Press, New York, 1993

The aim of the present study was to assess over an extended period the effect of psychosocial stress among individuals with minimal socioeconomic differences. The effect of psychosocial stress on the immune system was studied among married couples living in a kibbutz (communal settlement). The choice of kibbutz residents ensured a relative uniformity of factors that may affect the immune system. They share similar socioeconomic conditions, consume a similar diet, dwell in similar housing, and are cared by the same health care system. The effect of psychosocial stress was studied in Kibbutz residents over a one and a half year period and correlated with the level of cytotoxic NK activity and with NK cell phenotypic markers. Preliminary results of the first phase of the study were presented previously (12).

MATERIALS AND METHODS

Subjects Tested

Forty-six healthy, married couples with children, residing for at least ten years in a Kibbutz, were studied. Repeated analysis was carried out on 38 couples. The mean age of the males was 45.8 years while that of the females was 44.1 years.

All participants were asked to report on any infectious symptoms, chronic medication, smoking, alcohol and coffee consumption. Psychosocial variables were assessed by various questionnaires. These included a validated new stressful life event scale for kibbutz members (13), which is a modification and adaptation of Holmes and Rahe's list of life events (14). Other questionnaires assessed the demoralization score (which measures psychological distress), social support systems (measured by a newly validated questionnaire) (15), and hostility (16). Family function was determined using the validated Hebrew version of FACES III of Olson et al., (17). This questionnaire assesses two aspects of family function-cohesion and adaptability. An additional test was used for assessment of family hardiness (18).

Peripheral Blood Lymphocytes (PBL)

Venous blood was collected in the clinic of the kibbutz with preservative-free heparin. The blood samples were taken in the morning (between 7:30 and 8:30) from 6 to 8 individuals (i.e., from 3 to 4 couples), and reached the laboratory within one hour after venipuncture. Mononuclear cells were isolated by Ficoll-Hypaque barrier centrifugation. The cells in the interface were collected, washed twice in normal saline, and resuspended in RPMI-1640 medium supplemented with 10% heat inactivated fetal calf serum (FCS).

NK Assay

The procedure used for the assay of NK-activity was described previously in detail (12). K562 cells suspended fn normal saline at a concentration of 10^6 cells/ml were labeled for 1 hr at 37°C with 150-200 uCi ^{51}Cr (sodium chromate, Nuclear Research Center, Beer Sheva, Israel). The labeled cells were suspended in RPMI-1640 medium, supplemented with 10% heat inactivated FCS. NK cytotoxic assays were performed at effector to target ratios varying from 50:1 to 6:1. Effector cells suspended in 50 µl RPMI-1640 supplemented with 10% FCS were introduced in triplicates into microplate wells. To each well was then added 25 µl of target cell suspension, containing 5 x 10^3 ^{51}Cr-labeled K562 cells. Variation of effector to target cell ratio was achieved by varying the number of effector cells suspended in 50 µl medium, from 2.5 x 10^5 to 0.3 x 10^3. In each assay, wells containing labeled target cells alone, without effector cells, were kept as controls to determine the spontaneous ^{51}Cr release. Microplates were incubated for 4 hr at 37°C in incubators containing an atmosphere of 5% CO_2. At the end of the incubation the microplates were centrifuged at 1000 r.p.m. and aliquots of the supernatant fluids of each well were collected. The radioactivity of the supernatant fluids was determined in a gamma counter (Packard, Auto-Gamma Spectrometer). The percent specific ^{51}Cr release was calculated as follows:

$$\frac{\text{cpm experimental release - cpm spontaneous release}}{\text{cpm total release - cpm spontaneous release}} \times 100$$

The spontaneous release ranged from 8-12% of the total radioactivity.

Monoclonal Antibodies

The Leu-7 (HNK-1, CD 57) and Leu- llb (CD 16) monoclonal antibodies, reacting with human NK- cells, were purchased from Becton Dickinson (Mountain View, CA). FITC-labeled goat anti-mouse immunoglobulin was purchased from Bio-Yeda (Rehovot, Israel). The T8 (CD8) and T4 (CD4) monoclonal antibodies, purchased from Coulter Immunology, Hialeah, FL were used in the second phase of the study. In double labeling experiments phycoerythrin-conjugated T8 (CD8, Coulter Immunology) and fluorescein isocyanate-conjugated Leu-7 (CD57), purchased from Becton-Dickinson, Mountain View, CA., were used.

Immunofluorescent Assays

For indirect immunofluorescent assays, monoclonal antibodies at a volume of 0.01 ml were added to 0.05 ml of a suspension of PBL at a concentration of 10^7 cells/ml. After 45 min. incubation on ice, the cells were washed twice with cold RPMI-1640 medium. FITC-goat anti-mouse immunoglobulin, diluted 1:30 in phosphate buffered saline, was added at a volume of 0.1 ml to the cell sediments. The mixture was shaken and incubated for another 45 min. on ice, in the dark. The cells were again washed twice with cold RPMI-1640 medium, and resuspended in 1 ml 1% paraformaldehyde in normal saline, pH 7.0. The proportion of fluorescent lymphocytes was determined by microfluorometry using a fluorescence activated cell sorter (FACS scan, Becton-Dickinson).

For direct immunofluorescent assays and two-color flow cytometry, 10 µl of each of the two fluorescent monoclonal antibodies (PE - T8 and FITC - Leu-7) MoAbs were added to 50 µl cell suspension. The mixture of lymphocyte suspension and MoAbs was kept for 30 min at room temperature and was then centrifuged at 200 x g for 5 min. The pellet was washed twice with phosphate-buffered saline (PBS) containing 0.1% NaN3 and 0.1% bovine serum albumin. Finally, the cells in the washed pellet were resuspended in 1% paraformaldehyde and kept at 4°C until they were analyzed by flow cytometry.

Acquisition and analysis were carried out in a FACScan flow cytometer (Becton-Dickinson, Mountain View, CA) using the Consort 30 program. For each test, ten thousand cells were acquired. The lymphocyte population was gated according to their typical forward light scatter and right-angle light scatter. The immunofluorescent staining was determined by two-color flow cytometry, using the contour staining program of Consort 30.

RESULTS

1. Repeated assays of NK cell markers and of Psychological variables. A number of psychological tests were carried out repeatedly among the individuals in the study. There was a significant correlation between the results of the psychological tests administered repeatedly in the same individuals a year or more apart. Pearson's correlation coeficients for repeated tests were as follows: demoralization 0.66, family cohesion 0.48, family adaptation 0.46, $p < 0.05$ for all three tests. A similar overall stability was noted in repeated assays for cytotoxic NK activity and NK markers. Although in some individuals different results were obtained in tests performed after a year's interval, in most individuals both the cytotoxic NK activity and the proportion of cells expressing NK markers proved remarkably stable. The correlation coefficient for assays of cytotoxicity, expressed in lytic units, repeated in the same individuals a year or more apart, was $r = 0.47$, $p < 0.0005$. Similarly, the correlation between repeated determinations of the proportion of CD16+ cells (Leull+ cells) carried out a year or more apart, was $r=0.62$, $p<0.0005$, while that for repeated values of CD57+ cells (Leu-7+) cells was $r= 0.57$, $p < 0.0005$.

2. Sex differences in the correlation between CD16+ and CD57+ PBL. The mean of the proportion of PBL expressing various cell surface markers, including NK associated markers, was similar in men and women. Table 1 shows the correlation between various immunological parameters tested. In both men and women there was a significant correlation between cytotoxic NK activity and the proportion of CD16+ PBL, but not of CD57+ PBL. A striking sex difference became apparent in the correlation between the expression of CD16 and CD57, two markers characteristic for human NK cells. In women there was a significant correlation between the proportion of CD16+ and that of CD57+ PBL, while no such correlation could be detected in men. This striking sex difference was observed repeatedly in assays performed over a year apart. The CD57+ cell population consists of two phenotypically distinct subsets, that of CD57+CD8+ double positive cells, which encompass both NK and T cells, and that of CD57+CD8- single positive cells, which consist almost exclusively of NK cells. In the second phase of the study, the proportion of CD16+ PBL was correlated with the two subsets of CD57+ PBL. In women, a nonsignificant positive correlation was found between the proportion of CD57+CD8+ PBL and that of CD16+ PBL ($r=0.23$, $p>0.05$). On the other hand, there was a highly significant correlation between the proportion of CD57+CD8- PBL and that of CD16+ PBL ($r= 0.62$, $p< 0.0005$). As noted above, in men there was no correlation between the proportion of the entire population of CD57+ cells and that of CD16+ cells. Upon dissection of the CD57+ population into the CD57+CD8- and the CD57+CD8+ subsets striking differences could now be detected in their correlation with CD16+ cells. In men, the CD57+ CD8+ cell subset showed a negative correlation with the population of CD16+ cells $r= (-0.27, p<0.05)$. In contrast, a significant positive correlation could now be detected between the proportion of CD57+CD8- PBL and that of CD16+ PBL ($r=0.46$, $p<0.005$). Thus, the striking difference between men and women in the correlation between CD57+ and CD16+ cells could be attributed in its entirety to a difference in the correlation between CD16+ NK cells and the CD57+CD8+ cell subset in the two sexes.

3. Correlation between Immunological and Psychological Parameters. Two approaches were used to correlate between immunological and psychological parameters.

Table 1. Correlation between immunological parameters

		CD16	CD57	CD4	CD8
Men	NK activity	0.53*	-0.23	-0.10	0.13
	CD16		0.01	0.02	-0.04
	CD57			-0.25	0.39*
	CD4				0.53*
Women	NK activity	0.58*	0.07	-0.16	0.04
	CD16		0.45*	-0.23	0.12
	CD57			-0.50	0.51*
	CD4				-0.62*

* $p < 0.05$

In one approach, changes in the various immunological parameters and in psychological characteristics observed in repeated tests in the same individuals were correlated. This approach attempts to determine whether changes in any psychological test during the period of observation were accompanied by parallel changes in any of the immune parameters. A significant positive correlation was found in husbands between changes in demoralization and the proportion of CD16+ lymphocytes ($r = 0.42$, $p < 0.05$). No such correlation was seen among women in the study. In both sexes changes in demoralization showed a nonsignificant correlation with cytotoxic NK activity. Changes in family cohesion showed a significant negative correlation with the proportion of CD16+ lymphocytes in women ($r = -0.34$, $p < 0.05$). Although not significant, the same inverse correlation was also found in husbands ($r = -0.33$). In a second approach various immunological parameters were correlated with psychosocial assays in individuals tested during the second phase of the study. Thus, rather than determining whether various psychological and immunological characteristics changed in parallel over time, this approach assessed whether differences in one parameter among the individuals tested are correlated with differences in another parameter. In men, a number of striking correlations between immunological and psychological parameters were noted (Table 2). Demoralization showed a significant correlation with the proportion of either CD16+ or CD57+ PBL, and a nonsignificant correlation with the proportion of CD8+PBL. A nonsignificant correlation was also noted between demoralization and cytotoxic NK activity. Hostility in men showed a positive correlation with NK activity and with the proportion of CD8+ PBL. Family cohesion was inversely correlated in men with both NK activity and the proportion of CD16+ PBL. Among men, family adaptation was inversely correlated with cytotoxic NK activity and with the proportion of CD8+PBL. Similarly, family hardiness was inversely correlated with NK activity, and with the proportion of CD16+ and CD8+ cells.

Table 2. Correlation between psychosocial and immunological parameters in man

Immunological parameter	Psychosocial parameter				
	Demoralization	Family cohesion	Family adaptability	Hostility (MMPI)	Family hardiness
NK activity	0.27	-0.50*	-0.45*	0.41*	-0.37*
CD16+ (Leull+)	0.55*	-0.45*	0.12	0.12	-0.31*
CD57+ (Leu 7+)	0.33*	0.03	0.07	-0.13	-0.17
CD8+	0.21	-0.03	-0.45*	0.32*	-0.34*
CD4+	0.21	0.11	0.11	-0.29*	0.31*
CD4/CD8 Ratio	-0.15	0.03	0.34*	-O.25*	0.32*

* $p < 0.05$

In women, a significant negative correlation was seen between family adaptability and the proportion of CD8+ PBL (Table 3). Unlike in men, there was no significant correlation between various other psychological immunological parameters among women.

Table 3. Correlation between psychosocial and immunological parameters in women

Immunological parameter	Psychosocial parameter				
	Demoralization	Family cohesion	Family adaptability	Hostility (MMPI)	Family hardiness
NK activity	0.16	-0.06	-0.23	0.23	-0.07
CD16+(Leull+)	0.27	-0.11	0.02	0.18	-0.23
CD57+(Leu 7+)	0.06	0.07	0.07	0.01	-0.10
CD8+	-0.02	-0.03	-0.30*	0.01	-0.02
CD4+	-0.07	0.03	0.05	-0.01	0.04
CD4/CD8 Ratio	-0.03	0.08	0.31*	0.06	0.08

* $p < 0.05$

DISCUSSION

The results of the present study reflect the complexity of the interactions between psycosocial factors and the immune system. On the one hand various NK associated traits showed a remarkable stability over a prolonged period of time. On the other hand, some psychological factors were found to correlate with the level of NK activity and with the number of PBL expressing cell surface markers characteristic for NK cells.

The relative stability of the various NK associated traits noted in the present study is in agreement with results of previous studies in which there was a strong correlation between repeated measures of NK cytotoxicity (8, 9, 19). Stable individual differences in NK cytotoxicity were noted by Aoki et al., (20). The stability of NK cell attributes may indicate that the level of NK cells may be determined by a stable physiological characteristic of each individual and by the individual's psychological trait and disposition. Numerous tests indicate, however, that various psychological factors may affect cytotoxic NK activity. These factors include depression (6), anxiety (8, 12), life changes, hassles, and stressful events (4, 5, 8, 9). We have previously noted that individuals in the present study who had a low coping ability had impaired NK activity (7, 12), and this was particularly striking for those diagnosed as having anxiety (12).

In the present study, demoralization in men was found to be correlated with an increased proportion of CDl6+ and CD57+ NK cells. Similarly, enhancement, rather than impairment, of NK activity was noted among healthy chartered accountants as compared with controls during the peak stressful periods of the tax season (21). Possibly chronic stress, may increase immune responsiveness.

Sex differences were noted in a number of parameters of NK cells. Thus, only in women was there a correlation between the level of CD16+ and CD57+ PBL. This sex difference could be traced to a marked difference in the correlation between the level of CD57+CD8+ and that of CDl6+ PBL. A marked difference was also noted in the correlation of NK cells to various psychological parameters. Further studies will be required to determine to what extent these differences are controlled by hormonal or psychological differences between men and women.

In men a striking inverse correlation was noted between parameters of family function and the NK system. Thus, the cytotoxic NK activity was increased with lower family cohesion, adaptability and hardiness. In parallel, the number of CDl6+ NK cells was inversely correlated in men with family cohesion and hardiness. In women, changes in values of family cohesion were inversely correlatad with changes in the proportion of CDl6+ PBL observed in repeated tests. In this respect it is of interest that studies on the role of family function in the course of chronic illness indicate that, contrary to expectations, patients in "strong" families are more vulnerable and their survival is shorter (22). In patients with end-stage renal disease treated by center-based hemodialysis strong family bonds predicted early death rather than prolonged survival. Reiss et al., (22) discussed the various deletorious psychological consequences of strong families that could account for the "weakness of strong bonds". While the population tested in the present study consisted of healthy individuals,it is tempting to suggest that strong family ties may exert an adverse effect on the NK system.

ACKNOWLEDGEMENTS

The expert technical assistance of Yael Keren-Zur, Rivka Hadar, and Chaviva Wiener are gratefully acknowledged. This study was supported in part by grants from the Goldhirsch Foundation and from Ministry of Science and Technology of Niedersachsen, FRG.

REFERENCES

1. B. S. Rabin, S. Cohen, R. Ganguli, D. T. Lysle, and J. E. Cunnick, Bidirectional interaction between the central nervous system and the immune system, *Crit. Rev. Immunol.* 9:279 (1989).
2. Y. Yodfat, and M. Schlesinger, Psychosocial factors and cell-mediated immunity, *Clin. Immunol. Newsletter* 10:157 (1988).
3. G. F. Solomon, Psychoneuroimmunology: interactions between central nervous system and immune system, *J. Neurosci. Res.* 18:1 (1987).
4. E. S. Locke, L. Kraus, J. Leserman, et al., Life change stress, psychiatric symptoms, and natural killer cell activity, *Psychosomatic Med.* 46:441 (1984).
5. J. K. Kiecolt-Glaser, R. Glaser, E. C. Strain, et al., Modulation of cellular immunity in medical students, *J. Behavioral Med.* 9:5 (1986).
6. M. Irwin, M. Daniels, T. L. Smith, E. Bloom, and H. Wiener, Impaired natural killer cell activity during bereavement, *Brain, Behavior, and Immunity* 1:98 (1987).
7. M. Schlesinger, and Y. Yodfat, Effect of psychosocial stress on natural killer cell activity, *Cancer Detection and Prevention* 12:9 (1988).
8. S. M. Levy, R. B. Herberman, A. Simons, T. Whiteside, J. Lee, R. McDonald, and M. Beadle, Persistently low natural killer cell activity in normal adults: Immunological, hormonal and mood correlates, *Natural Immunity and Cell Growth Regulation* 8:173 (1989).
9. R. B. Moss, H. B. Moss, and R. Peterson, Microstress, mood, and natural killer cell activity, *Psychosomatics* 30:279 (1989).
10. A. O'Leary, Stress, emotion, and human immune function, *Psychological Bull.* 108:363 (1990).
11. S. Cohen, D. A. J. Tyrrell, and A. P. Smith, Psychological stress and susceptibility to the common cold, *New Engl. J. Med.* 325:606 (1991).
12. M. Schlesinger, and Y. Yodfat, The impact of stressful life events on natural killer cells, *Stress Med.* 7:53 (1991).
13. Y. Yodfat, P. Shwartzman, V. Soskolne, and S. Bronner, Life events readjustment scale in a kibbutz, *Israel. J. Med.* (in Press) (1992).
14. T. H. Holmes, and R.H. Rahe, The social readjustment rating scale, *J. Psychosom. Res.* 11:213 (1967).
15. P. B. Dorenwend, B. S. Dorenwend, I. Levav, and P. Shrout, The psychiatric epidemiology research interview (in Hebrew), *Harefuah* 100:274 (1981).
16. W. Cook, and D. Medley, Proposed hostility pharisaic virtue scales for MMPI, *J. Appl. Psychol.*, 38:414 (1954).
17. D. H. Olson, J. Portner, and Y. Lavee, FACES III, Department of Family Social Science, University of Minnesota, St. Paul 1985.
18. I. Hamilton, H. I. McCubbin, and A. I. Thompson, Family assessment inventories for research and practice, University of Wisconsin, Madison, pp. 125-130 (1987).
19. T. L. Whiteside, and R. B. Herberman, The role of natural killer cells in human disease, *Clin. Immunol. Immunopathol.* 53:1 (1989).
20. R. Aoki, T. Usuda, H. Miyakoshi, K. Tamura, and R. B.Herberman, Low NK syndrome: Clinical and immunologic features, *Natural Immunity and Cell Growth Regulation* 6:116 (1987).
21. B. Dorian, P. Garfinkel, E. Keystone, et al., Occupational stress and immunity (Abstract) *Psychosom. Med.* 47:77 (1985).
22. D. Reiss, S. Gonzalez, and N. Kramer, Family process, chronic illness, and death, On the weakness of strong bonds, *Arch Gen. Psychiatry* 43:795 (1986).

MULTIPLE PATHOGENS MAY INDUCE GROWTH FACTOR CASCADE RESULTING IN KS

J. G. Sinkovics, J. E. Szakacs, and F. Gyorkey

Cancer Inst., St. Joseph's Hospital; and Depts. of Med. & Med. Microbiol., Univ. of S. Florida College of Med., Tampa, FL; H. Lee Moffitt Cancer Ctr. and Dept. of Pathol., University of S. Florida College of Med., Tampa, FL; Veterans Adm. Med. Ctr. and Depts. of Pathol. and Virol., Baylor College of Med., Houston, TX

INTRODUCTION

In this brief review a list of potential pathogens is provided that are associated with Kaposi's sarcoma (KS) and may contribute to the initiation and/or maintenance of growth of KS cells. For the end result, which is the characteristic appearance and grouping of KS cells, the same growth factors are needed in a set sequence and combination. However, the pathogens inducing these growth factors may be different. Induction of the same growth factors by diverse pathogens can result in the generation of endothelial cell growth and transformation in sequence recognized as various subtypes of KS. Indeed there has to be an initiator of growth factor release from CD4 lymphocytes other than HIV in classical (Mediterranean) KS. On the other hand, HIV infection alone is not enough to induce KS: patients with hemophilia acquiring HIV infection through blood products die with AIDS but without developing KS.

A scenario for the regression of KS lesions can be envisioned as this phenomenon may proceed along several lines: 1. differentiation from elongated back to epithelioid phenotype of endothelial cells; 2. cytotoxicity of KS cell-specific T lymphocytes as this population expands under the effect of IL-2 when KS cells switch off the production of TGFß; and 3. TNFα and/or ß (lymphotoxin) delivering signals accepted by KS as those inductory to programmed cell death (apoptosis).

POTENTIAL AND SUSPECTED PATHOGENS

Cytomegalovirus (CMV)

This widely spread virus can induce the expression of FcR in fibroblasts and macrophages (1). HIV-antibody complexes captured by FcR enter CMV-infected macrophages and initiate HIV replication but without cell death. These macrophages harbor and spread HIV and serve as sources of monokines that may influence neighboring cells. Another effect of CMV is induction of topoisomerase II overexpression (2).

Herpesviruses accept inserted genes from other viruses. Examples are human adenovirus-associated virus type 2 *rep* gene in human herpes virus type 6 (3) or reticuloendotheliosis retrovirus genomic insertion in Marek's herpesvirus (4). Certain human CMV isolates contain sequences related to avian retroviral oncogene v-*myc* (5), but no systematic study exists on CMV isolates from KS if these isolates harbor inserted retroviral genomic sequences.

The association of CMV with KS is common and very well documented as mature virions, unenveloped viral nucleocapsids, viral antigens, viral genomic DNA and CMV-RNA are frequently present in KS lesions and patients with KS are strongly seropositive for CMV (6-9). The association of CMV with AIDS-KS is especially conspicuous since these patients commonly have CMV viremia (10). Yet it is not clear if CMV actually transforms endothelial cells into KS cells or if it induces growth factors in leukocytes, macrophages and endothelial cells that lead to cellular transformations characteristic of KS. No systematic study exists in which growth factors induced by CMV were analyzed. In African patients with endemic HIV-KS, electron microscopy, *in situ* hybridization and Southern blot hybridization all failed to detect CMV DNA (11), suggesting that KS in these patients can develop without the presence of CMV.

Despite its most intimate contact with KS cells in AIDS (9), CMV can not at the present time be considered as the causative agent of KS, but it appears to remain one of its strongest, but not essential, contributors.

Hepatitis B (HBV)

In an 80-year-old man with KS, HBV episomal (not integrated) DNA was detected in his tumor and skin cells while he was seronegative for HBV (12). This virus is commonly associated with AIDS but no systematic search for its genome in AIDS-KS cells has as yet been made.

Papovavirus BK

DNA genomic fragments of this virus were detected in 4 of 13 endemic African KS tissues and in none of 7 classical KS tissues. The early region of the BK genome can recombine with c-H-*ras*. The gene product protein of the recombinant gene was sarcomagenic in hamsters (13). Patients with AIDS are known to harbor this papovavirus and to succumb to multifocal leukoencephalopathy. No systematic study exists to show if recombinants of BK early region gene with c-H-*ras* were formed as a contributory factor to certain cases of Kaposi's sarcomagenesis.

Human Papillomavirus (HPV)

With the sensitive polymerase chain reaction, the E6 region of the HPV-16 genome could be readily detected in AIDS-KS cells (14). HPV DNA sequences were detected in 11 of 69 skin lesions of KS of patients with AIDS; in 3 of 11 KS lesions from HIV$^-$ homosexual men; and in 5 of 17 KS lesions of the HIV$^-$ classic disease. Thus, the incidence does not prove an essential etiologic role of HPV-16 in KS, but it may suggest that this virus has a contributory role in the generation of these lesions.

Retroviral Particles

Budding type C retroviral particles were seen in AIDS-KS cells (15), but such particles also appeared budding from normal vascular endothelial cells of the same patients. These retroviral particles could not be identified as HIV by morphological criteria. Preliminary *in situ* hybridization studies also failed to identify them as HIV-1 or HTLV-1.

In a cluster of Greek patients with KS, no evidence for HIV infection and for immunosuppression was found. The lesions were formed by lymphatic epithelial cells and dense infiltrates of CD4 T lymphocytes. KS cells contained cytoplasmic tubuloreticular structures (*vide infra*) and displayed budding retroviral particles (16). These patients circulated no antibodies for HIV-1 and 2 or HTLV-1. Their KS cells expressed ras p21 oncoprotein and c-*myc* and c-*erb*B2 oncogenes (17). These rare findings have not as yet been duplicated in patients with classical or endemic HIV^- KS.

Cytoplasmic Tubuloreticular Structures (TRS)

When first found in abundance in systemic lupus erythematosus, these structures were likened to unenveloped ribonucleoprotein strands of paramyxo- or retroviruses (18). Later, similar structures were found in cells of reticuloendotheliosis (hairy cell leukemia) (19) and in AIDS-KS cells (20). Similar structures can be induced by exposure to interferon-α and ß but not by γ in lymphocytes (21). Studies in which these structures would have been extracted from the cells, concentrated by centrifugation and then examined histochemically and for biological activity do not exist.

Tat

Male transgenic mice carrying HIV *tat* gene grow vascular tumors resembling those of human KS (22). The HIV *tat* gene product protein Tat is a biologically highly active polypeptide (23) which is mitogenic to vascular endothelial cells (24) and may serve as one of the initiator growth factors for AIDS-KS cells (*vide infra*).

Bacterial Angiomatosis

Rickettsial agents closely related to Rochalimaea quintana induce proliferative vascular lesions in the skin and viscera (hepatosplenic) of immunodeficient patients, including those with AIDS (25). These lesions may occur independently and concurrently with KS; they appear to be similar to, but distinguishable from, early KS lesions (26).

Mycobacteria

M. avium-intracellulare is commonly present in AIDS-KS lesions (27). This pathogen induces the release of IL-6 from human monocytes and large granular lymphocytes (28). IL-6 is a growth factor for KS cells (*vide infra*).

Mycoplasma

An AIDS-associated mycoplasma strain (*Mycoplasma fermentans seu incognitus*) is pathogenic in certain monkeys and occasionally in humans even without explicit immunosuppression (29). This agent enhances the cytocidal effect of HIV-1 on CD4 lymphocytes (30) and contributes to apoptotic death of these cells (see L. Montagnier *et al.* in this volume). Its contribution to the growth or regression of KS lesions is unknown.

GROWTH FACTORS (GF)

GF for KS cells derive from three major sources

1. from retrovirally infected CD4 lymphocytes (in AIDS-KS); or from immunologically overstimulated lymphocytes (in endemic African KS); or from immunosuppressed T cells (in iatrogenic KS of organ transplant recipients). Experimental proof exists only for GF secreted by retrovirally infected CD4 lymphocytes (31, 32).

2. KS cells themselves produce a number of GF that promote short term (bFGF, GM-CSF, IL-1ß, PDGF, TGFß) (31, 33) and sustained growth. The class of latter GF includes IL-6 (34) and KS bFGF (35, 36). Overexpression of a member of the *int-hst* gene family is responsible for the production of KS bFGF which works as a mitogen for endothelial cells (35). K-*fgf-hst* transferred by retroviral vector induced abundant capillary proliferation and angioma formation (37). Since AIDS-KS cells also express the gene for muscle α-actin, these cells function at the level of precursor vascular endothelial and/or smooth muscle cells (38).

It now appears that leukemia inhibitory factor or oncostatin M (OM) is the initiator GF that is produced by both retrovirally infected T lymphocytes and KS cells themselves (32, 39). OM is an initiator of IL-6 production and it uses the signal transducing subunit of the IL-6 receptor gp130 (40).

3. Monocytes-macrophages infiltrating KS lesions are potential sources of those GF that interact with endothelial cells: IL-1, TNFα and others (41). HIV replication in already infected monocytes-macrophages is suppressed by retinoic acid and TGFß, except when these cells are pretreated with retinoic acid or TGFß and infected with HIV thereafter; in this latter case, HIV replication is enhanced by the GF (42, 43).

INHIBITORS

Substances are known that suppress growth of normal and transformed endothelial cells. Corticosteroids and their derivatives (44); heparin and its analogues, especially pentosan polysulfate (45) and protamines; penicillamine and depletion of copper (46); suramine (46); platelet factor 4 (47); interferons α and ß (44); polysaccharide peptidoglycans (especially those from *Arthrobacter* strain AT-25) (47); mycelial protein-bound polysaccharides (especially those of *Coriolus versicolor*) (48); and the fumagillin antibiotics (46) all are potent inhibitors of normal and tumoral angiogenesis. This effect on the targeted endothelial cell is achieved at multiple levels: protooncogene-oncogene deactivation (49); GF suppression; differentiation induction; induction of programmed cell death (apoptosis) (50); and mobilization of cell-mediated immunity against transformed target cells.

REGRESSION OF KS

The mechanism of growth of this tumor is now understood to a great extent. It is not known how it regresses. Scenarios may be construed to challenge the investigators for proof or disproof. These lesions consist of cells undergoing sequential transformation. Pathologists do not recognize attributes of malignancy in early lesions of KS. Quite well differentiated lesions may grow in immunosuppressed patients with AIDS, whereas undifferentiated lesions grow in immunocompetent patients with classical KS (51). The early lesion may reverse by re-differentiation. Interferons α may

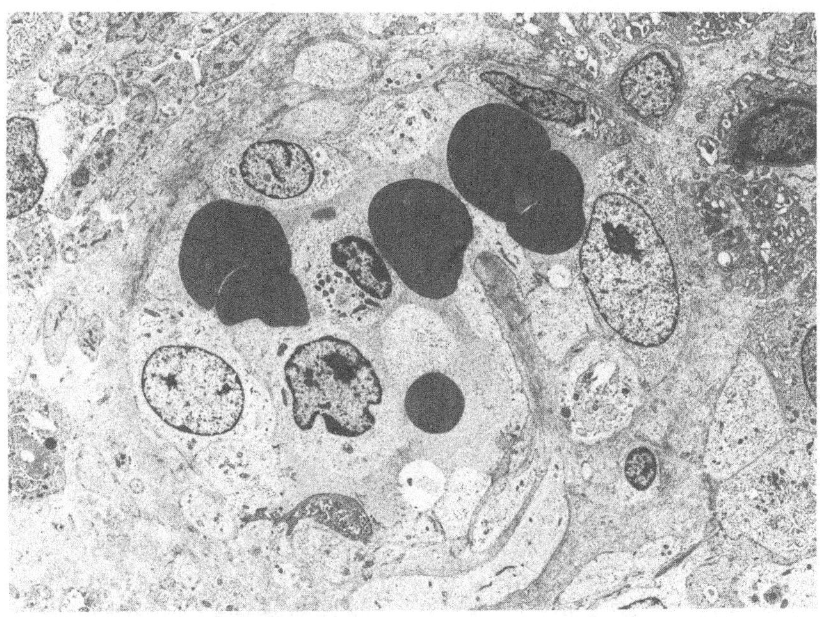

Fig. 1. KS cells undergoing apoptosis with condensation of chromatin at the periphery of nuclei in a 75 yr old man with classical KS showing fusiform sarcomatous growth pattern without vascular differentiation (EM X3300 and X 7800

deactivate some members of the *int* gene family leading to cessation of KS-FGF secretion, thus depriving KS cells from a major GF (52). Malignantly transformed KS cells protect themselves from cytotoxic lymphocytes and their IL-2-expanded clones by secreting the IL-2 antagonist TGFß. Switching off TGFß secretion could render these cells vulnerable to cytotoxic lymphocytes. At this point, TNFα of macrophage origin or TNFß (lymphotoxin) of T lymphocyte origin may induce programmed cell death (apoptosis). Apoptotic KS cells were observed in regressing lesions (Figs 1-3).

SUMMARY

While lipopolysaccharide endotoxin is the most prominent inducer of the kine-cascade (TNFα, IL-1, 4, 6, 8) that leads to shock and multiple organ failure, bacterial exotoxins and products of certain gram positive bacteria can induce the same end results. We theorize that more than one pathogen can induce the sequence of protooncogene activation and growth factor release that results in the formation of KS. If KS has its own unique viral etiology, this virus has not as yet been isolated or identified but we continue to search for it. However, it is entirely possible that these lesions do not have a single well-defined etiologic agent but are the result of multiple agents cooperating in a set sequence. An endogenous, or apathogenic exogenous, retrovirus may replace HIV for initiator growth factor induction in CD4 cells in the classical (Mediterranean) or iatrogenic disease; and other pathogens co-exist or sequentially replace each other in the African endemic disease; whereas an array of viral pathogens (prominent among them CMV) take over growth factor induction in endothelial cells proliferating in response to the initiator growth factor (oncostatin M) released from HIV-infected CD4 lymphocytes in AIDS-KS.

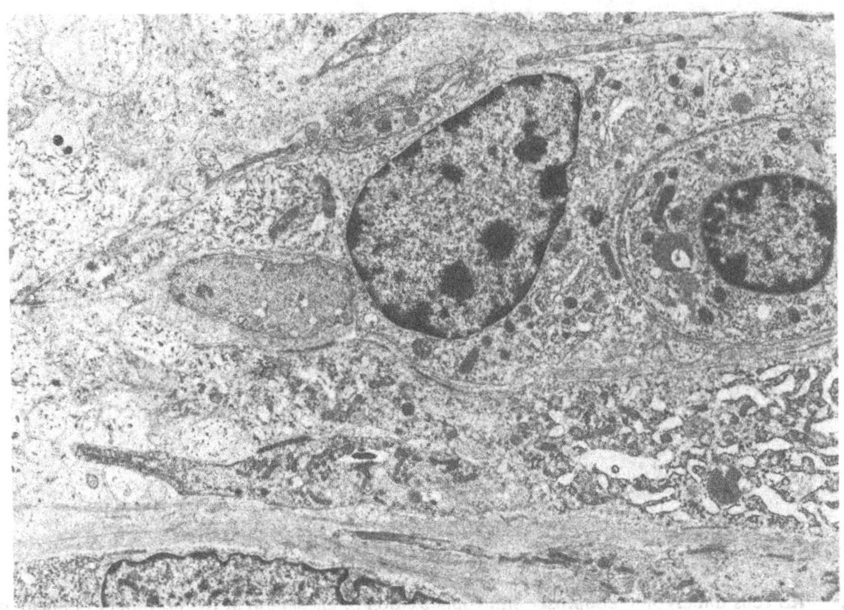

Fig. 2. KS cells undergoing apoptosis with condensation of chromatin at the periphery of nuclei in a 75 yr old man with classical KS showing fusiform sarcomatous growth pattern without vascular differentiation (EM X3300 and X 7800).

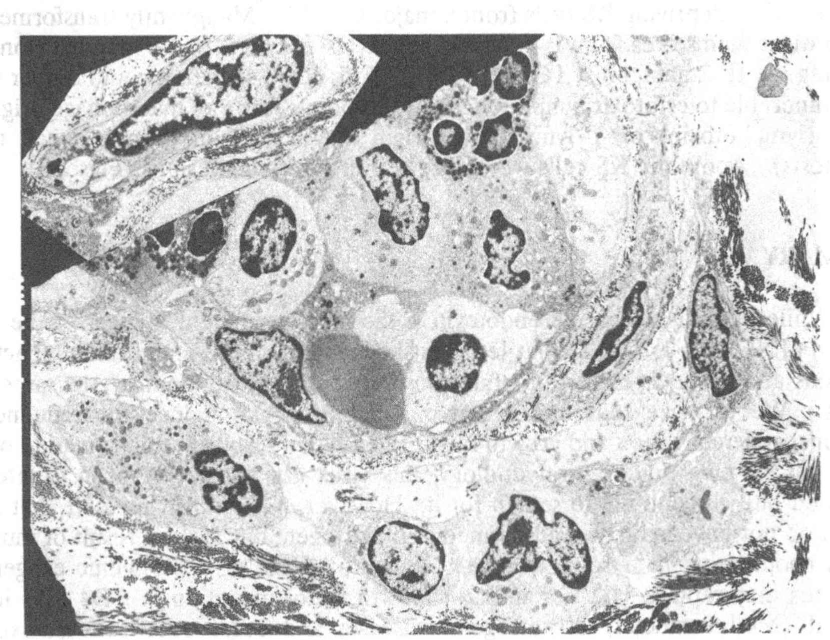

Fig. 3. Regressing KS lesion showing KS cells in the process of apoptosis in a man with AIDS-KS who is receiving interferon alpha therapy (EM X 6250)

REFERENCES

1. A. McKeating, P.D. Griffiths, R.A. Weiss, HIV susceptibility conferred to human fibroblasts by cytomegalovirus-induced Fc receptor, *Nature* 343:659 (1990).
2. J. D. Benson, E.S. Huang, Human cytomegalovirus induces expression of cellular topoisomerase II, *J. Virol.* 64:9 (1990).
3. B. J. Thomas, S. Efstathion, R.W. Honess, Acquisition of the human adeno-associated virus type-2 rep gene by human herpesvirus type-6, *Nature* 351:78 (1991).
4. R. I. Short, D. Jones, R. Kost, R. Witter, H-J Kung, Retrovirus insertion into herpesvirus *in vitro* and *in vivo*, *Proc. Nat. Acad. Sci.* USA 89:991 (1992).
5. D. H. Spector, J.P. Vacquier, Human cytomegalovirus (strain AD169) contains sequences related to the avian retrovirus oncogene v-myc,*Proc. Nat. Acad. Sci.* USA 80:3889 (1983).
6. I. Boldogh, E. Beth, E-S Huang, S.K. Kyalwazi, G. Giraldo, Kaposi sarcoma. IV. Detection of CMV DNA, CMV RNA and CMNA in tumor biopsies, *Internat J. Cancer* 28:469 (1981).
7. G. Giraldo, E. Beth, E-S Huang, Kaposi's sarcoma and its relationship to cytomegalovirus (CMV) III. CMV DNA and CMV early antigen in Kaposi's sarcoma, *Internat J. Cancer* 26:23 (1980).
8. D. H. Spector, S.B. Shaw, C.J. Hock, D. Alvans, T. Mitsuyasu, M. Gottlieb, Association of human cytomegalovirus with Kaposi's sarcoma, *in*: "Acquired Immune Deficiency Syndrome," M.S. Gottlieb, J.C. Groopman, eds., Proc Schering Corp UCLA Symposium, Allen R. Liss, New York, pp 109 (1984).
9. H. L. Ioachim, B. Dorsett, J. Melamed, V. Adsay, E.A. Santagada, Cytomegalovirus, angiomatosis and Kaposi's sarcoma: new observations of a debated relationship, *Modern Pathol.* 5:169 (1992).
10. F. Gyorkey, J.G. Sinkovics, R.J. Luchi, J.D. Small, P. Craig, R. Rossen, P. Gyorkey, J. Melnick, Kaposi's sarcoma in lymph nodes of patients with cytomegalovirus viremia, *Proc. Am. Assoc. Cancer Res.* 23:280 (Abstr. 1106) (1982).
11. R. F. Ambinder, C. Newman, G.S. Hayward, R. Bigger, M. Melbye, L. Kesters, E.V. March, P. Piot, P. Gigase, P.B. Wright, T.C. Quinn, Lack of association of cytomegalovirus with endemic African Kaposi's sarcoma, *J. Infect. Dis.* 156:193 (1987).
12. A. Siddiqui, Hepatitis B virus DNA in Kaposi sarcoma, *Proc. Natl. Acad. Sci.* USA 80:4861 (1983).
13. Y. O. Huang, J.J. Li, M.G. Rush, B.J. Poiesz, A. Nicolaides, M. Jacobson, W.G. Zhang, E. Coutavas, M.A. Abbott, A.E. Friedman-Kien, HPV-16-related DNA sequences in Kaposi's sarcoma, *Lancet* 339:515 (1992).
14. G. Barbanti-Brodano, M. Pagnani, P.G. Balboni, Studies on the association of Kaposi's sarcoma with ubiquitous viruses, *in*: "AIDS and Associated Cancers in Africa, G. Giraldo, E. Beth-Giraldo, N. Clumeck, M-R Gharbi, S.K. Kyalwazi, G. de The, eds., Karger, Basel, pp 175 (1988).
15. F. Gyorkey, J.G. Sinkovics, J.L. Melnick, P. Gyorkey, Retroviruses in Kaposi sarcoma cells in AIDS, *New Engl. J. Med.* 311:1183 (1984).
16. K. Rappensberger, E. Tschachler, E. Zonzits, R. Gillitzer, A. Hatzakes, A. Kaloterakis, D.L. Mann, T. Popow-Kraupp, R.J. Bigger, R. Berger, J. Stratigos, K. Wolff, G. Stingl, Endemic Kaposi's sarcoma in human immunodeficiency virus type 1-seronegative persons: demonstration of retrovirus-like particles in cutaneous lesions, *J. Invest. Dermatol.* 95:371 (1990).
17. D. A. Spandidos, A. Kaloterakis, M. Yiagnisis, A. Varatsas, J.K. Field, Ras, c-myc and c-erbB2 oncoprotein expression in non-AIDS Mediterranean Kaposi's sarcoma, *Anticancer Res.* 10:1619 (1990).
18. F. Gyorkey, J.G. Sinkovics, K.W. Min, P. Gyorkey, A morphologic study on the occurrence and distribution of structures resembling viral nucleocapsids in collagen diseases, *Am. J. Med.* 53:148 (1972).
19. J. G. Sinkovics, Tubuloreticular structures (TRS) in hairy cell leukemia, *J. Biol. Resp. Modif.* 6:573 (1987).
20. F. Gyorkey, J.G. Sinkovics, P. Gyorkey, Tubuloreticular structures in Kaposi's sarcoma, *Lancet* 2:984 (1982).
21. S. A. Rich, T.R. Owens, L.E. Bartholomew, J.U. Gutterman, Immune interferon does not stimulate formation of alpha and beta interferon-induced human lupus type inclusions, *Lancet* 1:127 (1983).
22. J. Vogel, S.H. Hinrich, R.K. Reynolds, P.A. Luciw, G. Jay, The HIV tat gene induces dermal lesions resembling Kaposi's sarcoma in transgenic mice, *Nature* 335:606 (1985).
23. B. R. Cullen, The HIV-1 Tat protein: an RNA sequence-specific processivity factor, *Cell* 63:655 (1990).
24. B. Ensoli, G. Barillari, S.Z. Salahuddin, R.C. Gallo, F. Wong-Staal, Tat protein of HIV-1 stimulates growth of cells derived from Kaposi's sarcoma lesions of AIDS patients, *Nature* 345:84 (1990).
25. D. A. Relman, J.S. Loutit, T.M. Schmidt, S. Falkow, L.S. Tompkins, The agent of bacillary angiomatosis, *New Engl. J. Med.* 323:1573 (1990).

26. T. A. Steeper, H. Rosenstein, J. Weiser, S. Inanipudi, D.C. Snover, Bacillary epithelioid angiomatosis involving the liver, spleen and skin in an AIDS patient with concurrent Kaposi's sarcoma, *Am. J. Clin. Pathol.* 97:713 (1992).
27. T. S. Croxson, D. Ebanks, D. Mildvan, Atypical mycobacteria and Kaposi's sarcoma in the same biopsy specimens, *New Engl. J. Med.* 308:1476 (1983).
28. D. K. Blanchard, M.B. Michelin-Norris, C.A. Pearson, C.S. Freitag, J.Y. Djeu, Mycobacterium avium-intracellulare induces interleukin-6 from human monocytes and large granular lymphocytes, *Blood* 77:2218 (1991).
29S-C Lo, S. Tsai, J.R. Benish, J.W. Shih, D.J. Wear, D.M. Wong, Enhancement of HIV-1 cytocidal effects in CD4$^+$ lymphocytes by the AIDS-associated mycoplasma, *Science* 251:1074 (1991).
30S-C Lo, C.L. Buckholz, D.J. Wear, R.C. Hohm, A.M. Marty, Histopathology and doxycycline treatment in a previously healthy non-AIDS patient systemically infected by *Mycoplasma fermentans* (incognitus strain), *Modern Pathol.* 4:750 (1991).
31. B. Ensoli, G. Barillari, R.C. Gallo, Cytokines and growth factors in the pathogenesis of AIDS-associated Kaposi's sarcoma, *Immunol. Reviews* 127:147 (1992).
32. B. C. Nair, A.L. DeVico, S. Nakamura, T.D. Copeland, Y. Chen, A. Patel, T. O'Neil, S. Oroszlan, R.C. Gallo, M.G. Sarngadharan, Identification of a major growth factor for AIDS-Kaposi's sarcoma cells is oncostatin M, *Science* 255:1430 (1992).
33. J. Corbeil, L.A. Evans, E. Vasak, D.A. Cooper, R. Penny, Culture and properties of cells derived from Kaposi sarcoma, *J. Immunol.* 146:2972 (1991).
34. S. A. Miles, A.R. Rezai, J.F. Sabazar-Gonzalez, M. Vander Meyden, R.H. Stevens, D.M. Logan, R.T. Mitsuyasu, T. Taga, T. Hirano, T. Kishimoto, O. Martinez-Maza, AIDS Kaposi sarcoma-derived cells produce and respond to interleukin 6, *Proc. Natl. Acad. Sci.* USA 87:4068 (1990).
35. P. Delli Bovi, A.M. Curatola, F.G. Kern, A. Greco, M. Ittmann, C. Basilico, An oncogene isolated by transfection of Kaposi's sarcoma DNA encodes a growth factor that is a member of the FGF family, *Cell* 50:729 (1987).
36. L. Xerri, J. Hassoun, J. Planche, V. Guigou, J-J Grob, P. Parc, D. Birnbaum, O. de Lapeyriere, Fibroblast growth factor gene expression in AIDS-Kaposi's sarcoma detected by in situ hybridization, *Am. J. Pathol.* 138:9 (1991).
37. O. Brüstle, A. Aguzzi, D. Talarico, C. Basilico, P. Kleihues, O. Wiestler, Angiogenic activity of the K-fgf-hst oncogene in neural transplants, *Oncogene* 7:1177 (1992).
38. H. A. Weich, S.Z. Salahuddin, P. Gill, S. Nakamura, R.C. Gallo, J. Folkmann, AIDS-associated Kaposi's sarcoma-derived cells in long-term culture express and synthesize smooth muscle alpha-actin, *Am. J. Pathol.* 139:1251 (1991).
39. S. A. Miles, O. Martinez-Maza, A. Rezai, L. Magpantay, T. Kishimoto, S. Nakamura, S.F. Radka, P.S. Linsey, Oncostatin M as a potent mitogen for AIDS-Kaposi's sarcoma-derived cells, *Science* 255:1432 (1992).
40. D. P. Gearing, M.R. Comeau, D.J. Friend, S.D. Gimpel, C.J. Thut, J. McGourty, K.K. Brasher, J.A. King, S. Gillis, B. Mosley, S.F. Ziegler, D. Cosman, The IL-6 signal transducer gp130: an oncostatin M receptor and affinity converter for the L1F receptor, *Science* 255:1434 (1992).
41. L. F. Fajardo, H.H. Kwan, J. Kowalski, S.D. Prionas, A.C. Allison, Dual role of tumor necrosis factor-α in angiogenesis, *Am. J. Pathol.* 140:539 (1992).
42. G. Poli, A.L. Kinter, J.S. Justement, P. Bressler, J.H. Kehrl, A.S. Fauci, Retinoic acid mimics transforming growth factor ß in the regulation of human immunodeficiency virus expression in monocytic cells, *Proc. Nat. Acad. Sci.* USA 89:2689 (1992).
43. J. A. Turpin, M. Vargo, M.S. Meltzer, Enhanced HIV-1 replication in retinoid-treated monocytes, *J. Immunol.* 148:2539 (1992).
44. J. Folkmann, How is blood vessel growth regulated in normal and neoplastic tissue? *Cancer Res.* 46:467 (1986).
45. A. Wellstein, G. Zugmaier, J.A. Califaro, F. Kern, S. Paih, M.E. Lippman, Tumor growth dependent on Kaposi's sarcoma-derived fibroblast growth factor inhibited by pentosan polysulfate, *J. Nat. Cancer Inst.* 83:716 (1991).
46. Editorial. Exploiting angiogenesis, *Lancet* 337:208 (1991).
47. T. E. Maione, G.S. Gray, J. Petro, A.J. Hunt, A.L. Donner, S.I. Bauer, H.F. Carson, R.J. Sharpe, Inhibition of angiogenesis by recombinant human platelet factor-4 and related peptides, *Science* 247:77 (1990).
48. S. Kumar, Control of tumor growth: endothelial cell as an alternative target, *Anticancer Res.* 10:1443 (1990).
49. S. S. Brenn, D. Zagzag, A.M.C. Tsanaclis, S. Gately, M-P Elkouby, S.E. Brien, Inhibition of angiogenesis and tumor growth in the brain, *J. Pathol.* 137:1121 (1990).

50. B. Robaye, R. Mosselmans, W. Fiers, J.E. Dumont, P. Galand, Tumor necrosis factor induces apoptosis (programmed cell death) in normal endothelial cells *in vitro*, *J. Pathol.* 138:447 (1991).
51. J. E. Szakacs quoted in J.G. Sinkovics, Kaposi's sarcoma: its oncogenes and growth factors, *Crit. Rev. Hem-Onc.* 11:87 (1991).
52. J. G. Sinkovics, Interferons: antiangiogenesis agents, *Can. J. Inf. Dis. 3:Suppl. X* 1 (1992).

EXPOSURE TO THE ABUSED INHALANT, ISOBUTYL NITRITE, COMPROMISES BOTH ANTIBODY AND CELL-MEDIATED IMMUNITY

Lee S.F. Soderberg[1] and John B. Barnett[2]

Dept. of Microbiol. and Immunol., College of Medicine, University of Arkansas for Medical Sciences, Little Rock, AR[1] and Dept. of Microbiol. and Immunol., West Virginia Univ. School of Med., Morgantown, WV[2]

INTRODUCTION

Isobutyl nitrite is a drug of abuse popular among male homosexuals (1). Frequent abuse of nitrite inhalants has been correlated with seropositivity to human immunodeficiency virus (HIV) (2) and with the incidence of Kaposi's sarcoma among AIDS patients (3). Inhalation studies by Lynch, Lewis, and collaborators (4, 5) and by McFadden and Maickel (6) using animals showed that isobutyl nitrite at occupational exposure levels, 300-400 ppm 7-8 hr/day, had little toxic or immunotoxic consequences. Abusers, however, expose themselves to doses in excess of 1500 ppm for shorter duration (10-20 inhalations over several hours, often on a daily basis (1, 7). We previously reported (8, 9) that mice exposed to isobutyl nitrite in an inhalation chamber for 45 min per day for 14 days to 900 ppm isobutyl nitrite had severely compromised T-dependent antibody responses. In the present study, this was extended to examine dose effects and the time to recovery. In addition, it is reported that such exposure also severely compromised cell-mediated immunity.

MATERIALS AND METHODS

Isobutyl Nitrite Treatment

Isobutyl nitrite, obtained at 97% purity from the National Center for Toxicological Research (NCTR), Jefferson, AR, was stored at 4 °C under nitrogen. Isobutyl nitrite was vaporized in a flask and quantified with a halothane monitor (Puritan-Bennet, model 222, Datex, Tewkesbury, MA) calibrated for isobutyl nitrite. Female, 6-8 week old C57BL/6N mice (NCTR, Jefferson, AR) were exposed to isobutyl nitrite in an inhalation chamber for 45 min per day for 14 days. Groups of 5 mice were assayed for immune activity at various intervals after the last exposure to isobutyl nitrite.

Drugs of Abuse, Immunity, and AIDS, Edited by
H. Friedman *et al.*, Plenum Press, New York, 1993

Immune Assays

For mitogen assays, triplicate spleen cell cultures at 2 x 10^5 cells/microculture were stimulated with 3 μg/ml concanavalin A (Con A, Sigma, St. Louis, MO). Cells were labelled with 1 μCi/culture ^{3}H-thymidine over the final 4 hr of 72 hr cultures. For mixed lymphocyte reactions (MLR), triplicate cultures of responder spleen cells were mixed with irradiated (2000 cGy) allogeneic (BALB/c) stimulator spleen cells at a 1:1 ratio. After 72 hr incubation, MLR cultures were labeled with ^{3}H-thymidine for 18 hr. Cultures were filtered and radioactivity was counted. Significance was determined by t-test, using the mean CPM of 5 individual animals. The data are reported as the mean percent of control values.

For the plaque-forming cell (PFC) assay, mice were immunized intravenously with 200 μl of a 20% suspension of sheep red blood cells 5 days prior to the day of assay. A standard slide assay in triplicate was used to measure specific antibody-forming cells. Significance was determined by t-test, using the mean PFC of 5 individual animals.

Spleen cells were primed for cytotoxic T lymphocyte (CTL) activity by incubating spleen cells with P815 target cells for 5 days. Specific cytotoxicity for ^{51}Cr-labelled P815 cells was then measured in triplicate using a standard 4 hr chromium release assay. Significance was determined by t-test, using the mean percent lysis of 5 individual animals.

RESULTS

Mice were exposed to isobutyl nitrite in an inhalation chamber for 45 min per day for 14 days. Mice were assayed for immune responsiveness at various times after the last exposure. As reported previously for 24 (8) and 72 hr (9) after exposure, mice exposed to isobutyl nitrite had significant reductions in spleen cellularity, T cell responses to mitogenic and allogeneic stimulation, and T-dependent antibody responses early after exposure (Figure 1). The number of viable cells per spleen was reduced by 20%. T cell proliferative responses to the mitogen, Con A, were reduced by 30-35% and to allogeneic stimulation in MLR were reduced by 50% in mice exposed to isobutyl nitrite. The number of specific T-dependent antibody-forming cells (PFC) induced in mice exposed to isobutyl nitrite was reduced by 70% compared with mice exposed to air. There was little, if any, improvement in responsiveness in the first 3 days after termination of treatments. However, by 7 days, all of the parameters tested returned to normal levels.

The immunotoxicity produced by exposure to isobutyl nitrite inhalation was dose dependent. Mice were exposed to various doses of the inhalant for 45 min/day for 14 days and immunoassays were performed 3 days later. As in Figure 1, antibody induction was reduced to 32% of control levels at the 900 ppm dose. At 750 ppm, antibody induction was significantly improved and was 55% of control levels. At 300 ppm, isobutyl nitrite was found to have no effect. This is in agreement with earlier reports using longer dosing periods (5, 6). Unexpectedly, at a dose of 600 ppm, the inhalant consistently enhanced antibody responsiveness. At this intermediate level, responses were approximately 80% above control values.

The induction of specific CTL is important to resistance to viral infections and to tumor cell growth. As shown in Table 1, exposure to isobutyl nitrite severely compromised this cell-mediated immune mechanism. Exposure to the nitrite inhalant reduced specific CTL induction at all effector to target cell ratios, by up to 40%.

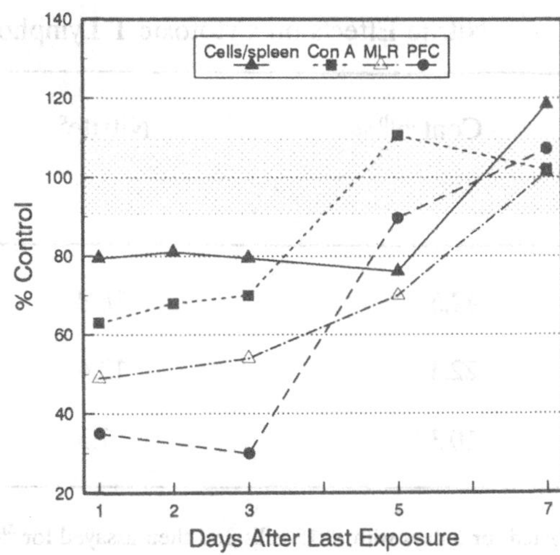

Fig. 1. Recovery of immune reactivity following exposure to isobutyl nitrite. Groups of 5 mice were exposed to 900 ppm isobutyl nitrite or air for 45 min/day for 14 days and assayed at various times thereafter. Spleen cells were stimulated with 3 μg/ml Con A or with a 1:1 ratio of allogeneic stimulator cells. For the PFC assay, mice were immunized with sheep red blood cells 5 days prior to the standard antibody-forming assay.

DISCUSSION

The present studies indicate that habitual inhalation of isobutyl nitrite may lead to impaired cell-mediated as well as humoral immune responses. Both the induction of specific antibody to a T-dependent antigen and the induction of T cell mediated cytotoxicity were compromised in mice exposed to high doses of isobutyl nitrite by inhalation. T cell proliferative responses to mitogenic and allogeneic stimulation were reduced by about 30% and 50%, respectively, suggesting that the inhalant produced a T cell defect. We previously reported (9) that similar exposure did not affect B cell mitogenic responses to lipopolysaccharide and preliminary data suggest that T-independent antibody responses were also unaffected.

Previous studies of isobutyl nitrite toxicity reported little or no toxicity at inhalation doses (300-400 ppm) and duration (6-7 hr/day for up to 18 wk) relevant to occupational exposure (4-6). The present data using briefer exposure periods also suggest that isobutyl nitrite was not immunotoxic at 300 ppm. At higher doses (750 and 900 ppm), more reflective of the exposures of abusers, the inhalant caused dose dependent immunosuppression. Interestingly, at an intermediate dose (600 ppm), antibody responses were significantly enhanced. Similar biphasic responses have been well documented following radiation and chemotherapeutic drug exposures and have been attributed to the exquisite sensitivity of T suppressor cells (10).

The immunotoxicity of subchronic exposure (14 days) was not permanent. While immunocompetence did not improve until 5 days after termination of treatments, all parameters tested returned to approximately normal levels by 7 days. This would suggest that habitual exposure to nitrite inhalants could render an individual immunocompromised even during hiatuses in exposure. However, the immune system recovers rapidly when exposures are totally stopped.

Table 1. Nitrite Effects on Cytotoxic T Lymphocyte Induction

Effector/target cell ratio[a]	Control[b]	Nitrite[c]	% Reduction in activity
50:1	42.5	26.8	37
25:1	22.4	13.4	40
12:1	10.3	7.3	29

[a]Spleen cells were incubated for 5 days with P815 cells and then assayed for ^{51}Cr release at the designated effector to target cell ratios.
[b]Data are expressed as percent lysis.
[c]Mice were exposed to 900 ppm isobutyl nitrite, 45 min/day for 14 days and harvested for sensitization 3 days later.

Acknowledgments

The authors wish to thank Michael Shaw and Denise Rose for their able technical assistance. This work was supported by USPHS NIDA grant DA06662.

REFERENCES

1. H. W.Haverkos and J. Doughtery, Health hazards of nitrite inhalants, *Amer. J. Med.* 84:479 (1988).
2. A. R.Moss, D. Osmond, P. Bacchetti, J.-C. Chermann, F. Barre-Sinoussi and J. Carlson, Risk factors for AIDS and HIV seropositivity in homosexual men, *Amer. J. Epidem.* 125:1035 (1987).
3. H. W.Haverkos, P.F. Pinsky, D.P. Drotman and D.J. Bregman, Disease manifestation among homosexual men with acquired immunodeficiency syndrome: A possible role of nitrites in Kaposi's sarcoma, *Sex. Trans. Dis.* 12:203 (1985).
4. D. W.Lynch, , W. J. Moorman, J.R. Burg, F.C. Phipps, T. R. Lewis and A. Khan, Subchronic inhalation toxicity of isobutyl nitrite in BALB/c mice. I. Systemic toxicity, *J. Toxicol. Env. Hlth* 15:823 (1985).
5. D. M.Lewis, W. A. Koller, D. W. Lynch and T. J. Spira, Subchronic inhalation toxicity of isobutyl nitrite in BALB/c mice. II. Immunotoxicity studies, *J. Toxicol. Env. Hlth* 15:835 (1985).
6. D. P.McFadden, and R.P. Maickel, Subchronic toxicology of butyl nitrites in mice by inhalation, *J. Appl. Toxicol.* 5:134 (1985).
7. K. R. Romeril, and A.J. Concannon, Hienz body haemolytic anaemia after sniffing volatile nitrites, *Med. J. Aust.* 1:302 (1981).
8. L. S. F.Soderberg, J.B. Barnett, and L.W. Chang, Inhaled isobutyl nitrite impairs T cell reactivity, *Adv. Exp. Med. Biol.* 288:265 (1991).
9. L. S. F. Soderberg, and J.B. Barnett, Exposure to inhaled isobutyl nitrite reduces T cell blastogenesis and antibody responsiveness, *Fund. Appl. Toxicol.* 17:821 (1991).
10. R. E. Anderson, and N.L. Warner, Ionizing radiation and the immune response, *Adv. Immunol.* 24:215 (1974).

NATURAL KILLER CELLS AND *CRYPTOCOCCUS NEOFORMANS*

Juneann W. Murphy

University of Oklahoma Health Sciences Center
Department of Microbiology and Immunology
Oklahoma City, Oklahoma

Drugs of abuse that affect natural and acquired immune defenses could definitely alter an individuals susceptibility to life-threatening fungal infections. Although specific studies in which drugs of abuse have been used will not be reported here, it is anticipated that the ensuing discussion of the natural effector cells and their potential for limiting fungal infections may suggest how such drugs, especially those that alter natural killer (NK) cell and T cell functions, predispose an individual to infections with the yeast-like organism, *Cryptococcus neoformans.*

It is well established that a combination of natural and acquired immune defenses are responsible for protection against systemic fungal infections. This is certainly the case for cryptococcosis, a disease caused by the eukaryotic microorganism, *C. neoformans. C. neoformans* is an organism with a rigid cell wall that is surrounded by a polysaccharide capsule. This organism is distributed ubiquitously in nature and is frequently found in a desiccated state in debris around pigeon roosts. When the cryptococcal cells become aerosolized, humans and animals who inhale the organism may develop pulmonary cryptococcosis which can range from an asymptomatic disease to a mild respiratory infection with pneumonia-like symptoms. In normal, healthy individuals, the disease is generally limited to the lungs and is resolved there. In contrast, individuals who have compromised host defenses especially those with reduced T lymphocyte function, are extremely susceptible to disseminated cryptococcosis. AIDS patients are examples of individuals who are very susceptible to systemic cryptococcosis. Prior to AIDS there were only about 300 cases of cryptococcosis in the United States (1). Now the number of cryptococcal infections is much higher with 7% of the AIDS patients having the disease (2). In fact, cryptococcosis is one of the leading life-threatening diseases in AIDS patients (2, 3). Use of drugs that suppress lymphocyte functions, whether the functions are direct-killing mechanisms or lymphokine-mediated mechanisms, could produce another group of individuals who are extremely susceptible to life-threatening fungal infections such as cryptococcosis.

From both human and animal studies, it is clear that lymphocytes, especially CD4$^+$ T lymphocytes are essential in host defense against *C. neoformans* (3-8); however phagocytic and natural killer cells also play a role in eliminating cryptococci from the body (9, 10). The specific mechanisms by which these various effector cell populations

Drugs of Abuse, Immunity, and AIDS, Edited by
H. Friedman *et al.*, Plenum Press, New York, 1993

contribute to clearance of this encapsulated yeast have not been completely elucidated. It appears that the natural effector cells alone are probably not capable of completely eliminating the organism, and the host must develop an effective cell-mediated immune response specific to *C. neoformans* to effectively clear the infection (10-13). It is not yet clear how the T lymphocytes interact to mediate protection against cryptococci, but if this was understood then it may be possible to identify susceptible individuals and to devise appropriate preventions and therapies for affected individuals.

For a number of years, my laboratory has been studying the effects of natural killer cells on cryptococci. We have shown that murine natural killer cells interact with this eukaryotic organism in a manner somewhat similar to the way NK cells interact with tumor or viral infected-cell targets (14-19). The sequence of stages in NK cell interactions with tumor targets has been described as binding, programming, delivery of the lethal hit, target cell death, and recycling (20). We have found that a similar series of stages occurs in NK cell-*C. neoformans* interactions (14-19). That is, NK cells first bind to the cryptococcal cells and the binding is Mg^{++} dependent (14). The binding initiates a programming state in the NK cells which leads to exocytosis of the NK cell cytolytic components (16). The programming stage is Ca^{++} dependent with both tumor and cryptococcal targets (14). Exocytosis of lytic material by the NK cells results in cryptococcal target cell death (17). It has been shown with the tumor targets that NK cells release the target cell and then recycle to another target (20). We have not directly shown that recycling occurs with cryptococcal targets; however, we have some data that suggest recycling may occur.

Some differences in NK cell interactions with cryptococcal targets as compared to tumor cell targets have been observed. NK cells bind to cryptococci through numerous microvilli; whereas, NK cells bind to tumor targets by long stretches of membrane-membrane contact (18). This difference in the physical binding characteristics of NK cells to cryptococcal and tumor targets might have been expected considering that cryptococci are very rigid cells which have as their outer layer a capsule and thick cell wall in contrast to the membrane bound tumor cell target (18). Another difference we have noted is in the time it takes for murine NK cells to bind to cryptococci as compared to the time needed to form firm conjugates with YAC-1 tumor targets (18). It has been reported, and we have confirmed, that murine NK cells will maximally bind to YAC-1 cells in 20 min; whereas, 2 hr is required for murine NK cells to bind maximally to cryptococcal targets (18, 21). YAC-1 targets are lysed within 5-10 min after NK cells bind, but cryptococcal cells are shown to be killed only after an additional 4 hr following binding (18, 21). The overall sequence of events in NK cell-mediated killing of cryptococcal targets is considerably slower than are the events in NK cell-mediated lysis of tumor targets. The granules of the NK cells contain the components that are lytic for tumor targets as well as the components that kill cryptococcal targets; however, the granules are slower in killing cryptococcal targets as compared to YAC-1 targets (15). Cytolysin which has been identified as a major lytic factor in the NK cell granules is also effective in killing cryptococci (15).

My laboratory has had some interest, as have others, in whether or not human NK cells inhibit the growth of *C. neoformans*. Miller et al. (22) have shown that human NK cells inhibit the growth of *C. neoformans* in the presence but not in the absence of anticryptococcal antibody. Those investigators used an effector to target (E:T) ratio of 100:1 in their studies (22). We have recently assessed the anticryptococcal activity of human NK cells and found that anticryptococcal activity can be detected in the absence of anticryptococcal antibody at a much lower E:T ratio of 2:1 (23).

Our source of human NK cells for these studies was peripheral blood from normal healthy donors at the Oklahoma Blood Institute. Buffy coats were centrifuged on Ficoll to obtain the mononuclear cell fraction. In some cases the mononuclear cells were incubated on plastic Petri dishes and the adherent cells were collected as a monocyte-enriched fraction. In other cases, the mononuclear cell fraction was passed over nylon wool to remove the monocytes/macrophages and B lymphocytes, and the nylon wool nonadherent (NWN) cells were collected as a source of NK and T cells. The NWN cells were further fractionated into a large granular lymphocyte (LGL)-enriched pool and a T cell-enriched fraction by centrifugation on discontinuous Percoll gradients. By flow cytometry, we found that the NWN fractions were comprised of >75% T cells based on the presence of CD3 on the surface of the cells, 3-10% NK cells as indicated by the expression of surface CD16, <5% monocytes or $CD15^+$ cells, and no Ig^+ or B cells. The LGL fraction was enriched for NK cells (25-50% $CD16^+$ cells); however, the LGL-enriched fractions were contaminated with 50-75% $CD3^+$ cells or T lymphocytes. The T cell-enriched fractions were greater than 95% $CD3^+$ cells with the remaining 5% being mainly $CD16^+$ cells (23).

Preliminary experiments were done with the various mononuclear cell fractions to determine the optimal E:T ratio for assessing anticryptococcal activity, and we found that a 100:1 ratio was optimal with the monocyte fraction, and a 2:1 ratio routinely displayed positive anticryptococcal activity with the NWN, LGL-enriched and T cell-enriched fractions as effector cells in an 18 h cryptococcal growth inhibition assay. The level of NK cell activity for each of the cell fractions was determined with the standard assay of ^{51}Cr-release from K562 tumor targets. NWN populations of human lymphocytes as effector cells at an E:T ratio of 50:1 with K562 targets displayed on an average 30% NK cell activity; whereas, the mean NK cell activities of the LGL- and the T-cell-enriched fractions were 43% and 24%, respectively (23). Although there was an enrichment in NK cell activity in the LGL population and a reduction in the T cell-enriched fraction, these changes were not reflected in the anticryptococcal activities as measured by effector cell-cryptococcal target cell conjugate formation and growth inhibition of *C. neoformans* with the two fractions. Furthermore, the fractions highly enriched for T cells and depleted of most NK cells displayed as much anticryptococcal activity as did the NK cell-enriched fractions (23). These data suggested that freshly isolated human T cells as well as NK cells can directly interact with cryptococci and inhibit the growth of the organism.

Considering that the mouse NK cells characteristically bound to cryptococci through numerous microvilli, the physical characteristics of human effector cell interactions with cryptococci were assessed with scanning and transmission electron microscopy. As would be expected with a phagocytic cell fraction, the monocytes or plastic adherent cells surrounded the cryptococcal cells with their extended membranes and internalized the organism (23). In contrast, many of the effector cells in the LGL fraction bound to the cryptococcal target cells with numerous microvilli, an association that was reminiscent of that of murine NK cells with cryptococci (Figure 1A and B). In the transmission electron micrographs, it was evident that the microvilli of the human cells were capable of penetrating the cryptococcal capsule (Figure 1C and D). When the preparations containing the T cell-enriched populations and cryptococcal targets were examined, still a different type of cell-cell interaction was observed. Effector cells in the T cell-enriched fraction bound to cryptococcal targets at the edges of folded membrane protrusions (Fig. 2). It was also noted that the cryptococcal cells were never internalized when the LGL- or T cell-enriched populations were used as effector cells. On the basis of the lack of phagocytosis as well as physical characteristics of the cell-cell associations, the lymphocyte interactions with cryptococcal cells were clearly different from those of the monocytes. Furthermore, the physical interactions of the cells in the NK-enriched populations appeared to be distinguishable from the cell-cell interactions

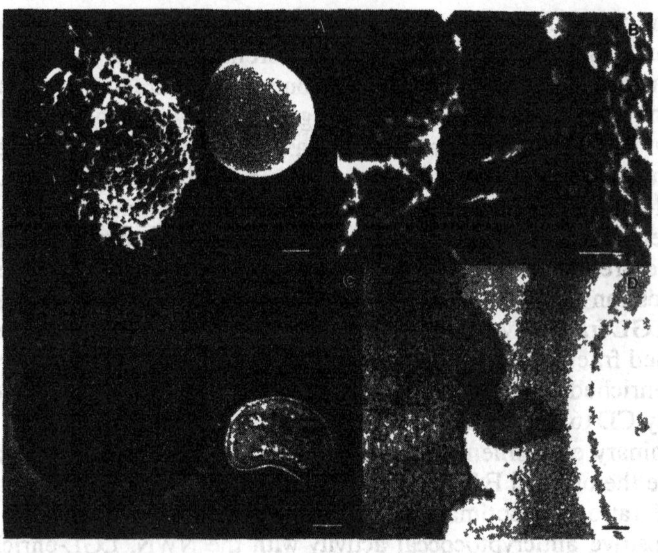

Fig. 1. **Human large granular lymphocytes (LGL) (left side of photographs) bound to *Cryptococcus neoformans* cells (right side of photographs). (A) Scanning electron micrograph; (B) higher magnification of the cell-cell contact area in A; (C) transmission electron micrograph of a thin section through a human LGL-*C. neoformans* conjugate; and (D) higher magnification of the contact area in C This figure is reproduced from Ann. Rev. Microbiol. 45:509-538, 1991 (10).**

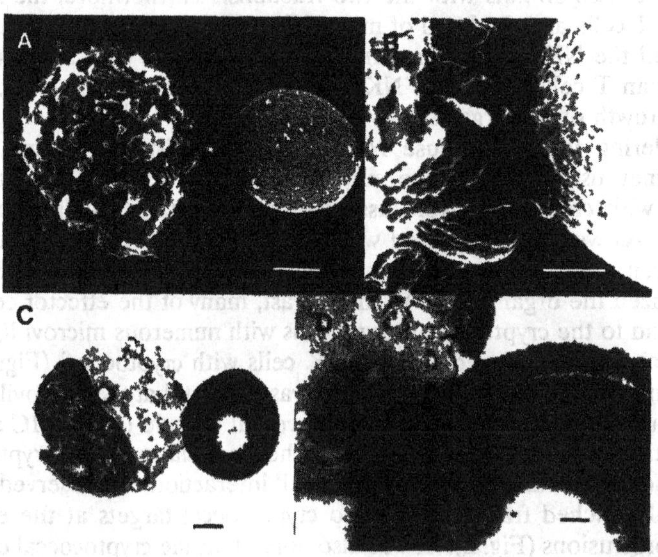

Fig. 2. **Human T lymphocytes (left side of photographs) bound to *Cryptococcus neoformans* cells (right side of photographs). (A) Scanning electron micrograph; (B) higher magnification of the cell-cell contact area in A; (C) transmission electron micrograph of a thin section through a human T cell-*C neoformans* conjugate, and (D) higher magnification of the contact area in C.**

when T lymphocyte-enriched fractions were used as effector cells with cryptococcal target cells. Further studies will be necessary to determine if human NK and T cells do indeed have different forms of physical interactions with *C. neoformans* target cells. It is clear however from the electron microscopy studies that human lymphocytes directly bind to *C. neoformans* cells and that two different types of cell-cell interactions are involved (Figs. 1 and 2) (23).

To confirm that freshly isolated human NK cells as well as T cells were capable of limiting *C. neoformans* growth, cell populations enriched for monocytes, LGL or T cells were significantly depleted of monocytes, NK cells or T cells prior to performing conjugate and growth inhibition assays with *C. neoformans* target cells. When anti-CD15 antibody and complement were used to remove monocytes, the anticryptococcal activity of the monocyte fraction was significantly diminished; however, the anticryptococcal activities of similarly treated LGL- and T cell-enriched fractions were unaffected (23). These results confirmed that contaminating monocytes in the LGL- and T cell-enriched populations were not responsible for inhibiting cryptococcal growth. Depletion of NK cells from the various effector cell populations with anti-CD16 and complement significantly reduced the anticryptococcal activity of the LGL-enriched fraction but had no effect on the ability of the T cell-enriched fraction to limit the growth of cryptococci. The anti-CD16 and complement treatment was shown to be effective in depleting NK cells by assessing the NK cell activity before and after antibody and complement treatment using a ^{51}Cr release assay with K562 target cells. Together, these data indicate that freshly isolated human NK cells when assayed at a 2:1 effector to target cell ratio with cryptococcal target cells were able to inhibit the growth of the organism. Furthermore, the data suggest that freshly isolated normal human T cells were also capable of inhibiting cryptococcal growth (23).

To confirm that human T cells could limit cryptococcal growth, two methods were used to deplete T cells from the effector cell populations. First, T cells were removed by rosetting with sheep red blood cells (SRBC) for 1 hr at 29°C. After treating an LGL fraction that had 78% T cell contamination and 32% anticryptococcal activity with SRBC, the nonrosetting cells which contained only 4% CD3$^+$ cells displayed only 9% anticryptococcal activity. When the T cell-enriched fraction that contained 86% T cells was subjected to SRBC, 8% CD3$^+$ cells remained in the nonrosetting fraction and the anticryptococcal activity of that fraction was reduced from 46% to 5%. These data add further support to the contention that human T cells can inhibit the growth of cryptococci. Second, T cells were depleted by treating the effector cell populations with anti-CD3 and complement. Removal of T cells in this fashion from the T cell-enriched fractions also significantly diminished the anticryptococcal activity adding more evidence that human T cells have anticryptococcal activity (23).

In conclusion, two populations of freshly isolated human lymphocytes were shown to directly bind to and inhibit the growth of *C. neoformans* cells in vitro when the effector and target cells were mixed at a ratio of 2:1. One might predict that this anticryptococcal activity demonstrated by human lymphocytes could be in part responsible for the effective natural resistance against cryptococci that is apparent in most healthy humans. Since *C. neoformans* is ubiquitous, it is difficult to know whether or not the T cell reactivity that was observed in these studies is a result of natural resistance or due to previous sensitization of individuals to cryptococci. Irrespective of these details, the data emphasize that human lymphocytes have direct inhibitory activity against *C. neoformans*. Thus, it would be expected that any drug which significantly diminishes NK cell and/or T lymphocyte activities may predispose an individual to disseminated cryptococcosis, a potentially fatal disease.

Acknowledgements

This work was supported by a U. S. Public Health Service grant AI18895 from the National Institutes of Allergy and Infectious Diseases. Electron microscopy was performed at the Samuel Roberts Noble Electron Microscoope Laboratory, Norman, OK. The assistance of Bill Chissoe, Diane Hurd, and Phillip Dang in preparation of the electron micrographs is greatly appreciated.

REFERENCES

1. J . Vandepitte, Clinical aspects of cryptococcosis in patients with AIDS, *in*: "Mycoses in AIDS Patients," H. V. Bossche, D. W. R. Mackenzie, G. Cauwenbergh, J. V. Cutsem, E. Drouhet, and B. Dupont, eds., pp. 115, Plenum Press, New York (1990).
2. S. L. Chuck, and M. A. Sande, Infections with *Cryptococcus neoformans* in the acquired immunodeficiency syndrome, *N. Engl. J. Med.* 321:794 (1989).
3. J. A. Kovacs, A. A. Kovacs, M. Polis, W. C. Wright, V. J. Gill, C. U. Tuazon, E. P. Gelmann, H. C. Lane, R. Longfield, G. Overturf, A. M. Macher, A. S. Fauci, J. E. Parrillo, J. E. Bennett and H. Masur, Cryptococcosis in the acquired immunodeficiency syndrome, *Ann. Intern. Med.* 103:533 (1985).
4. J. O. Hill, CD4$^+$ T cells cause multinucleated giant cells to form around *Cryptococcus neoformans* and confine the yeast within the primary site of infection in the respiratory tract, *J. Exp. Med.* 175:1685 (1992).
5. J. O. Hill, and A. G. Harmsen, Intrapulmonary growth and dissemination of an avirulent strain of *Cryptococcus neoformans* in mice depleted of CD4$^+$ or CD8$^+$ T-cells, *J. Exp. Med.* 173:755 (1991).
6. G. B. Huffnagle, J. L. Yates and M. F. Lipscomb, Immunity to a pulmonary *Cryptococcus neoformans* infection requires both CD4$^+$ and CD8$^+$ T cells, *J. Exp. Med.* 173:793 (1991).
7. C. H. Mody, M. F. Lipscomb, N. E. Street and G. B. Toews, Depletion of CD4$^+$ (L3T4$^+$) lymphocytes *in vivo* impairs murine host defense to *Cryptococcus neoformans*, *J. Immunol.* 144:1472 (1990).
8. T. S. Lim, J. W. Murphy and L. K. Cauley, Host-etiological agent interactions in intranasally and intraperitoneally induced cryptococcosis in mice, *Infect. Immun.* 29:633 (1980).
9. J . W. Murphy, Natural host resistance mechanisms against systemic mycotic agents, *in*: "Functions of the natural immune system," C. W. Reynolds and R. H. Wiltrout, eds., pp. 149, Plenum Publishing Corp., New York. (1989).
10. J . W. Murphy, Mechanisms of natural resistance to human pathogenic fungi, *Ann. Rev. Microbiol.* 45:509 (1991).
11. M. F. Lipscomb, T. Alvarellos, G. B. Toews, R. Tompkins, Z. Evans, G. Koo and V. Kumar, Role of natural killer cells in resistance to *Cryptococcus neoformans* infections in mice, Am. J. Path. 128:354 (1987).
12. M. R. Hidore, and J. W. Murphy, Correlation of natural killer cell activity and clearance of *Cryptococcus neoformans* from mice after adoptive transfer of splenic nylon wool-nonadherent cells, *Infect. Immun.* 51:547 (1986).
13. M. R. Hidore, and J. W. Murphy, Natural cellular resistance of beige mice against *Cryptococcus neoformans*, *J. Immunol.* 137:3624 (1986).
14. M. R. Hidore, and J. W. Murphy, Murine natural killer cell interactions with a fungal target, *Cryptococcus neoformans*, *Infect. Immun.* 57:1990 (1989).
15. M. R. Hidore, N. Nabavi, C. W. Reynolds, P. A. Henkart and J. W. Murphy, Cytoplasmic components of natural killer cells limit the growth of *Cryptococcus neoformans*, *J. Leuk. Biol.* 48:15 (1990).
16. M. R.Hidore, T. W. Mislan and J. W. Murphy, Responses of murine natural killer cells to binding of the fungal target *Cryptococcus neoformans*, *Infect. Immun.* 59:1489 (1991).
17. M. R. Hidore, N. Nabavi, F. Sonleitner and J. W. Murphy, Murine natural killer cells are fungicidal to *Cryptococcus neoformans*, *Infect. Immun.* 5:1747 (1991).
18. J . W. Murphy, M. R. Hidore and N. Nabavi, Binding interactions of murine natural killer cells with the fungal target *Cryptococcus neoformans*, *Infect. Immun.* 59:1476 (1991).
19. N. Nabavi, and J. W. Murphy, *In vitro* binding of natural killer cells to *Cryptococcus neoformans* targets, *Infect. Immun.* 50:50 (1985).

20. S. R. Targen, and R. L. Deem, NK-target cell interactions in binding, triggering, programming, and lethal hit of NK cytotoxicity, *in*: "Mechanisms of Cytotoxicity by NK Cells," R. B. Herberman and D. M. Callewaert, eds., pp. 155-172, Academic Press, Orlando, Fla. (1985).
21. J . C. Roder, R. Kiessling, P. Biberfeld and B. Andersson, Target-effector interaction in the natural killer (NK) cell system, II. The isolation of NK cells and studies on the mechanism of killing, *J. Immunol.* 121:2509 (1978).
22. M. F. Miller, T. G. Mitchell, W. J. Storkus and J. R. Dawson, Human natural killer cells do not inhibit growth of *Cryptococcus neoformans* in the absence of antibody, *Infect. Immun.* 58:639 (1990).
23. J . W. Murphy, M. R. Hidore, and C. S. Wong, Direct interactions of human lymphocytes with the yeast-like organism, *Cryptococcus neoformans*, *J. Clin. Invest.* (in press) (1993).

INDEX

Acetaldehyde, 160
Acquired immunity, 69–70
Acquired immunodeficiency syndrome (AIDS)-dementia complex (ADC), 184
Acquired immunodeficiency syndrome (AIDS) embryopathy, 213
Acquired immunodeficiency syndrome (AIDS)-related complex (ARC), 205
ACTH, *see* Adrenocorticotropic hormone
α-Actin, 258
Acute monoblastic leukemia, 108
ADC, *see* Acquired immunodeficiency syndrome (AIDS)-dementia complex
Adenylate cyclase-cyclic adenosine monophosphate (cAMP), 115, 117
Adrenal hormones, 1, 3, 4, 7, 14
Adrenal medulla, 231, 232
Adrenocorticotropic hormone (ACTH), 1, 2, 226, 230, 231, 232
AFCs, *see* Antibody forming cells
AIDS, *see* Acquired immunodeficiency syndrome
Alanine aminotransferase (ALT), 155
Alcohol, *see* Ethanol
Alpha-adrenergic receptors, 232
Alveolar macrophages
- cocaine and, 135–142
- ethanol and, 153
- marijuana and, 67

Alzheimer's disease care givers, 228
Anal intraepithelial neoplasia, 221, 222
Anal squamous cell carcinoma, 221
Androgens, 149
Anemia, 192
Antibiotics, 74, *see also* specific types
Antibody forming cells (AFCs), 116, 122, 124
Anti-CD3 antibodies
- cocaine and, 127–133
- marijuana and, 74, 75, 76, 77
- stress and, 226

Anti-CD16 antibodies, 249, 273
Anti-CD57 antibodies, 249
Anti-CR1 antibodies, 166
Anti-CR3 antibodies, 166
Anti-*Cryptosporidium* antibodies, 176
Anti-FcR II antibodies, 166
Anti-FcR III antibodies, 166
Antigen presentation, 135
Anti-L3T4 antibodies, 74, 97, 99–100, 102
Anti-Ly2 antibodies, 74, 99–100, 102
Antinociception, 30–31, 32
Apoptosis, 255, 257, 258, 259
ARC, *see* Acquired immunodeficiency syndrome (AIDS)-related complex
Arginine, 110–111
Arthrobacter strain AT-25, 258
Aspartate aminotransferase (AST), 155
Astrocytes, 182, 184, 213, 214
Astrocytomas, 108
Ataxia Telangiectasia, 111
Autonomic nervous system (ANS), 3, 226
Azidothymidine (AZT), 197, 203, 204, 206, 208, 222

Bacterial angiomatosis, 257
Bacterial infections, *see also* specific types
- ethanol and, 153–157
- marijuana and, 67–71
- morphine and, 41

Basal cell skin carcinoma, 221
Basic fibroblast growth factor (bFGF), 258
B cells
- *C. neoformans* and, 271
- ethanol and, 154, 175
- FIV and, 197
- immunotherapy and, 205
- isobutyl nitrite and, 267
- marijuana and, 67
- morphine and, 47
- in seronegative IVDUs, 242, 243, 245
- stress and, 2, 4, 228

B103 cells, 97, 100, 103
Benzanthracene, 110
Benzathine penicillin chemotherapy, 81
Benzopyrene, 110
Beta-adrenergic agonists, 227
Beta-adrenergic antagonists, 3
Beta-adrenergic receptors, 227, 232
Beta-endorphin, *see* β-Endorphin
bFGF, *see* Basic fibroblast growth factor
Bisexuals, 211, 219, 235, 236
Bleomycin, 111
Blood-brain barrier, 58, 214
Blood products, 255
Blood transfusions, *see* Transfusion-associated infections
Bone marrow cells
- FIV and, 194

Bone marrow cells (*cont'd*)
HD and, 220
morphine and, 29–32, 49
morphine binding sites on, 31–32
Bone marrow transplantation, 206
Bovine serum albumin (BSA)
cocaine and, 137
ethanol and, 166
marijuana and, 89, 90, 92, 97
morphine and, 36
Brain, 14, 22, 41
immune cells of, 182, 183–184
Brain cancer, 221
Breast cancer, 221
BSA, *see* Bovine serum albumin

Calcium, 62, 165, 270
cytosolic free, 127, 129–132
cAMP, *see* Cyclic adenosine monophosphate
Cancer, 9, *see also* specific types
Candida albicans, 47, 49, 240
Candida glabrata, 240
Candida krusei, 240
Candidiasis, 225, 235, 238, 240
Cannabinoid receptors, 115–119
Carcinomas, 192, *see also* specific types
Catecholamines, 3, 7, 58, 227, 228, 231, 232
Cats, *see* Feline immunodeficiency virus
CD4/CD8 ratio
ethanol and, 154
morphine and, 35
in seronegative IVDUs, 243
stress and, 227, 228
CD2 cells, 35, 228, 241, 243, 245
CD3 cells, *see also* Anti-CD3 antibodies
C. neoformans and, 271, 273
marijuana and, 100, 102
MIMP and, 205
stress and, 227, 228
CD4 cells, 236, 238, 239, 240, *see also* CD4/CD8 ratio
AZT and, 222
bone marrow cell proliferation and, 32
C. neoformans and, 269
CIN and, 220
cocaine and, 181, 182
ethanol and, 175, 177
FIV and, 192, 193
immunotherapy and, 203, 204, 207, 208
KS and, 255, 257, 258, 259
morphine and, 35, 36, 37–38, 182
opiates and, 23, 24, 181
in seronegative IVDUs, 241, 242–243, 245
stress and, 228, 229, 249, 251
CD8 cells, *see also* CD4/CD8 ratio
ethanol and, 175, 177
FIV and, 192, 193
immunotherapy and, 207
morphine and, 35, 36, 37–38
opiates and, 23
in seronegative IVDUs, 241, 243, 245
stress and, 228, 230, 231, 232, 247, 249, 250, 251, 252, 253
CD11b cells, 166, 167
CD15 cells, 271, 273
CD16 cells, 167, 247, 249, 250, 251, 253, 273
CD18 cells, 166, 167
CD20 cells, 228, 243
CD21 cells, 243
CD25 cells, 205
CD26 cells, 228, 243, 245
CD29 cells
morphine and, 35, 36, 37–38
in seronegative IVDUs, 241, 242, 245
stress and, 228
CD32 cells, 167
CD35 cells, 166
CD45RA cells, 228, 242, 243
CD56 cells, 227, 228, 230, 231, 242
CD57 cells, 247, 249, 250, 251, 253
cDNA, 97, 98, 100, 104, 115
Cell-mediated immunity, 21
cocaine and, 135
isobutyl nitrite and, 265–268
KS and, 258
marijuana and, 67, 110
stress and, 2, 4, 226, 227
Central nervous system (CNS)
marijuana and, 115, 117
morphine and, 184
morphine-binding sites and, 61, 62, 63, 64, 65
perinatal AIDS and, 214
Central nervous system (CNS) toxoplasmosis, 235
c-*erb*B2 genes, 257
Cervical intraepithelial neoplasia (CIN), 219, 220–221, 222
Cf25, 206
cGMP, *see* Cyclic guanosine monophosphate
Chediak-Higashi syndrome, 42
Chemiluminescence measurement, 136, 137, 141
Chemotaxis, 49, 153, 165, 226
Chemotherapy, 81, 197, 206, 220, 267
Chorioamnionitis, 212, 215
c-H-*ras* gene, 256
Chromosomal damage
heroin and, 21–22
marijuana and, 111
CIN, *see* Cervical intraepithelial neoplasia
Circle of Willis, 213
Cirrhosis, 172
Classical (Mediterranean) Kaposi's sarcoma (KS), 255, 256, 259
CMV, *see* Cytomegalovirus
Cocaine
crack, 211, 213
cryptosporidiosis facilitation by, 143–149
cytoplasmic alkalinization and, 132
cytosolic free calcium and, 127, 129–132
HIV-1 replication and, 181–185
metabolites of, 121–126, *see also* specific types
perinatal AIDS and, 211, 212, 213, 215
respiratory burst and, 135–142, 182
T cell proliferation and, 127–133
Codeine, 64
Co-factor hypothesis, 181, 183

Co-factors, 195
Colon cancer, 111, 221
Complement, 137, 166, 167, 273
Concanavalin A (Con A)
ethanol and, 154, 165, 177
immunotherapy and, 205, 207
isobutyl nitrite and, 266
marijuana and, 74, 75, 76
morphine and, 53, 54, 55, 56, 57
opioids and, 15
stress and, 226
Condylomata accuminata, 221
Coping sequence, 9–11
Coriolus versicolor, 258
Corticosteroids, 2, 3, 16, 226, 227, 258
Corticosterone, 2
Corticotropin, *see* Adrenocorticotropic hormone
Corticotropin releasing factor (CRF), 8
Corticotropin releasing hormone (CRH), 1, 226
Cortisol, 226, 229–230, 231, 232
Coumarin, 166
CP-55,940, 115, 116, 117, 118
CP-56,667, 116, 117, 118
Crack cocaine, 211, 213
Crandell feline kidney fibroblasts, 193, 196
CR1 cells, 166
CR3 cells, 166
CRF, *see* Corticotropin releasing factor
CRH, *see* Corticotropin releasing hormone
Cryptococcal meningitis, 225, 235, 238, 240
Cryptococcosis, *see Cryptococcus neoformans*
Cryptococcus neoformans, 235, 269–273
Cryptosporidiosis, 235
cocaine and, 143–149
ethanol and, 175–178
Cryptosporidium parvum, *see* Cryptosporidiosis
CTLL cells, 74, 205
CTLs, *see* Cytotoxic T lymphocytes
Cyclic adenosine monophosphate (cAMP)
cannabinoid receptors and, 115, 116, 117, 119
ethanol and, 165
morphine and, 35, 36, 37–38
stress and, 226, 227
Cyclic guanosine monophosphate (cGMP), 165
Cyclooxygenase, 160
Cyclophosphamide, 82, 207
Cytochrome P-450, 121, 124
Cytokines, *see also* specific types
cocaine and, 136, 181–185
ethanol and, 159–164
marijuana and, 68, 70, 73, 110
morphine and, 35, 42
opiates and, 181–185
opioids and, 14
perinatal AIDS and, 214
stress and, 1, 4
Cytomegalovirus (CMV)
cocaine and, 183
immunotherapy and, 204
KS and, 255–256
morphine and, 183, 184
stress and, 228
Cytomegalovirus (CMV) esophagitis, 235
Cytomegalovirus (CMV) placentitis, 212, 215
Cytomegalovirus (CMV) retinitis, 235
Cytoplasmic alkalinization, 132
Cytoplasmic tubuloreticular structures, 257
Cytosolic free calcium, 127, 129–132
Cytotoxic T lymphocytes (CTLs)
isobutyl nitrite and, 266
marijuana and, 96, 98, 100, 101, 102, 103
morphine and, 35

DAGO, 62
DAMGO, 16
DCF, *see* Dichlorofluorescein
DCFH-DA, *see* 2′,7′-Dichlorofluorescin diacetate
DDC, 204
DDI, 204
Delayed-type hypersensitivity, 4, 15, 41
Delta opioid receptors, 13, 16, 61
Dermatitis, 23
Dexamethasone, 3–4
Dextran sulfate, 97
Dextrorphan, 62, 63
Diarrhea
cryptosporidiosis and, 144, 145, 149, 175, 178
FIV and, 192
Dichlorofluorescein (DCF), 166
2′,7′-Dichlorofluorescin diacetate (DCFH-DA), 166, 167
Diethyl dithiocarbamate (DTC), 203
Dimethyl sulfoxide (DMSO), 68, 69, 70, 74, 82, 83, 84, 85, 90, 91, 116
Dithiotheitol (DTT), 63, 65
DMSO, *see* Dimethyl sulfoxide
DNA, 110–111, 226, 256
DPDPE, 16
Drug abuse, *see* Intravenous drug users
DTC, *see* Diethyl dithiocarbamate
DTT, *see* Dithiotheitol
Dynorphin, 13, 30–31, 49

EBV, *see* Epstein-Barr virus
Ecgonine HCl, 136, 141
Ecgonine methylester HCl, 136, 140, 141
ELISA, *see* Enzyme-linked immunosorbent assay
Encephalitis, 225
Endemic African Kaposi's sarcoma (KS), 258, 259
Endocrine system, 7, 225–232
Endocrine umbrella, 206, 207
β-Endorphin, 13, 15, 49, 58
bone marrow cell proliferation and, 30, 31
cAMP and, 37
marijuana and, 73
morphine-binding sites and, 61, 63, 65
stress and, 229
Endothelial cells
CMV and, 256
ethanol and, 160–161, 162
KS and, 255, 258
perinatal AIDS and, 213, 214
env gene, 197

Enzyme-linked immunosorbent assay (ELISA), 129, 197, 242
Epidemiology, 235–240
Epinephrine, 226, 227, 232
Epithelial cells, 257
Epstein-Barr virus (EBV), 204, 228
Erythrocytes, *see* Red blood cells
Erythroxylon coca, 135
Esophagitis, 225, 235
Estrogens, 149
Ethanol, 165–168
  bacterial infections and, 153–157
  cryptosporidiosis and, 175–178
  cytokines and, 159–164
  head and neck cancer and, 107
  L. pneumophila and, 169–172
Etorphine, 31
European Collaborative Study, 212

FACES III, 248
FACS analysis, *see* Fluorescence activated cell sorter analysis
Factor VIII, 214
FAIDS, *see* Feline acquired immunodeficiency syndrome
FBS, *see* Fetal bovine serum
FcR II, 167
FcR III, 167
FCS, *see* Fetal calf serum
Feline acquired immunodeficiency syndrome (FAIDS), 192, *see also* Feline immunodeficiency virus
Feline immunodeficiency virus (FIV), 189–201
  clinical manifestations of, 192
  as co-factor model, 195
  as HIV chemotherapy model, 197
  as HIV pathogenesis model, 193–195
Feline leukemia virus, 195
Ferricytochrome c, 162
Fetal bovine serum (FBS), 89, 90, 92, 116
Fetal calf serum (FCS), 63, 74, 96, 248
Fetal development, 135, *see also* Perinatal acquired immunodeficiency syndrome
Fibroblast growth factor (FGF), 258
Fibroblasts, 96, 193, 196, 255
FIV, *see* Feline immunodeficiency virus
Flow cytometry, 74
Fluconazole, 240
Fluorescence activated cell sorter (FACS) analysis, 36, 75, 97, 99, 166
FLV, *see* Friend leukemia virus
Follicular hyperplasia, 192
Forskolin, 35, 37, 116, 117, 119
Friend leukemia virus (FLV), 189, 190, 205–206
Fumagillin antibiotics, 258

Gamma globulin, intravenous, 203
Gamma glutamyl transpeptidase, 214
Gastrointestinal candidiasis, 238
Gender, MAIDS and, 149, *see also* Women
Giardia muris infections, 178
Glial cells, 184
Glucocorticoids, 1–4, 14, 227
Glucose-1 transporter, 214
Glutamine, 96
Glutathione, 63
GM-CSF, *see* Granulocyte-macrophage-colony stimulating factor
Goat-anti-rabbit antibody, 166, 249
gp41, 204, 205, 214
gp120, 204
gp130, 258
gp160, 204
G-proteins, 115, 119
Gram-negative bacteria, 67, 70
Gram-positive bacteria, 259
Granular lymphocytes, 226, 257, 271, 272, 273
Granulocyte-macrophage-colony stimulating factor (GM-CSF), 203
  ethanol and, 155
  KS and, 258
  morphine and, 29–30, 32
Granulocytes, 41, 153, 205
Granulomas, 155
Growth factors, 255–260
Growth hormones, 2
Guinea pigs, 95, 169

Hairy cell leukemia, 257
Hamsters, 81–82, 83, 84
HD, *see* Hodgkins disease
Head and neck cancer, 221
  immunotherapy for, 207
  marijuana and, 107–111
Helper T cells, 1, 4, 235
Hemophilia, 255
Heparin, 258
Hepatic necrosis, 155
Hepatitis, 21, 172
Hepatitis B staphylococcal infection, 235
Hepatitis B vaccine, 206
Hepatitis B virus, 256
Hepatocytes, 172
Hepatotoxicity
  of cocaine, 141
  of ethanol, 155–156, 159–161, 165
HEPES, 89, 96, 116, 137
Heroin, 14, 17–18, 21–22, 23, 26, 35
  HIV-1 replication and, 181
  perinatal AIDS and, 211, 213
  syncytia formation and, 41
Herpes simplex encephalitis, 225
Herpes simplex virus (HSV), 204, 228, 235
Herpes simplex virus type 1 (HSV1), 96–104
Herpes simplex virus type 2 (HSV2), 95, 101
Herpesviruses
  Marek's, 256
  marijuana and, 95–104
  perinatal infections and, 212
  swine, 25
Herpes virus type 6, 256
Herpes zoster, 235
Heterosexual transmission, 211, 235, 236, 238
Hippocampus, 3

Histocompatibility antigens, class II, 43, 49
Histoplasmosis, 235
HIV, *see* Human immunodeficiency virus
Hodgkin's disease (HD), 219–220
Hofbauer cells, 213
Homosexuals, 221
  epidemiology of infection in, 235, 236
  isobutyl nitrite used by, 265
  KS in, 219, 256
  stress in, 225–232
  syphilis in, 81
HPA, *see* Hypothalamic-pituitary-adrenal axis
HPV, *see* Human papilloma virus
hst gene family, 258
HSV, *see* Herpes simplex virus
HTLV, *see* Human T cell lymphotropic virus
HU-210, 116, 117
HU-211, 116, 117
Human adenovirus-associated virus type 2, 256
Human immunodeficiency virus 2 (HIV-2), 257
Human immunodeficiency virus 1 (HIV-1) replication, 181–185
Human immunodeficiency virus 1 (HIV-1) spectrum disease, 225–232
Human immunodeficiency virus (HIV) vaccine, 190, 197, 200, 204
Human papilloma virus (HPV), 108, 220, 256
Human T cell lymphotropic virus (HTLV), 242
Human T cell lymphotropic virus I (HTLV I), 195, 241, 257
Human T cell lymphotropic virus II (HTLV II), 241
Humoral immunity
  cocaine and, 135
  isobutyl nitrite and, 265–268
  marijuana and, 67, 110
  stress and, 2, 4, 226
Huntington's disease, 9
Hydrocortisone, 205
N-Hydroxynorcocaine, 141, 142
Hypothalamic-pituitary-adrenal axis (HPA), 41
  stress and, 1–4, 226
Hypothalamus, 8, 14, 226

Iatrogenic Kaposi's sarcoma (KS), 258, 259
IBMX, *see* 3-Isobutyl-1-methyl xanthine
Ibuprofen, 160
IFN, *see* Interferon
Ig, *see* Immunoglobulin
IL, *see* Interleukin
Immunization, 67
Immunofluorescent assays, 249
Immunoglobulin A (IgA), 175, 177, 178
Immunoglobulin G (IgG), 38, 166, 167, 192
Immunoglobulin M (IgM), 38, 154
Immunotherapy, 203–208
IMREG-1, 203, 204
Imuthiol, 203
Indomethacin, 205, 207
In situ hybridization, 256, 257
Interferon (IFN), 73, 204, 205, *see also* specific types
Interferon-α (IFN-α), 14, 154, 203, 257, 258
Interferon-β (IFN-β), 154, 257, 258
Interferon-γ (IFN-γ)
  bone marrow cell proliferation and, 31–32
  ethanol and, 153, 154
  KS and, 257
  marijuana and, 90
  morphine and, 42, 47, 49, 53, 54, 55, 56, 57
  stress and, 4, 226
Interleukin-1 (IL-1), 206–208
  KS and, 258, 259
  marijuana and, 110
  morphine and, 31, 32, 42, 47, 49
  stress and, 226
Interleukin-2 (IL-2), 203, 206–208
  AZT and, 204
  cocaine and, 127, 128–129, 130–132
  ethanol and, 154
  KS and, 255, 259
  marijuana and, 73, 74, 75, 77, 78, 79, 110
  MIMP and, 205
  morphine and, 42, 47, 53, 54, 55, 56, 57
  stress and, 4
Interleukin-3 (IL-3), 32
Interleukin-4 (IL-4)
  bone marrow cell proliferation and, 32
  ethanol and, 178
  KS and, 259
  morphine and, 42, 47
  stress and, 4
Interleukin-5 (IL-5), 4, 42, 47
Interleukin-6 (IL-6)
  ethanol and, 169–172
  KS and, 257, 258, 259
  morphine and, 42, 47, 49
  opioids and, 14
  stress and, 4
Interleukin-8 (IL-8), 259
int gene family, 258
Intravenous drug users (IVDUs), 14, 181, 183, 221
  epidemiology of infection in, 235, 236
  HD and, 219
  hepatitis in, 21
  KS and, 220
  seronegative, 241–246
In vitro studies
  of cannabinoid receptors, 116
  of cocaine, 122
  in immunotherapy, 206–207
  of morphine, 41–50, 58
In vivo studies
  of cocaine, 122
  of ethanol, 153–157
  in immunotherapy, 207–208
  of MIMP, 205
  of morphine, 58
Ionomycin, 131
3-Isobutyl-1-methyl xanthine (IBMX), 116, 117
Isobutyl nitrite, 265–268
Isoprinosine, 203, 204, 205
Isoproterenol, 231, 232
IVDUs, *see* Intravenous drug users

Kaposi's sarcoma (KS), 219–220
classical (Mediterranean), 255, 256, 259
endemic African, 258, 259
growth factor cascade resulting in, 255–260
iatrogenic, 258, 259
isobutyl nitrite and, 265
regression of, 258–259
Kappa opioid receptors, 13, 15, 16, 17
K562 cells, 242, 248, 271, 273
K-*fgf-hst* gene, 258
Kibbutz members, 247–253
Kubler-Ross, E., 9
Kupffer cells
ethanol and, 155, 159, 160, 161, 162, 164
morphine and, 181

Lactation, 212
Laryngeal papillomatosis, 235
L929 cells, 96–97, 103
Lectins, 21, 182–183, *see also* specific types
Legionella pneumophila
ethanol and, 169–172
marijuana and, 67–71
Leprosy, 4
Leu-7 antibodies, 249
Leu-11b antibodies, 249
Leu-enkephalin, 13, 49
Leukemia, 108, 225, 257
Leukemia inhibitory factor, *see* Oncostatin M
Leukocyte migration inhibitor factor, 226
Leukocytes, 22, 53, 64, 95, 256, *see also* Polymorphonuclear leukocytes
Leukoencephalopathy, 213, 256
Leukopenia, 192, 203
Leukopheresis, 62
Leukoplakia, 235
Levorphanol, 62
Life events scale, 248
Lipopolysaccharide (LPS), 42
ethanol and, 154, 162–164, 172, 177
KS and, 259
marijuana and, 89, 92–93
MIMP and, 205, 206
morphine and, 53, 54, 55, 56, 57, 184
Listeria monocytogenes
ethanol and, 155–156
marijuana and, 67, 101
MIMP and, 206
LP-BM5 murine leukemia virus, 190, *see also* Murine acquired immunodeficiency syndrome
cocaine and, 143, 144, 145, 146, 148, 149
ethanol and, 175, 176, 177
LPS, *see* Lipopolysaccharide
L3T4 cells, 75, *see also* Anti-L3T4 antibodies
Luminol, 137
Lung cancer, 111, 221
Ly2 cells, 75, 77, 78, *see also* Anti-Ly2 antibodies
Lymphadenopathy, 192
Lymph nodes
cryptosporidiosis and, 144
marijuana and, 82
morphine and, 53, 54, 56
Lymphocytes, *see also* specific types
cocaine and, 123
ethanol and, 169
FIV and, 194
HD and, 220
isobutyl nitrite and, 266
KS and, 257
marijuana and, 74, 92, 95
morphine and, 53–54, 58, 184
perinatal AIDS and, 212
SIV and, 24
stress and, 2, 229–230, 231–232
Lymphocytosis, 192, 241
Lymphokines, 29, 226, 269, *see also* specific types
Lymphomas, 219, 220, 222
Lymphopenia, 1–2
Lymphosarcomas, 192
Lymphotoxins, 226

Macrophage-colony stimulating factor (MCSF), 29–32
Macrophage migration inhibitor factor, 226
Macrophages
C. neoformans and, 271
CMV and, 255, 256
cocaine and, 135–142
ethanol and, 153, 154, 155, 162, 165, 169–172
FIV and, 194
KS and, 258
marijuana and, 67, 73, 89–93, 95, 103
MIMP and, 205
morphine and, 41, 42, 43, 47, 49, 50, 184
opiates and, 25
opioids and, 15
respiratory burst of, *see* Respiratory burst
stress and, 226, 228
MACS, *see* Multicenter AIDS Cohort Study
MAIDS, *see* Murine acquired immunodeficiency syndrome
Major histocompatibility gene complex (MHC), 103
Malaria, 220
Marek's herpesvirus, 256
Marijuana, 73–79
bacterial infections and, 67–71
head and neck cancer and, 107–111
herpesviruses and, 95–104
receptors of, 115–119
splenocytes and, *see* under Splenocytes
syphilis and, 81, 82–87
TNF-α inhibition by, 89–93
Marinol, 73
Maternal-fetal interface, 212, 213, 215
MCSF, *see* Macrophage-colony stimulating factor
Megakariocytes, 194
Melanoma, 221
Meningitis, 225, 235, 238, 240
Meningoencephalitis, 225
β-Mercaptoethanol, 63
2-Mercaptoethanol, 74
Met-enkephalin, 13, 49

Methadone, 26, 58, 64
bone marrow cell proliferation and, 31
fetal development and, 215
for seronegative IVDUs, 241, 242, 243–245
Meth A tumor, 206
Methyl inosine monophosphate (MIMP), 205–206
N-Methylmorphine, 58
MHC, *see* Major histocompatibility gene complex
Mice, *see also* Murine acquired immunodeficiency syndrome cannabinoid receptors and, 115–119
cocaine and, 121–126, 136–142, 143–149
ethanol and, 153–157, 165, 169–170, 171, 175–178
immunotherapy and, 205–206, 207
isobutyl nitrite and, 265–270
marijuana and, 68–71, 73–79, 89–93, 95, 98, 99–100, 102, 103
morphine and, 41–50
opioid receptors and, 16–17
Microcephaly, 213
Microglia, 182, 184, 214
MIMP, *see* Methyl inosine monophosphate
Mineralocorticoids, 3–4
Mitogens, *see also* specific types
isobutyl nitrite and, 267
marijuana and, 75, 77, 95
morphine and, 35, 38, 41, 53
stress and, 226, 228, 229, 230
Molluscum contagiosum, 235
Monkeys, 35–39, *see also* Simian immunodeficiency virus
Monoclonal antibodies, 242, 249, *see also* specific types
Monocytes
C. neoformans and, 271, 273
cocaine and, 182
ethanol and, 153, 170
KS and, 257, 258
morphine and, 49
opiates and, 25
perinatal AIDS and, 212
respiratory burst of, *see* Respiratory burst
in seronegative IVDUs, 241
stress and, 226
Monokines, 255
Mononuclear cells, 41, 155, 242, *see also* Peripheral blood mononuclear cells
Morphiceptin, 63, 65
Morphine, 14, 15–18, 21, 241
bone marrow cells and, 29–32, 49
compartment-specific effects of, 53–58
HIV-1 replication and, 181–185
in vitro studies of, 41–50, 58
in vivo studies of, 58
low-dose effects of, 35–39
SIV and, 22–26
Morphine-binding sites
on bone marrow cells, 31–32
on T cells, 61–65
mRNA, 104
Multicenter AIDS Cohort Study (MACS), 228
Mu opiate agonists, 62–63
Mu opioid receptors, 13, 15, 16, 42, 43, 61–62, 65
Murine acquired immunodeficiency syndrome (MAIDS), 189
cocaine and, 143–149
ethanol and, 175–178
Mycelial protein-bound polysaccharides, 258
Mycobacteria, 169, 170, 235, 257
Mycoplasma, 204, 257
Myelodysplasias, 192
Myeloid neoplasms, 192

Naloxone, 14, 15
bone marrow cell proliferation and, 29–30
cAMP and, 37
morphine-binding sites and, 61, 62, 63, 64, 65
Naltrexone, 16, 17
dose-dependent blocking action of, 53, 54, 57, 58
in vitro studies of, 42, 43, 47
Napthalenes, 110
Natural killer (NK) cells
C. neoformans and, 269–273
ethanol and, 153, 169
immunotherapy and, 205
marijuana and, 73, 102, 103
morphine and, 22, 35, 38, 41, 54, 55, 57
opiates and, 25
opioids and, 15
in seronegative IVDUs, 241, 242, 243, 245
stress and, 226, 227, 228, 229, 230, 231, 247–253
Nerve growth factor, 213
Neuroblastoma cells, 100, 103, 117, 181
Neurominidase, 63
Neurotransmitters, 3, 95–96
Neutralizing antibodies, 197
Neutropenia, 192
Neutrophils, 73
NHL, *see* Non-Hodgkin's lymphoma
Nitrosamines, 110
NK cells, *see* Natural killer cells
Nocardiosis, 235
Non-Hodgkin's lymphoma (NHL), 219
Non-opiate binding site, 61
Nor-binaltorphimine, 16, 17
Norcocaine, 121, 124, 141, 142
Norepinephrine, 226, 227, 230, 231–232
Norphiceptin, 62
Northern blot analysis, 96, 97–98, 100, 103–104
NPT 15392, 205
NPT 16416, 205
N18TG2 neuroblastoma cells, 117

OAM study, *see* Opiate-AIDS-monkey study
Oligodendrocytes, 213
Oncostatin M (OM), 258, 259
Opiate-AIDS-monkey (OAM) study, 22–26
Opiates, *see also* specific types
HIV-1 replication and, 181–185
SIV and, 21–26
withdrawal from, 24–25

Opioid receptors, 13–18, 41
delta, 13, 16, 61
kappa, 13, 15, 16, 17
morphine immunomodulatory effects and, 53–58
mu, 13, 15, 16, 42, 43, 61–62, 65
Opioids, 13–18, *see also* specific types
bone marrow cell proliferation and, 29–32
Opportunistic infections, *see also* specific types
HD and, 220
immunotherapy and, 203
opiates and, 21, 26
Oral candidiasis, 240
Oral carcinoma, 221
Oral hairy leukoplakia, 235
Organ transplantation, 220, 258
Oropharyngeal candidiasis, 238

Pancreatic cancer, 221
p24 antigens, 23, 182, 214
Papovavirus BK, 256
Parenchymal cells, 160–161, 162
PBLs, *see* Peripheral blood lymphocytes
PBMs, *see* Peripheral blood mononuclear cells
P815 cells, 266
PCFs, *see* Plaque forming cells
PCR, *see* Polymerase chain reaction
PDGF, *see* Platelet derived growth factor
Peanut agglutinin (PNA), 154
Penicillamine, 258
Penicillin, 96
Pentazocine, 31
Pentosan polysulfate, 258
PEPSCAN analysis, 197
Perinatal acquired immunodeficiency syndrome (AIDS), 211–215
Peripheral blood lymphocytes (PBLs)
morphine-binding sites and, 62
stress and, 1, 2, 3, 248, 249, 250, 251, 252, 253
Peripheral blood mononuclear cells (PBMs)
C. neoformans and, 270–271
cocaine and, 181–184
FIV and, 189, 194
marijuana and, 110
methadone and, 58
morphine and, 35–39, 49, 181–184
in seronegative IVDUs, 241
Peritoneal macrophages
cocaine and, 135–142
ethanol and, 153
PHA, *see* Phytohemagglutinin
Phagocytes, 167
C. neoformans and, 269
cocaine and, 135, 136, 141
ethanol and, 153, 159
morphine and, 21, 47, 49
opiates and, 25
in seronegative IVDUs, 241
Phentolamine, 232
Phorbol ester, 165
Phorbol myristate acetate (PMA), 49, 160, 161, 164
Phospholipase C, 63
Phycoerythrin, 249
Phytohemagglutinin (PHA)
cocaine and, 127–133, 182–183
immunotherapy and, 205, 207
marijuana and, 74, 75, 76, 110
morphine and, 58, 182–183
morphine-binding sites and, 62, 63
opioids and, 15
in seronegative IVDUs, 241, 242, 243, 245
stress and, 1, 226, 227, 228, 229, 230, 231
Pituitary gland, 14, 232
Pituitary hormone secreting cells, 206
Placentitis, 212, 215
Plaque forming cells (PFCs)
isobutyl nitrite and, 266
MIMP and, 205
morphine and, 42, 43, 44, 47, 48, 49
stress and, 227
Plasminogen activator, 226
Platelet derived growth factor (PDGF), 258
PMA, *see* Phorbol myristate acetate
PMNs, *see* Polymorphonuclear leukocytes
PNA, *see* Peanut agglutinin
Pneumocystis carinii pneumonia, 225, 235, 238, 240
Pokeweed mitogen (PWM)
MIMP and, 205
in seronegative IVDUs, 241, 242, 243, 245
stress and, 228, 229, 231
Polyethylene glycol, 204
Polymerase chain reaction (PCR), 194, 256
Polymorphonuclear leukocytes (PMNs), 42
ethanol and, 153, 155, 162, 165–168, 169
marijuana and, 110
in seronegative IVDUs, 241
Polysaccharide peptidoglycans, 258
Primary central nervous system (CNS) lymphoma, 219
Primary infections, 67, 70
Procaine, 123
Prodynorphin, 13
Proenkephalin, 13
Prolactin, 2, 73
Promiscuity, 211
Proopiomelanocortin, 13
Propionibacterium acnes, 103
Propranolol, 232
Prostaglandins, 204, 205
Prostitution, 211
Protamines, 258
Protein kinase C, 207
Proteolytic enzymes, 63
Prothymocytes, 205
PWM, *see* Pokeweed mitogen
Pyramidal cells, 3

Rabbits, 81, 82, 83–84, 85, 86
Radiation therapy, 107, 206, 220, 267
ras p21 oncoprotein, 257
Rats
ethanol and, 153, 154, 165
marijuana and, 97, 103–104
morphine and, 41, 53–58
stress in, 1–2

RD1, 36
Reactive oxygen intermediates, 141
Recall antigens, 241
Red blood cells, 29, *see also* Sheep red blood cells
Renal disease, 192, 253
Renal transplantation, 220
rep gene, 256
Respiratory burst, 135–142, 182
Reticuloendotheliosis, 256, 257
Retinitis, 235
Retinoic acid, 258
Retroviral particles, 256–257
RNA, 110–111, 226, 256
RNase, 197
Rochalimaea quintana, 257
RPMI-1640, 248, 249
  cannabinoid receptors and, 116
  cocaine and, 122, 128
  marijuana and, 74, 82, 89, 96
  morphine-binding sites and, 63

Salmonella, 89, 206
SDS, *see* Sodium dodecyl sulfate
Secondary immunity, 69–70
Septic shock, 70
Seronegative intravenous drug users (IVDUs), 241–246
Serum proteins, 89–93
Sex hormones, 2, 149
Sheep red blood cells (SRBCs)
  C. neoformans and, 273
  cocaine and, 122, 123
  ethanol and, 154
  MIMP and, 205
  morphine and, 41–50
  stress and, 227
Short-loop negative feedback system, 232
Simian immunodeficiency virus (SIV), 21–26, 201
SIV, *see* Simian immunodeficiency virus
Smoking, 107, 110, 111, 221
SOD, *see* Superoxide dismutase
Sodium azide, 36, 97, 166
Sodium dodecyl sulfate (SDS), 97–98
Solid tumors, 219–222
Southern blot hybridization, 256
Sperm, 204
Spleen weight
  cryptosporidiosis and, 143, 144, 145
  immunotherapy and, 207
  morphine and, 45, 47
Splenocytes
  cannabinoid receptors and, 115–119
  cocaine and, 121–126
  ethanol and, 153, 154, 177
  isobutyl nitrite and, 266
  marijuana and, 73–79, 97, 99–100, 102
  MIMP and, 205
  morphine and, 41, 42, 43, 46, 47, 48, 49, 53, 54, 55, 57
  morphine-binding sites on, 61–62, 64, 65
  stress and, 3, 4, 7, 232
Squamous cell carcinoma of the anus, 221
Squamous cell head and neck cancer, *see* Head and neck cancer
SRBCs, *see* Sheep red blood cells
Staphylococcus albus, 67
Stem cells, 29, 30–31
Steroids, 7
Streptomycin, 96
Stress
  HIV-1 spectrum disease and, 225–232
  HPA and, 7–11, 226
  in kibbutz members, 247–253
Stress hormones, 226–227, 228–230, *see also* specific types
Sulfur compounds, 63
Superoxide anions
  cocaine and, 141
  ethanol and, 159–164, 165
  in seronegative IVDUs, 241
Superoxide dismutase (SOD), 161, 162
Suppressor T cells, 2, 43, 232
Suramine, 258
Swine herpesvirus, 25
Sympathetic nervous system (SNS), 230, 231–232
Sympathoadrenomedullary system, 226
Syncytia formation, 41
Syphilis, 81–87, 235
Systemic lupus erythematosus, 257

Tamoxifen, 149
tat gene, 257
T-cell leukemia, 225
T-cell lymphoma, 225
T-cell rosette formation, 15, 22, 41, 95, 110
T cells, *see also* specific types
  C. neoformans and, 269–270, 271–273
  cocaine and, 127–133
  ethanol and, 154–155
  FIV and, 197
  heroin and, 41
  immunotherapy and, 203–208
  isobutyl nitrite and, 266, 267
  KS and, 255, 258
  marijuana and, 67, 73, 95, 102, 110
  methadone and, 58
  morphine and, 41, 43, 47
  morphine-binding sites on, 61–65
  opiates and, 21–22, 24
  opioids and, 15
  in seronegative IVDUs, 242
  stress and, 2, 3, 226, 227, 228, 232, 250
Testicular cancer, 221
Tetanus toxin, 15–16, 41, 226
δ-9-Tetrahydrocannabinol (THC), *see* Marijuana
TGF, *see* Transforming growth factor
Th1 cells, 4
Th2 cells, 4
THF, *see* Thymic humoral factor
Three-Mile Island, 227, 228
Thy 1.2 cells, 154, 207
Thymic humoral factor (THF), 204
Thymidine, 74, 128, 205, 266
Thymocytes, 62, 65, 143, 154

Thymopentin, 203, 204
Thymus gland, 3, 4, 206, 207, 227
Thyroid hormones, 2
T-lymphocytosis, 203
TNF, *see* Tumor necrosis factor
TNP-ficoll, 154
Topoisomerase II, 255
Toxoplasmosis
  epidemiology of, 225, 235, 238, 240
  FIV and, 195
Transforming growth factor-β-(TGF-β)
  cocaine and, 182–183
  KS and, 255, 258, 259
  morphine and, 182–183, 184, 185
Transfusion-associated infections
  epidemiology of, 235, 236, 238
  KS and, 220
Transplacental infection, 211–215
Treponema pallidum subsp. *pallidum*, 81–87
Tropoblasts, 213
Tuberculosis, 235, 238, 240
Tumoral angiogenesis, 258
Tumor necrosis factor (TNF), *see also* specific types
  bone marrow cell proliferation and, 32
  ethanol and, 159, 162
  marijuana and, 68, 70, 71
  opioids and, 14
Tumor necrosis factor-α (TNF-α)
  cocaine and, 182, 183
  ethanol and, 153, 154, 155
Tumor necrosis factor-α (*cont'd*)
  KS and, 255, 258, 259
  marijuana inhibition of, 89–93
  morphine and, 182, 183, 184, 185
Tumor necrosis factor-β (TNF-β), 255

U1 cells, 182

Vaccines, 67
  hepatitis B, 206
  HIV, 190, 197, 200, 204
  syphilis, 81
Vasculitis, 212, 215
Villitus, 213
Vimentin, 49
v-*myc* gene, 256

WEHI-164 cells, 68, 90, 91
Western blot analysis, 197
Wilcoxon Sign Rank tests, 242
Women
  epidemiology in, 236, 238
  stress in, 252, 253

YAC-1 cells, 53, 270
Yaws, 82
Y chromosome, 149

Zidovudine, *see* Azidothymidine
Zinc, 206–208

9780306445668